1 MONTH OF
FREE
READING

at

www.ForgottenBooks.com

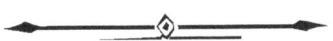

By purchasing this book you are eligible for one month membership to ForgottenBooks.com, giving you unlimited access to our entire collection of over 700,000 titles via our web site and mobile apps.

To claim your free month visit:

www.forgottenbooks.com/free711249

ISBN 978-0-483-27903-2
PIBN 10711249

This book is a reproduction of an important historical work. Forgotten Books uses state-of-the-art technology to digitally reconstruct the work, preserving the original format whilst repairing imperfections present in the aged copy. In rare cases, an imperfection in the original, such as a blemish or missing page, may be replicated in our edition. We do, however, repair the vast majority of imperfections successfully; any imperfections that remain are intentionally left to preserve the state of such historical works.

CLINICAL LECTURES

ON

SURGERY,

DELIVERED AT THE HOSPITAL OF LA CHARITÉ.

BY

L. GOSSELIN,

PROFESSOR OF CLINICAL SURGERY IN THE FACULTY OF MEDICINE, PARIS,
SURGEON TO THE CHARITÉ AND ROTHSCHILD HOSPITALS, MEMBER
OF THE INSTITUTE (ACADEMY OF SCIENCES), PRESIDENT OF
THE ACADEMY OF MEDICINE, MEMBER OF THE
CHIRURGICAL SOCIETY, COMMANDER OF
THE LEGION OF HONOR, ETC.

TRANSLATED FROM THE FRENCH .

BY

LEWIS A. STIMSON, M.D.,

SURGEON TO THE PRESBYTERIAN HOSPITAL, PROFESSOR OF PATHOLOGICAL ANATOMY IN
THE MEDICAL FACULTY OF THE UNIVERSITY OF NEW YORK.

WITH TWENTY-ONE ILLUSTRATIONS.

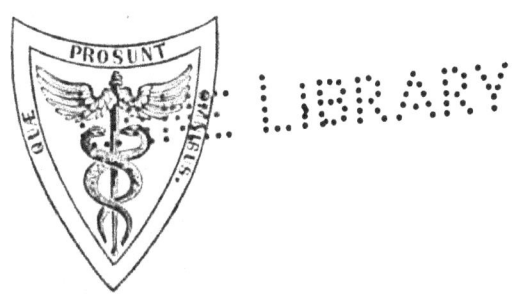

PHILADELPHIA:

HENRY C. LEA.

1878.

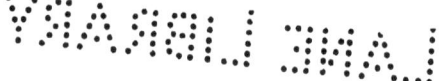

PHILADELPHIA:
COLLINS, PRINTER,
705 Jayne Street.

PREFACE.

THE lectures of which these are a part were delivered by Professor Gosselin during the first five years following his advancement to the position occupied so long by Velpeau. The surgical service of La Charité, which for more than two hundred years has been connected with medical instruction at Paris, now belongs to the ranking chair of Clinical Surgery in the École de Médecine, and a position in one of its three wards is the prize awarded each year to the student who passes the best examination for the internat. Professor Gosselin himself, after having risen through all the subordinate positions, and having gained each promotion by a competitive examination, stands now, since the death of Velpeau, at the head of the surgical section of the Faculty.

In the preface to the first edition of his lectures, Professor Gosselin has explained the three motives which led to their publication. The first was the desire to exemplify his conception of the proper method of clinical instruction, that in which a patient is taken as the text of a lecture in which everything relating to the etiology, symptomatology, prognosis, and treatment of the affection is properly developed and illustrated, so far as possible, by the patient himself. The second was to show to what extent the acquisitions of modern scientific research are applicable to the treatment of disease; and the third, to publish his own original opinions upon certain questions, especially those he had not treated of in previous works.

In making a selection of the lectures for translation the choice was guided by two considerations: 1st, to take those which would be most serviceable and of the greatest interest to the profession in America ; and, 2d, to take those upon subjects with which the author is more particularly identified, those in which he has done much original and valuable work. Among the latter may be especially mentioned the study of the different forms of osteitis, of certain forms of arthritis, of the ultimate results of fracture of the limbs, and of the influence of adolescence upon the pathogeny and prognosis of certain affections. The only important deviation from the original arrangement occurs in Part IV., which is made up of a section upon Surgical Septicæmia, and of two lectures taken from a section upon Gunshot Wounds.

The translation was made in Paris, during a prolonged service in Professor Gosselin's wards, and contains several corrections and revisions made for it by him. It is hoped that the opportunities thus afforded have insured an exact rendering of the author's thoughts.

LEWIS A. STIMSON.

New York, June, 1878.

ERRATA.

Page 153, 13th line from top, for *with* read *without.*
"   172, 11th "   "   bottom, for *an* read *no.*
"   220, 1st "   "   top, for *esteo-* read *osteo-.*

CONTENTS.

PART I.

SURGICAL DISEASES OF YOUTH.

PART II.

FRACTURES OF THE LIMBS.

PART III.

TRAUMATIC OSTEITIS AND NECROSIS.

PART IV.

TRAUMATIC FEVER, PYÆMIA, AND SEPTICÆMIA.

PART V.

DISEASES OF THE ARTICULATIONS.

PART VI.

PHLEGMONS, ABSCESS, FISTULA.

'CLINICAL LECTURES

ON

SURGERY.

PART I.

SURGICAL DISEASES OF YOUTH.

LECTURE I.

INGROWN TOE-NAIL AND ITS TREATMENT.

Considerations upon the diseases of youth—Distinction between lateral onychia, semilunar onychia, and sub-ungual onychia—Origin of lateral onychia or ingrown toe-nail—Etiology—Influence of age, social position, sex, inappreciable general cause—Treatment—Local anæsthesia by means of ice and salt.

GENTLEMEN: I never fail, whenever the occasion presents itself, to call your attention to the influence exerted by age upon the development, course, and prognosis of surgical diseases, and the consequences of the operations necessitated by them.

The surgical pathology of childhood has already been made the subject of special studies, and if that of old age has not been treated of in separate works, yet our authors have not omitted to mention whatever there is of importance in its relations with the diseases of each organ and system.

In most of the descriptions which have been handed down to us, the classical authors have taken the adult age as the type. They have noted certain details peculiar to infancy and old age, but have forgotten the period of adolescence, the limits of which, without being rigorously determined, lie between the ages of 15 and 25 years, a period in which occur the development of puberty and the completion, sometimes rapid and irregular, of the growth of the skeleton.

I do not claim that this age is exposed to diseases which are developed during no other. I know, on the contrary, and I shall often have occasion to tell you, that most of those of which it offers examples are quite frequent in childhood, and that some are also seen in the adult. I claim only that certain diseases are notably more frequent during youth than at other ages, and that the prognosis and treatment are thereby affected to an extent which our predecessors did not notice, and upon which my attention has been fixed for a certain number of years.

I shall presently operate before you upon a young man 16 years old, who offers you an example of one of the diseases of youth, an ingrown toe-nail.

His history, in brief, is this: His constitution is good, and he has not recently had any serious disease. For the last two years he has been employed in a pastry-cook shop, and compelled to remain on his feet a great part of the day. Four months ago he noticed an excoriation at the outer side of the nail of the great toe of the left foot. He took no care of it, and continued to walk. But the excoriation increased; and, as it was lodged in the cutaneous groove which receives the edge of the nail, it is probable that it was kept open by the irritation constantly excited in it by this edge. The oozing grew more and more abundant, and the sore at last became the seat of smarting pains, which were more severe in the evening. Suppuration also increased when the patient had walked all day. When he woke in the morning, the pain and swelling were very moderate. On different occasions the swelling increased, was accompanied by a redness which spread over the dorsal surface of the toe, and the patient was compelled to keep the bed for twenty-four hours. Another time the redness was accompanied by a little fever, and appears to have assumed the character of an angeioleucitis. No serious treatment has been given it; and the young man, after another exacerbation which compelled him to stop his work, decided to ask us for the attentions necessary to a complete cure.

I shall say no more about the functional symptoms; they are those of which I have just spoken. They are light, are accompanied by no alteration of important functions, and might have been borne much longer were it not that they interfered with his walking and thus prevented the exercise of his calling.

As to the physical symptoms, they also are very simple; you have noticed them when comparing the left toe with the right one, which is healthy. They consist in a rather hard and, as it were, hypertrophied swelling of the cutaneous rim which is found at the outer side of the nail, and in the existence of a narrow solution of continuity, elongated, granulating, reddish, and suppurating, which occupies the entire depth and the anterior two-thirds of the lateral groove corresponding to the edge of the nail. As there is some tumefaction, this groove is deeper than usual. Pushing aside the cutaneous rim, we see that the small vegetating wound extends not only to the bottom of the groove, but also around the edge of the nail, and is continued under it, if not throughout its whole extent, at least over that portion where the attachments of the nail to the skin are not very firm; and this portion is larger than usual, because the ulceration has destroyed part of the skin which established the connection.

There is no doubt as to the diagnosis: we have here to deal with the disease described under the name of *ingrown toe nail*, one which I sometimes call *lateral ulcerated onychia*, in distinction from two other rarer varieties: semilunar ulcerated onychia (extending all around the nail), and sub-ungual ulcerated onychia. The term ulcerated onychia has the advantage of denoting that it is not the nail which is diseased, that it is the neighbouring skin which has been excoriated, and that this excoriation is kept up by the edge of the nail, which acts upon it as a foreign body. I wish I could tell you exactly how the ulceration begins in such a case, and especially how it began in the case of this young man. But I have never had the opportunity to see the beginning. It may be that it is simply traumatic, the skin which corresponds to the edge of the nail having been cut at a certain moment by this edge, either naturally sharp, or rendered so by careless trimming of the nail, which in addition may have brought the edge against a part of the skin which is thinner and less protected by the epidermis than those portions which are normally in contact with it.

It may also be that the origin is pathological, that it may have begun in a moist erythema or slight herpes aggravated and ulcerated by the pressure of the edge of the nail. I have been consulted by two patients who had had for a few days the slight skin disease which I have just mentioned. I made them keep the room, take a warm foot-bath, and place, morning and evening, some subnitrate of bismuth in the groove of the nail. In a few days the disease disappeared; but I have asked myself whether, if no care had been taken, and if the patients had continued to walk, it might not have ended in an ingrown nail.

Whichever of these may be the origin, we can still draw two conclusions to direct the prophylaxis: the first is that we must advise every one, and especially adolescents, for they are chiefly exposed to this trouble, not to cut off that part of the nail which covers the sub-ungual cuticle, or, if you prefer, not to carry the section beyond the epidermic adhesions of the border of the nail, so as not to bring this border, made a little sharper by the trimming, into contact with a part of the skin which is thin and unprovided with epidermis. The second is that pressure from below upwards, while walking, forces the already more or less altered skin against this edge, and that consequently rest is necessary to increase the chances of a cure when the patient decides not to undergo an operation.

But if we are not quite sure of the anatomical pathogeny of the ingrown toe-nail, we know very well the conditions which favour its development and act as predisposing causes. These conditions, which have certainly affected our patient, are three in number: age, social position, and sex.

1. *Age.*—The patient is 16 years old. You may think it is only chance which has given us this occasion to see an ingrown toe-nail upon a person of this age. No; on the contrary, it is very common in adolescents. For the last ten years I have kept a record of all the

cases of incurvation of the nail of the great toe[1] which I have treated. Fifty-four of these were upon boys (I will speak of the girls in a moment), and are thus grouped according to the ages.

I saw none before the age of 14 years. I do not claim that it does not exist, but I believe it to be very rare. My table begins at 14½ years:—

Patients 14½ and 15 years of age .	2		Patients 23	.	.	.	2
" 16	12		" 24				1
" 17	8		" 25				2
.. 18	6		26				1
.. 19	6		.. 29				1
.. 20	7		.. 30				2
.. 21	2						—
" 22	2						54

You see then that from 14½ to 20 years we have 41 cases; from 21 to 25 years 9 cases; from 26 to 30 years 4 cases. It must also be noted that in one of my two patients aged 30 years, the disease began when he was only 18 years old. I was right then in telling you that adolescence predisposes to this disease.

But how explain this influence of age? I do not hide from you that this is a difficulty which we shall encounter in some of the other diseases of youth. I suppose we must consider it due to rapid growth, in consequence of which the nail becomes a little too large for the surrounding skin, or, the toe being compressed in shoes which have become too small, the edge of the nail is pressed too firmly against the cutaneous fold. You see, gentlemen, I do not exclude the other local causes, just as I admitted a moment ago the possible intervention of general ones. But the existing local causes, the rapid growth of the nail, the lengthening of the foot, pressure upon it by shoes that have become too small, enable us to understand why incurvation of the nail is more likely to occur during the period of growth than at any other time.

2. *Social Position.*—My 54 patients belonged to my hospital practice. In private practice I have treated only two young men for ingrown toe-nail. This is doubtless due to the fact that youths of the labouring classes take less care of themselves at the beginning, walk and fatigue themselves more, and, above all, do not supply themselves soon enough, when growing rapidly, with new shoes in which the toe would have more room.

3. *Sex.*—Its influence is proved again by figures. During the ten years I have treated in all ten women, seven of them in the hospital, three in private practice. As in the case of the males, here too we see the influence of adolescence, for eight of my patients were between the ages of 15 and 22.

1 was	.	15 years old.		1 was	.	19 years old.
2	. .	16 " "		2	. .	22 " "
2	. .	17 " "				

Of the last two, one was 30 years old, but the disease began at the age of 13 years; the other was 43 years old.

---

[1] Ingrown toe-nail occurs much more rarely on the other toes, and is then due to a general rather than to local causes. I speak now only of that of the great toe.

If you ask me why growing girls are less exposed to ingrown toe-nail than boys are, I answer, without, however, being too affirmative on this point, that I attribute it to this, that in general girls walk and fatigue themselves less, take rather better care of themselves, and do not so often grow rapidly.

But must we not also admit some general cause in this etiology? Let me explain. There are appreciable general causes, and others which are inappreciable. I have found more of the former in the 64 cases which I have treated. You have heard me speak sometimes of syphilitic onychia. But you notice, or you will notice hereafter, that in such cases the ulceration, instead of being limited to the edge of the nail, extends all around the matrix and sometimes to the sub-ungual dermis; also that the great toe is not alone affected, the others are attacked at the same time. In the real ingrown toe-nail, that of youth, the disease occupies exclusively the lateral border of the nail and the great toe. I should also tell you that it is much more frequent on the outer[1] than on the inner side, and that when it occupies the latter the former is almost always affected at the same time. In the statistics which I have carefully kept on this point, I find the inner side alone affected only three times, both sides of the same nail four times, and in the forty-seven other cases the outer side alone.

As to the other general cause which we meet with so often in the diseases of youth as well as in those of infancy, scrofula, I have had no reason to think it has affected my patients.

There remain then the inappreciable general causes. Without de-fining them, we are obliged to admit their influence in many diseases; it is likewise probable that they exist in this one. This will explain the occasional development of an ingrown toe nail during adult life, that is to say during a period when the predisposing causes of which I have spoken exist to a much less degree or not at all, also why in certain youths both sides of the nail are affected, and in others both feet either at the same time or successively. I have occasionally seen ingrown toe-nail, appear, sometimes on the great toe, sometimes on one of the others, during convalescence after an acute disease or in the course of a chronic one, under conditions, in short, where it was impossible to lay it to the charge either of growth, or walking, or even the fatigue of standing. These cases are not included in my statistics. I attribute them to one of these inappreciable and unnamed general causes, and in any case they deserve separate study, since their treat-ment should not be the same, and an operation should be considered useless and even dangerous.

This slight affection is certainly not serious, since it compromises neither health nor life. It has only the inconvenience of making it painful to walk and thereby interfering with the business of those who gain their livelihood by walking or standing most of the day. An-other peculiarity, and one which has especially interested the surgeons, is its tendency to return, even after serious operations, but the notions

---

[1] Referring to the median line of the body, not of the foot.

which I have given you upon the influence of age diminish greatly
the importance of this fact. The ingrown nail of youths may return,
but only during the period of life which predisposes to it. Youth
once passed, the trouble does not return after treatment. Suppose
then, that, in spite of your care, one or two relapses take place while
your patient is between 16 and 22 years of age. After that time you
may be sure the trouble will not re-appear. Moreover, we possess
means which protect even the adolescent from a return of the affection.

Treatment.—There are few surgical diseases for which so many
local treatments have been proposed. I have counted as many as
seventy-five of them, all suggested by honourable surgeons moved by
the desire to protect the patients from relapses; they had not learned
that relapses cease with the period of youth. Of these means, some
are simple, and consist of dressings repeated once or twice each day;
others, of partial or complete extraction of the nail; others, of varied
and complicated operations with the knife or caustics, generally
supplemented by the extraction of more or less of the nail. I shall
describe only the three principal methods and the two or three processes to which I advise you to give the preference in your practice.

1ST METHOD. *Dressings.*—This method, to which I attach the name
of Fabrizio d'Aquapendente, an Italian surgeon of the 16th century
who wrote a large work on surgery, consists in interposing between
the nail and the ulceration a foreign body, which separates them from
one another and prevents the second from being continually irritated
by the first. For this purpose Fabrizio used lint, as we do also to-day.

A few months ago you saw me treat in this way a woman who
came every other day to the consultation, and who for various reasons
was not willing to allow the nail to be torn out. I passed every time
with a spatula a few threads of lint under the outer edge of the nail.
I took pains to press it past the edge and well under the nail, and
then completed the dressing with another pad of lint, which I placed
on the upper surface of the corresponding cutaneous ridge, and kept
in place by means of a strip of diachylon plaster wrapped two or three
times around the toe so as to press the pad well under the ridge.
After six weeks, during which this dressing was renewed every other
day, the ulceration was cicatrized, the tumefaction about it diminished,
and the edge of the nail sufficiently separated from its cutaneous
groove. I told the patient to wear broad shoes and not to cut the
nail short, especially on the outer side. Since then I have not seen
her, but have heard that there has been no return of the trouble.

Instead of lint you may use a strip of tin (Desault); or of lead
(Boyer); or even of cork.

I advise you, gentlemen, to familiarize yourselves with one of these
dressings, and, in my opinion, the simplest is the one with lint. You
may have occasion to use it in the earlier stages, or in the later ones
when the patients have the time to take care of themselves, and are
able to remain six or eight weeks without walking, or walking but
little. For this interposition of a foreign body is not easily borne
when the pressure upwards, which is produced by walking or standing,

constantly forces the inflamed skin against it; and, although not so sharp and irritating as the edge of the nail, it is still in a certain measure a cause of irritation.

I have not thought of employing this treatment for this patient, because it requires too much time, and because confinement to the bed or to the room is undesirable at his age. I may also add that these dressings have the inconvenience of being quite painful at the moment of application and for an hour or two thereafter. And, finally, this mode of treatment is one of those which expose the most to a return of the trouble. You will see it succeed on persons in easy circumstances, especially women, who not only can give themselves the needed time and rest, but, once cured, can favour themselves and walk but little. Our young man, on the contrary, is obliged to gain his living by his legs, and as soon as he is cured he will have to begin at once to walk, so that the chances of an early return of the affection would be great.

2D METHOD. *Simple Extraction.*—This operation, which is applied sometimes to the whole of the nail, sometimes only to the half which is ingrown, is intended to remove the body which acts as an irritant, and give the little fungoid ulceration time to heal. Of course, the nail grows again, for in removing it we do not destroy that portion of the skin which produces it, and notably the deep posterior fold called the *matrix.* I will describe in a moment the method of extraction which I prefer, before performing the combined operation of which it forms part.

This method has the real advantage that it can be performed without pain, and is followed by a prompt cure, for at the end of five or six days, during which rest and a protecting dressing alone are needed, the raw surface has become dry and the ulceration healed. But, unfortunately, it is often followed by a return of the trouble. I cannot give the exact figures, but I remember to have seen in the service of Velpeau a certain number of patients who returned at short intervals to undergo the operation a second, third, or fourth time. As I have already told you, I know that after a while adolescence ends, and with it the tendency to the reproduction of the disease; but still it is an inconvenience which we should seek to avoid as much as possible, and in this respect the combined operations are a little more successful.

3D METHOD. *Combined Operations.*—These are the ones by which it is proposed to remove both the edge of the nail and the cutaneous ridge upon which the fungoid granulations are found. For this purpose some authors have recommeded caustics; others have combined extraction of the nail with excision of the fleshy parts. To this last operation I give the preference, but, after tearing out the nail, I cut off only a portion of the ridge, so as to have a wound which is smaller, will cicatrize more promptly, and is less likely to give rise to erysipelas or angeioleucitis, and, moreover, is sufficiently removed from the articulation of the two phalanges to avoid the chances of provoking suppurative arthritis. I propose, also, to remove on the affected side a considerable portion of the matrix, so that the new nail may be much narrower than the old one. You understand that this reduction of the breadth of the nail diminishes the chances of a relapse, which are greater the nearer the edge of the nail is to the bottom of the groove in which it lies. I have several times measured the new nail a few months after this operation, and have always found it narrower than that of the other foot. I have already published my method of performing this operation,[1] and I shall now execute it before you in the following manner:—

1st Time.—To prevent pain I shall make use of a freezing mixture composed of equal parts of pounded ice and salt. The mixture will be made just before it is to be applied, and will be placed in a small bag made of thin muslin. I shall place this bag upon the dorsal surface and the sides of the great toe, cover it with a compress, and leave it in place for two minutes, when I shall remove it to see if anæsthesia has been obtained. If I find the skin still red and sensitive I shall re-apply the mixture and leave it until sensibility is entirely deadened.

I recommend this mode of anæsthesia in this operation, because, since the parts upon which we are to operate are superficial, it is useless to seek to dull the sensibility of the deeper ones, as we have to do when our incisions are carried beyond the limits of the skin, and consequently we are not embarrassed by the pre-occupations of general anæsthesia produced by inhalation. Local anæsthesia may be obtained by refrigeration with ether, but this process requires more time and does not produce so complete a result; and as the operation we are to perform is very painful, we must deaden sensibility as completely as possible.

2d Time.—Standing at the foot of the bed, and at the affected side, and having seized the toe firmly with my left hand, I shall pass one of the blades of a strong pair of scissors on its side under the nail as far back as the matrix, then turning the edge upwards, and closing the scissors quickly, I shall divide the nail lengthwise into two equal parts. Then with a stout pair of forceps I shall seize each piece in turn and tear it out. Sometimes the nail is friable and breaks; then of course the fragments must be successively removed. Do not forget that for this purpose you need a very strong pair of forceps, one whose blades will not twist under the violent effort you will have to make.

3d Time.—This consists in the excision of a strip of skin, leaving a wound which, though small, comprises in front a portion of the cutaneous ridge and abnormal vegetations, and behind the external lateral portion of the matrix. For this I shall take a bistoury, and make, behind, at the junction of the transverse and lateral portions of the matrix, a transverse incision one-quarter of an inch long through the entire thickness of the skin, and then carry it along the summit of the lateral cutaneous ridge to its anterior extremity. I shall then

---

[1] Gosselin, Sur le Traitement de l'Ongle incarné, Gazette Hebdomadaire, 1853, tome i. p. 7.

dissect inwards the flap thus formed, so as to include in it the entire length and thickness of the sub-ungual dermis for a breadth of nearly one-quarter of an inch, that is, its antero-lateral portion and the corresponding piece of the posterior portion or matrix.

I shall finish with a protective dressing made of a cloth covered with cerate, lint, compresses, and a narrow band. This dressing will be renewed every day for eight or ten days, at the end of which time the patient will be able to leave his bed, and perhaps the hospital.

During the last year you have seen me treat several patients in this way. In no case did any complication occur. In all the little wound healed, and the dermis dried in a length of time which varied from eight to fifteen days. When the patients left us they had no nail, but they could wear a shoe and walk by placing a rag or a little carded cotton over the toe. In only one of my sixty-four cases was the cure delayed by an angeioleucitis of the foot and leg, followed by small multiple abscesses along the course of the lymphatic vessels, and although delayed the cure was still obtained.

Upon none of the patients whom we have had this year have we as yet seen any return of the affection. But I have already told you that my method, although it removes the ulcerated skin and diminishes the breadth of the nail, still does not always prevent a relapse. In only five of my sixty-four cases has the disease returned, three boys and two girls, but I have had no example of a second return. Consequently the most unlucky have had to undergo the operation only twice. I have seen again several of them who had then passed the age of 25 years, and in whom the affection had not returned, and I have yet to see a relapse in any of my patients who have passed the period of youth.

LECTURE II.

SUB-UNGUAL EXOSTOSIS OF THE GREAT TOE.

Description of antecedents and symptoms—Diagnosis—Importance of age and sex; it is a disease of youth, more common in girls than in boys—Anatomical characteristics—Analogy to epiphysary exostosis, and to naso-pharyngeal polyps—Treatment—Possible relapse—Cessation of this tendency after adolescence.

GENTLEMEN: I have here a small piece which I removed the day before yesterday in your presence from the great toe of a girl 20 years old. She was a dressmaker who had been admitted into the hospital a few days before to be treated for a tumour as large as a small nut occupying the interior and superior surface of the left great toe at its which I have given you upon the influence of age diminish greatly the importance of this fact. The ingrown nail of youths may return, but only during the period of life which predisposes to it. Youth once passed, the trouble does not return after treatmen. Suppose then, that, in spite of your care, one or two relapses take place while your patient is between 16 and 22 years of age. After that time you may be sure the trouble will not re-appear. Moreover, we possess means which protect even the adolescent from a return of the affection.

Treatment.—There are few surgical diseases for which so many local treatments have been proposed. I have counted as many as seventy-five of them, all suggested by honourable surgeons moved by the desire to protect the patients from relapses; they had not learned that relapses cease with the period of youth. Of these means, some are simple, and consist of dressings repeated once or twice each day; others, of partial or complete extraction of the nail ; others, of varied and complicated operations with the knife or caustics, generally supplemented by the extraction of more or less of the nail I shall describe only the three principal methods and the two or three processes to which I advise you to give the preference in your practice.

1ST METHOD. *Dressings.*—This method, to which I attach the name of Fabrizio d'Aquapendente, an Italian surgeon of the 16th century who wrote a large work on surgery, consists in interposing between the nail and the ulceration a foreign body, which separates them from one another and prevents the second from being continually irritated by the first. For this purpose Fabrizio used lint, as we do also to-day.

A few months ago you saw me treat in this way a woman who came every other day to the consultation, and who for various reasons was not willing to allow the nail to be torn out. I passed every time with a spatula a few threads of lint under the outer edge of the nail. I took pains to press it past the edge and well under the nail, and then completed the dressing with another pad of lint, which I placed on the upper surface of the corresponding cutaneous ridge, and kept in place by means of a strip of diachylon plaster wrapped two or three times around the toe so as to press the pad well under the ridge. After six weeks, during which this dressing was renewed every other day, the ulceration was cicatrized, the tumefaction about it diminished, and the edge of the nail sufficiently separated from its cutaneous groove. I told the patient to wear broad shoes and not to cut the nail short, especially on the outer side. Since then I have not seen her, but have heard that there has been no return of the trouble.

Instead of lint you may use a strip of tin (Desault); or of lead (Boyer); or even of cork.

I advise you, gentlemen, to familiarize yourselves with one of these dressings, and, in my opinion, the simplest is the one . . . . You may have occasion to use it in the earlier stages, or when the patients have the time to take care of t] able to remain six or eight weeks without walkin little. For this interposition of a foreign body ; when the pressure upwards, which is produced by

But I rejected such an opinion, and admitted an exostosis, for the following reasons :—

1st. *The Age.*—Although I have seen an example of sub-ungual exostosis in a woman 47 years old, it is none the less true that this, like ingrown toe nail, is a disease of youth. Dupuytren, who was the first in France to give a clear and methodical description of this affection, reports five cases in which the patients were from 20 to 25 years old, but in all of them the disease began at about the age of 18. Dupuytren, however, although mentioning the age of each of his patients, did not call attention to this fact. Legoupil,[1] on the other hand, clearly points out adolescence as one of the principal predisposing causes, for, he says, "most of the cases within my knowledge are confined between the ages of 15 and 20, and I found none who had passed their 26th year." It is certain that Legoupil speaks not of cases which he had himself observed, but of those which he found recorded, and, indeed, it is incontestable that almost all such belong to the end of the period of adolescence, although the authors do not call attention to this fact. Still it is easy to understand how this etiological idea may have escaped the notice of many persons. Subungual exostosis is rare, and each surgeon, having seen only a few examples, and having seen them only at long intervals, may have considered the similarity of age as the result of chance. As for me, I have preserved the record of only eight patients. Seven of these were aged as follows: two, 19 years old; two, 20; one, 21; one, 24; and one, 25; but in all the disease commenced one or two years before I saw them for the first time. I said just now that I had had one patient 47 years old; that proves that this, like ingrown toe-nail, may be developed in the adult; but it is exceptional, and we may consider it the rule that sub-ungual exostosis is a disease of youth.

2d. *Sex.*—Our patient was a young girl. Now, the analysis of the cases shows that, unlike ingrown toe-nail, this affection is more common among girls than among boys. Dupuytren's five cases were all girls. Legoupil points out that the ten cases of which he knew were all young girls. Of mine, five were girls, three were boys. Although in the printed records you find girls mentioned more often than boys, still you will meet with the mention of boys often enough to be authorized to believe that the proportion differs from that which exists for ingrown toe-nail. I can offer you no figures to prove this, since I have only eight personal cases, and that is insufficient to establish a rule. But connecting with my results the impression left upon me by reading published cases, I believe that relatively there are more boys affected with sub-ungual exostosis than there are girls affected with ingrown toe-nail. As to the diagnosis, however, the question remains the same. The sex was a circumstance favourable to the opinion that it was an exostosis rather than a cancer, and it was from this point of view that I was led to speak to you of the influence of sex. I am absolutely unable to explain this predilection for the female

---

[1] Malgaigne's Revue Médico-Chirurgicale, tome viii. p. 21 (1850).

sex, a predilection which you will not find in the other diseases of youth.

3d. As to the ulceration, the exudation, and the pains, which remind us of ulcerated cancer, you must remember that these incidents are quite frequent in sub-ungual exostosis. The cause is topographical; it is the pressure of the shoes while walking that occasions them. The pain is furthermore due to the sensibility, normally very great, of the sub-ungual dermis which is affected by the inflammation, to the ulceration, and the lack of protection by the nail, the limits of which are surpassed by the tumour and are generally much reduced by cutting, as in this case. This cutting off of the nail is all the easier because the nutritive trouble produced by the morbid growth is followed by the loosening of that part which covers it.

Perhaps if the tumour had been less voluminous it might at first have been taken for a simple ingrown nail. You noticed, however, and this is always the case in sub-ungual exostosis, that the vegetations were not lateral, but placed above and in front. I admit that the anterior edge of the nail may have contributed to their formation, and that consequently they may have had the same origin as those of ingrown toe-nail, but in primitive and uncomplicated ingrown toe-nail the affection is upon the side and not on top, and it is not accompanied by a tumefaction which raises the front part of the nail, and advances beyond the anterior edge, as is the case here.

The diagnosis having been made, we have to ask ourselves whether the etiological diagnosis ought not to be completed by the indication of some general cause other than the age and sex. You often hear us speak of syphilitic exostoses. I have examined and questioned this patient, and have not found, and have no reason to suspect, syphilitic antecedents. Even had I found them, I should doubtless not have attributed this exostosis to them, for my own experience and that of other surgeons have taught us that sub-ungual exostosis of the great toe, and that of the other toes, and also those of the fingers,[1] are not of syphilitic origin. The same is true for the other exostoses of young people, and we find in this circumstance another reason to justify the separate description of the diseases of youth upon which you hear me so often insist.

Pathological Anatomy.—Of what was this tumour composed? Before removing it I told you what it would probably prove to be, but now that we have the piece in our hands I can give you a more exact account. On the surface you see the sub-ungual dermis, below it, but intimately united with it, is a white layer, fibrous in appearance, one-eighth of an inch thick, which seems to the naked eye to be formed of dense fibro-cartilaginous tissue, but the microscope fails to discover any cartilaginous cells in it, and shows it to be formed in reality of very dense fibrous tissue. Under this, and again con-

[1] Sub-ungual exostosis may be developed upon the other toes and upon the fingers. All authors have pointed this out. I have had one example upon the third toe, and one under the nail of the index finger of the right hand. But it is infinitely more frequent on the great toe.

nected closely with it, you see a mass of bone, nearly one-quarter of an inch thick, formed in part by the abnormal growth, and in part by the portion of the phalanx from which it came. The tumour then was not a pure exostosis, it was an exostosis covered by fibrous tissue, or, if you prefer, an osteo-fibrous growth. In this respect it differs from other exostoses of youth, which are formed exclusively of bony tissue, and it has some analogy to naso-pharyngeal fibromas which spring from the bone, but are formed exclusively of fibrous tissue. That is to say, that in adolescents, and by the fact of the growth of the body, perversion of nutrition leads sometimes to an excess of bony tissue attached to the bones themselves, sometimes to an excess of fibrous tissue attached to the periosteum, sometimes to a simultaneous exaggeration of both bony and fibrous tissues It is this last variety which we have before us, and this was also the case in the other examples which I have had occasion to examine. There may be cases in which the exostosis is purely bony, but those which I have observed have been such that I am authorized to tell you that the tumour generally is mixed, that is to say, osteo-fibrous.

Treatment.—There is no reason to hope that these tumours can be removed by internal treatment, and I have no facts even which permit me to believe that, left to itself, the disease will get well by simple increase of age. I had then to offer to our patient only an operation, and this is the one you saw me perform. First I removed the nail after local anæsthesia by means of a mixture of ice and salt as in the operation of ingrown toe-nail; then I isolated the tumour by two curved incisions, and detached it with a strong bistoury, hollowing out a little the upper and anterior surface of the phalanx to a depth of about one-sixth of an inch. In doing this I proposed to remove together with the tumour all its roots of implantation, so as to protect the patient from a return of the affection. The bone offered but a slight resistance; if it had been harder I should have used the gouge and mallet. A simple dressing, the same as for an ingrown toe-nail, terminated the operation.

This operation differs from Dupuytren's in this, that he shaved off the base of the tumour horizontally with the blade of the bistoury, while I used the point, forcing it in first on the inner then on the outer side, holding the tumour, meanwhile, with pronged forceps. The bony substance resisted a little, but by using some force, I easily overcame it.

You will find in the books other modes of treatment. Liston (of London) and Lenoir (of Paris) preferred disarticulation of the outer phalanx, in order the more certainly to prevent a return of the trouble. Dr. Debrou, of Orleans, animated by the same desire, thought it sufficient to amputate in the continuity of the phalanx, forming a dorsal flap out of the sub-ungual dermis, and a plantar one. This skilful surgeon based his operation upon two dissections which had shown him that the origin and implantation were upon the anterior border of the phalanx, and extended so short a distance upon its upper surface that amputation at the point indicated might be made with the certainty of removing all the disease, and preventing its reproduction.

Gentlemen, I do not wish to exaggerate the danger of amputation in contiguity, and still less of that in continuity, but still this danger is certainly greater than that of the ablation to which I give the preference. The slight excavation which I made so as to pass beyond the limits of the disease, and to the usefulness of which I called attention in 1861,[1] appears to me quite sufficient to protect the patient from a relapse. At least in none of the eight persons upon whom I have operated in this way has the growth returned, and even if it should return once, I feel convinced that if the patient had reached the age of 25 or 26 years at the time of the second operation, another return would not take place, the age which predisposes to this kind of production having been passed.

LECTURE III.

NON-SPECIFIC EPIPHYSARY EXOSTOSIS OF YOUTH OR EXOSTOSIS OF DEVELOPMENT.

Description of the disease—Incurability by internal treatment—Operation useless, because the tumour is indolent and without danger, and will cease to grow after adolescence—Surgical intervention reserved for some exceptional cases.

GENTLEMEN: As we finished the visit this morning we were stopped by a young man, 19 years old, whose father came to ask my advice about a tumour situated upon the inferior and internal portion of his son's right knee. The tumour first appeared when the boy was 16 years old, it has grown little by little without causing any pain, but now that it has reached the size of a lady apple the young man and his parents begin to worry about it, and wish to know if it cannot be removed. You saw that the tumour was round, slightly knobbed, and so hard that there was no doubt about its being formed of bone. The skin that covers it is normally soft and movable. Seizing it with one hand, and fixing the leg solidly with the other, I recognized that the tumour was tightly adherent to and confounded with the inner tuberosity of the tibia.

Consequently I did not hesitate to pronounce the diagnosis exostosis, and you heard me add, exostosis of adolescence. By that I wished you to understand that there are developed in adolescents exostoses which are not due to a specific cause, but which are purely local lesions unaccompanied either by pains or marked functional troubles,

---

[1] Bulletin de la Soc. de Chirurgie, June 12, 1861.

and which will not disappear under the influence of a general treat-ment.

You often see in the surgical wards, and you will hereafter meet with in practice, patients bearing tertiary syphilitic exostoses. Sometimes they are young people, but more often they are adults, and in any case the diagnosis indicates at once the existence of a general cause, syphilis, under the influence of which the lesion has been produced, and behind this cause the possibility of a disappearance under the influence of an appropriate treatment.

On the other hand, you will often hear me call your attention to bony swellings which I call *hyperostoses*. I shall tell you that these hyperostoses sometimes follow osteitis of infancy or of youth, but in such a case last throughout the patient's life, and become from time to time the seat of fresh inflammatory action, and even of necrosis. I shall further show you that these hyperostoses may form on adults, especially after a fracture.

But in the case of this young man you see there has been no inter-vention either of the syphilitic cause or of an antecedent osteitis. We have here a very circumscribed, indolent, bony swelling, which is due to no appreciable cause, and which can be explained only by an aber-ration or excess of bony development at certain points of the skele-ton, at the time when the system·is working to complete this latter, an aberration comparable to that which causes the formation at the same age of sub-ungual exostosis and naso-pharyngeal polyps. Only, while in this case the production is exclusively bony, you remember that in sub-ungual exostosis it is osteo-fibrous, and in the naso-pharyngeal polyps exclusively fibrous.

I said that you would meet with analogous cases in your practice. You will find them oftener upon the lower than the upper limbs, and in the neighbourhood of the extremities rather than upon the body of the bone. In this connection I accept willingly the opinion uttered by M. Broca[1] before the Société de Chirurgie upon the origin of these exostoses in the border of the epiphysary cartilage, and more often upon the side than in front or behind, and with him I give them the name of epiphysary exostoses. But I should like to be sure that my learned colleague had had the occasion, which I, for my part, have not had, to verify the fact upon the cadaver. On some subjects you find many at a time. In a case presented by M. Marjolin[2] to the Société de Chi-rurgie, there were a great many of them, and they were symmetrical, that is, they occupied the same place and had the same size on the right and on the left. It is true that this was a child six years old; but although this lesion is generally seen during youth, yet like the other lesions of this age it sometimes occurs in children.

When the father asked me repeatedly what I thought should be done for the tumour, you heard me answer, "Nothing." The exos-tosis causes no functional trouble, no pain; if there were any chance that we might cause it to disappear by inoffensive external or internal

[1] Broca, Gazette des Hôpitaux, 1865, p. 295.
[2] Marjolin, Gazette des Hôpitaux, 1864, p. 344.

treatment, we would make the attempt, for it is disagreeable for any one, and especially for a young man, to bear a deformity. But we know and we have warned the patient that the tumour will not disappear under the influence of drugs, and that it may even increase a little until the skeleton is completed, that is, until the end of adolescence. Consequently I prescribed only some precautions in the hope of preventing too great growth. I advised him to avoid long walks and fatigue, and to cover the upper portion of the leg with cotton and duck, so as to protect the exostosis from external violence, or at least to diminish its effect.

Gentlemen, observe that we could get a radical cure only by a cutting operation. This operation, which would consist in dissecting back the skin, uncovering the base of the tumour, and removing it with a chain-saw or gouge, would certainly not be difficult of execution. But it would inevitably be followed by suppuration, for the wound would be too large to permit immediate union ; the suppuration would undoubtedly attack the bone itself, and the patient would have to run the risk of an acute suppurative osteo-myelitis, the danger of which disease I shall often have to point out to you.

At the beginning of my studies, in 1834, I saw Professor Roux remove by an operation of this kind an epiphysary exostosis of the lower portion of the femur of a strong, handsome young man 18 years old. Suppurative osteo-myelitis of the femur set in, and was complicated by pyæmia, which carried off the patient at the end of twenty days. Roux had performed the operation because he thought the tumour would grow until it caused intolerable pain and annoyance.

To-day surgeons ought to know that—the period of adolescence ended—tumours of this kind remain stationary, and, as a rule, cause no trouble in the functions of the affected part.

There are, however, exceptions. M. Broca has reported the case of a young man, 20 years old, whose exostosis was complicated by a cyst developed about it. This cyst grew so large that the surgeon thought an operation necessary, and removed both it and the bony tumour successfully. I think that perhaps in such a case puncture of the cyst, followed by an injection of the tincture of iodine, without touching the exostosis, might be sufficient. I should not be willing to remove the latter unless it interfered notably with the action of the muscles.

An English surgeon, M. Coote,[1] was led to operate by special reasons which, in any case where they should present themselves, would be a precise indication for surgical intervention. The patient, 26 years old, had had for many years an exostosis of the transverse process of the seventh cervical vertebra. The tumour, which was only as large as a good-sized nut, projected above the clavicle, pushed the subclavian artery forward, and forced upward and compressed the nerves of the brachial plexus. Hence numbness and coldness of the hand and fingers, and pain along the arm and in the shoulder. Removal of the tumour, which was, of course, difficult in this region, caused the disappearance of all these functional troubles.

---

[1] Coote, Union Médicale, 1861, tome xii. p. 188.

In 1857, at the Hôpital Cochin, I saw a still rarer exception. The patient, 51 years old, had had, since the age of 15 or 16, an exostosis upon the inner portion of the left femur. (Figs. 1 and 2.) It had

Fig. 1.   Fig. 2.

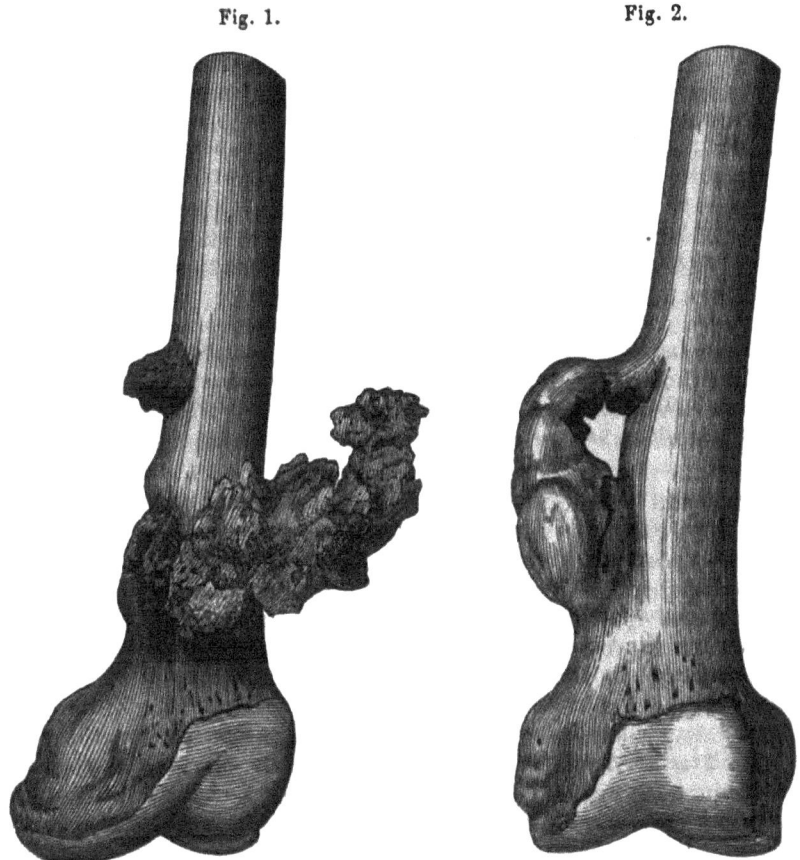

Arched exostosis of femur—broken.   Fragments in place.

never given him any trouble, when one day he was knocked down by a wagon, the wheel of which, passing over his thigh, fractured the exostosis. Its anatomical disposition was very unusual. Instead of a single implantation, which is habitual, it had two: the lower one very large, the upper one smaller. It had thus the form of a loop or of a large zygomatic arch.

The weight of the wagon caused a comminuted fracture of this exostosis, detaching it from its insertions, and at the same time a contused wound, which made the fracture compound.

Suppuration was abundant; the patient fell promptly into a dangerous hectic condition; I amputated through the thigh about the thirtieth day, and the patient was carried off by pyæmia.

With the exception then of such cases as these, fix in your minds this fact, that epiphysary or developmental exostoses may remain

2

without causing any inconvenience, that they cease to grow when adolescence ends, and that their removal offers dangers to which it is absolutely contra-indicated to expose the patient when the tumour is indolent and inoffensive.

<hr>

LECTURE IV.

SUFFOCATING AND REBELLIOUS NASO-PHARYNGEAL FIBROMA OR FIBROUS POLYP.

Hemorrhagic and suffocating form of fibroma—Large implantation upon the base of the skull—Signification of the word polyp—Palliative operations—Nélaton's operation—Cauterization by electrolysis—Nitric acid—Chloride of zinc—Increase —Exophthalmia, hemiplegia, their disappearance at the age of 25 years.

GENTLEMEN: We have just seen, as we completed the visit, a young man, 23 years old, whom I have treated in our wards for nearly two years for a naso-pharyngeal fibrous polyp which had become suffocating and hemorrhagic, and who appears now to be cured of this serious affection. His history is so instructive from all points of view, and especially with reference to the influence of age, that I wish to relate it to you again, and beg you to engrave it upon your minds.

This young man, Joseph Pellard, entered our wards for the first time the 21st of April, 1869. He was then 22 years old. He told us that since the age of 16 or 17 he had noticed a change in his voice, which had grown nasal, and a slight difficulty in breathing through his nose. During several years these functional symptoms troubled him so little that he paid no attention to them and consulted no one.

At about the age of 20 he bled frequently from the nose; but although the nasal tone had increased, and respiration through the nostrils was impossible, he was still able to live without treatment. After some time the epistaxes became more frequent, though not very abundant; each time the respiration became more embarrassed, and deglutition was difficult. The patient was then obliged to consult a physician, who sent him to me for the surgical treatment which he considered necessary.

The day we examined the patient for the first time, we found that he was large, well formed, and did not have the pale look of anæmic subjects, which proved that the quantity of blood lost had not been considerable. What struck us most was the frequency of his respirations, and the snoring sound which accompanied them. Questioned upon this point, the patient said he did not generally feel choked, but he was short of breath when walking, and for that reason could neither walk fast nor run.   He added that on two occasions, without apparent cause, he had had short attacks of suffocation.   His face was not deformed.

In order to examine the nostrils and nasal fossæ, I placed the patient before a window, introduced successively into each nostril Duplay's bivalve nasal speculum, and saw, at about three-quarters of an inch from the nostril, on each side, a round reddish body.   I told the patient to close the mouth and make a forcible expiration, and thus discovered not only that these round bodies were not pushed forward, but also that not a particle of air escaped through the nasal fossæ, and that consequently these latter were entirely obstructed. At the same time, I mentioned that the intra-nasal tumours had neither the flattened form nor the pinkish-gray colour of mucous polyps.

Carrying, then, my investigation into the pharynx, I saw at once that the soft palate was pressed forward.   I tried to press it back with my finger but was unable to do so, finding resistance upon the sides as well as in the median line.   Then depressing the tongue, I saw in the middle of the pharynx a round reddish body extending nearly half an inch below the edge of the palate, and evidently continuous with the resisting body above it.   Finally, passing the right index finger beyond the palate, I felt that this fleshy body occupied all the upper or nasal portion of the pharynx.   I could pass the end of my finger between it and the wall on the right side, but not on the left, but it was impossible to get behind, or above, or to move it, because it occupied the whole space, and seemed to be fixed upon the first cervical vertebræ.

By these physical and functional symptoms, I recognized one of those tumours so well studied recently by Professor Nélaton, which we know by the name of naso-pharyngeal polyps.

It was not a mucous polyp, because, in the first place, polyps of that kind do not ordinarily reach such a size, secondly, because it was redder, and above all, because its consistency was firmer.   All these points are characteristic of fibrous polyps.

The size of the tumour might have given rise to the idea of its being a cancer, and its resistance to the remedies employed during eighteen months might afterwards have confirmed this idea.   But there was no ulceration ; now, cancer of the nasal, buccal, and pharyngeal cavities, hardly reaches this size, and does not last so long without ulcerating.   On the other hand, cancer, especially cancer that progresses slowly (this tumour was at least five years old), is very rare at this age.

Finally, M. Nélaton's researches have taught us two things which ought to be utilized in the diagnosis.   The first is that naso-pharyngeal fibrous growths are seen especially upon young people, and the second is that they are seen almost exclusively upon boys and not upon girls.

The cases which I have met are entirely confirmative of these two opinions.   I have seen naso-pharyngeal fibromas only upon adoles-

cents and upon boys. I have read of some cases where the patients
were girls; but I am not sure that the diagnosis was correct.

Apropos of that, gentlemen, let me put you on your guard against
the titles given to many facts in books and periodicals published
before 1848. Up to that time they had not had occasion to make the
distinctions among naso-pharyngeal tumours which we make to-day,
and they gave the name of polyp to every growth which projected
into the naso-pharyngeal cavities, without occupying themselves with
the nature of the tissue of which the tumour was composed. We now
know that there are found in these regions, fibromas, epitheliomas,
and cancers, which resemble one another by many of their physical
and functional characters. Now, while the two latter may appear at
any age and in both sexes, the first present the two etiological peculiarities which I have just mentioned.

I will not go so far as to affirm that naso-pharyngeal fibrous polyps
never appear in girls. I only say that neither M. Nélaton nor I have
yet observed a positive example of it.

The age and sex, then, of our patient, favoured the opinion that
the tumour was a fibroma ; but I used the expression *polyp*. What
do we mean by this word, and is it rightly used here?

Clinically, we have long called polyps tumours developed and free
in those natural cavities of the body which communicate with the
exterior, and most of which are covered by a mucous membrane,
tumours of which one of the principal characteristics is that they are
attached by a pedicle, that is to say, by a portion which is smaller
than the free and prominent portion of the tumour. This word
"polyp" has the disadvantage of conveying no anatomo-pathological
idea. Modern surgery, however, has retained it for two reasons :
first, because the presence of the pedicle indicated by this word leads
to operations relatively easy (ligature, excision) and different from
those necessitated by the tumours of other regions ; second, because
the pedicle carries with it the idea of non-malignancy, that is, of not
being cancerous. I cannot tell you why it is so, but such is the fact,
and I formulate it thus : In the natural cavities cancerous tumours
are not pedicular ; only non-malignant tumours have a pedicle.

That, however, does not mean that non-malignant tumours always
have a pedicle, and in fact, in the case of a young man of whom I
am now speaking, I was authorized, for the reasons I have given
you, to admit a fibroma ; but I was by no means authorized the first
day, and you will see I have been less and less so ever since, to
admit a pedicle. I could not see one, and with my finger I could
feel only a small portion of the tumour free, while the latter was
absolutely immovable, and I thought I found a sort of fusion
between it and the corresponding portions of the skeleton, the basilar surface of the occipital and sphenoid, and the lower face of the
petrous portion of the temporal. If, then, the tumour was pedicellated,
it was impossible for me to determine it at first, and I was obliged to
reserve that part of the diagnosis until, the tumour having been
diminished in some way, I should be able to carry my finger around
it and see if the implantation was notably smaller than the free

portion. I will tell you now that my later explorations demonstrated the absence of a pedicle and the existence of a large base of implantation. Consequently it was not a polyp, in the rigorous acceptation of the word.

If you have heard me still use the expression, it has been because, on the one hand, it had this other signification, that in my opinion the growth was fibrous and consequently non-malignant, and, on the other hand, I was justified by usage. In the works which have been published in France upon this subject under the inspiration of Nélaton, especially in the theses of Drs. Perier and D'Ornellas, as well as in the discussions upon the subject, the word polyp has been habitually used to indicate every kind of naso-pharyngeal fibrous growth of adolescence.

Remember, nevertheless, to make this distinction, that among the tumours of this kind, some are distinctly pediculated, others are completely sessile, and I will show you hereafter the importance of this distinction for the treatment.

The anatomical diagnosis being thus established, naso-pharyngeal fibroma broadly implanted upon the upper wall of the pharynx, and projecting at the same time into the two nasal fossæ and into the inferior and middle regions of the pharynx, I completed it, by adding that the tumour interfered enough with respiration by blocking up the air passages to deserve the name of suffocating fibroma or polyp.

In this last quality lay the necessity for surgical intervention. But what was to be done?

I passed in review all the simple and compound operations which have been recommended for cases of this kind. I saw at once that a simple operation was impossible on account of the size of the tumour, and that it was necessary to select one of the complex and multiple ones which I was the first to distinguish as *preliminary, fundamental,* and *complementary.*[1]

The end proposed in these operations has been to separate the tumour completely at the point of implantation, in the hope of thereby removing it entirely and protecting the patient from relapse, which, according to the experience of Nélaton, confirmed afterwards by that of all surgeons, is very common in this disease, and has been attributed to the insufficiency of the removal. The reasoning, apparently correct, was this: Let the surgical intervention be such as will entirely remove or destroy all the roots of the tumour, and its reproduction will not take place. Some facts agreed with the theory, but others, and they were quite numerous, disagreed. Reproductions occurred in spite of all the care which had been taken to shave off the surface of implantation, to scrape it and to destroy all that could be considered as forming part of the tumour. To be convinced of this you have only to read the tables prepared by M. Michaux de Louvain in 1867.[2] He has collected twenty-seven cases of total re-

---

[1] Goselin, Traitement chirurgical des Polypes des fosses nasales et du pharynx. Thèse de Concours pour une Chaire de Médecine opératoire Paris, 1850.

[2] Michaux (de Louvain) Quelques Mots encore sur les Polypes fibreux naso-pharyngiens volumineux. Bulletin de l'Académie de Belgique, 3d série, tome i. in 4to.

section of the superior maxilla which resulted in eighteen complete successes, one incomplete, two *relapses*, and three deaths; and twenty-nine cases of removal with resection of the palatal arch, which gave twelve successes, five incomplete results, three unknown, four *relapses*, and five deaths. I am not at all sure that the successes given as complete remained such indefinitely; some of the patients may have had relapses after the surgeon had lost sight of them. But it is nevertheless true, according to the known results, that a relapse is possible after serious preliminary operations which permit the entire removal of the tumour.

I had then to determine whether, in order to save my patient from the death by suffocation which threatened him, I ought to perform a serious preliminary operation which would give me free access to the surface of implantation, so that I might attack the latter with cutting instruments, and afterwards, if neccessary, cauterize it. I had to choose between incision of the soft, followed by resection of the hard palate (Nélaton's method), and resection of the superior maxillary bone, as practised by Flaubert of Rouen, Robert, and Michaux.

I was but little tempted by the first, because, the surface of implantation being probably very large, I should have been unable to get an opening large enough to allow me to operate upon it properly. This preliminary operation, which has the great advantage of sparing the face and leaving the alveolar-dental arch intact, appears to me to be sufficient and preferable when the implantation is small, when it is limited, for example, to the basilar surface of the occipital bone; but it is certainly insufficient when the implantation is very large, as was the case here. With reference to the certainty of execution, the maxillary route was undoubtedly preferable. But besides the inevitable disfigurement which it causes, it is more serious and is more likely than the former to lead to purulent infection. I know that the statistics published by M. Michaux seem to prove the contrary, but remember, and this objection applies to all statistics based on observations gathered from journals, that all the cases, and especially the unfortunate ones, have not been published, and that consequently statistics of this kind, in spite of their apparent exactitude, do not definitely settle the question of the comparative danger of different operations. For my part, I am convinced by the results of resection of the upper maxilla for other affections than polyps, that this operation is more dangerous than resection of the palate. Moreover, in the present case it was not only the preliminary operation, but also the fundamental one, which was dangerous. This great tumour was very vascular, for it had frequently occasioned epistaxis, and there was reason to fear that if I attacked it with the bistoury, scissors, or hooks, the patient would die upon the table from hemorrhage.

Reflecting upon those dangers to which a complicated operation exposed the patient, I thought of the influence of age, and asked myself whether the patient, being twenty-two years old, was not near that period of life in which tumours of this kind have no tendency to be produced, and consequently none to reappear. I remembered that my learned friend and colleague, M. Legouest, had uttered formally, before the Société de Chirurgie in 1865, the opinion that naso-pharyngeal polyps might be treated by a simple and palliative operation until the period of their habitual formation had passed.

Furthermore, having, as I have just told you, no very precise notions as to the extent of the implantation, and not being willing to engage in a perilous operation without being better informed, I decided to confine myself at first to a palliative operation which should have a double object, that of relieving the patient from the danger of suffocation, and giving me more definite ideas as to the connections of the tumour by which my future action would be determined.

Having decided upon this plan, I proposed soon to put it into operation, when, on reaching the hospital on the morning of the 27th of April, I learned that the patient had had during the night a violent fit of suffocation which had nearly proved fatal. There was then no more time to be lost, and I performed the same day a palliative operation intended to prevent asphyxia.

The patient having been seated upon a chair in front of a window, I divided, as an indispensable preliminary operation, the soft palate along the median line, and resected a portion of the hard palate (Nélaton's method), and by the way thus opened I introduced a strong pair of polypus forceps, with which I seized the tumour and tried to draw it towards me, combining the movement of traction with that of rotation. After using considerable force I brought away a very small piece of the tumour; I tried again two or three times, without any success, and then taking a pair of pronged forceps I fixed them firmly in the morbid mass and cut beyond them with strong curved scissors; this time I brought away a piece as large as a walnut. I then repeated the manœuvre after giving the patient time to rest and spit.

The operation had not been very long, but the young man had lost considerable blood and felt weak, so I decided not to try to remove any more, and occupied myself with checking the flow of blood. For that purpose I touched the bleeding portions of the tumour several times with a brush dipped in a mixture of one part of perchloride of iron at 30° and three parts of water, and made the patient gargle his throat with a still weaker solution of the same preparation. The flow soon stopped, and the patient was able to walk back to his bed. The following days respiration was much freer, suffocation no longer threatened, and no accident consecutive to the operation endangered the life of the patient. In a word, my incomplete and palliative operation had had none of the unfortunate consequences which might have attended an attempt at a radical cure. Still we were far from a cure, and had even to expect an increase in the portion which had not been removed.

I should mention that the portion removed was examined, and found to consist of a fibrous framework and a rather large number of blood vessels.

Examining the patient daily, I discovered between the twentieth and thirtieth days that the tumour increased a little above the soft palate; without waiting for it to become sufficiently large to again interfere with respiration, I subjected the patient during the next two months to ten operations with the electrolytic apparatus. You remember that the arrangement of the currents in this apparatus is such that they produce a sort of chemical destruction and elimination of the tissues traversed by them, which, however, is not a real gangrene.

Those of you who assisted at those operations remember that they lasted ten or fifteen minutes and were quite painful, also that the eschars produced were small, and that the tumour increased again as soon as the elimination was finished. In short, after two months nothing had been gained or lost; the fibroma was no longer suffocating, and in no way did it compromise life, but it was still there, and I easily recognized every day, by passing my finger through the division of the soft palate, that the tumour was sessile and occupied a large surface, that it did not belong to the category of polyps, properly so called.

After two or three more weeks passed in observation I recognized that the tumour continued to increase, without, however, becoming large enough to again cause the suffocation which had so incommoded and threatened the patient at the time of his admission into the hospital. Furthermore, there was no flow of blood except on the days when the tumour was touched either for exploration or for electrization, and the general health remained good.

Anxious to keep the disease in this condition, that is, within the limits compatible with health, continuing to fear the consequences of a great curative operation, and hoping that one day or another the influence of age would make itself felt, I gave up electrolysis, which caused a good deal of pain and yielded only insufficient results, and I decided that thereafter the tumour should be attacked and destroyed as far as possible by means of caustics applied through the opening in the palate or through the nostrils. At first I used monohydrated nitric acid, carried through the division of the palate with all the precautions necessary to prevent its falling into the pharynx and œsophagus. This mode of cauterization had the advantage of causing but little pain and no loss of blood; but it had the disadvantage of destroying only the surface and not at all the parenchyma. For this reason I ultimately had recourse to the application of points and grains of chloride of zinc, giving to the caustic, which was well dried and composed of one-third chloride of zinc and two-thirds flour, the form and dimensions suitable to the passage through which I had to apply it. Three different times I attacked the nasal prolongations which had grown nearly down to the nostrils, and for that I used grains having the form and size of oats. For the pharyngeal portion, on the other hand, I used triangular points having a length of from one-half to three-quarters of an inch, and a breadth at the base of one-third of an inch. These points were applied by means of long polypus forceps, and I was careful to choose those whose points were the hardest. Notwithstanding the hardness of the tumour, I never had to make a preliminary incision with the point of the bistoury. I applied every time two or three of these points. The operation had the disadvantage of causing the blood to flow for from fifteen to thirty minutes. But as the patient ate well, and repaired rapidly, and as in fact the amount of blood lost each time was hardly more than three ounces, the disadvantage was not too great. I noticed only that the tumour became more and more vascular as it grew older.

Such was the condition of affairs during August and September; caustics had been applied ten different times, and had produced eschars of greater or less size. In short, the tumour was smaller than at first, but there was still the same extent of implantation and the same tendency to increase as soon as we ceased to employ the means of partial destruction. Wearied with his long stay in the hospital, and not considering himself ill enough to remain, the young man begged to be allowed to depart, promising to return if he did not get better.

He left us on the 18th of October, 1869, having obtained from his five months of treatment this important result, that our first palliative operations had saved his life, but with the chagrin of knowing that he was not cured, a chagrin that he felt very keenly, notwithstanding the hope we gave him of a cure at the end of adolescence.

When he returned two months later, the 30th of December, 1869, Pellard informed us that he had had no fresh hemorrhages, and that his health continued good, but that for some time he had felt that his respiration was again becoming affected. Furthermore, although he felt well, he had grown thin, and I pointed out to you a beginning of exophthalmia on the left side; I attributed it to this, that the left nasal prolongation had destroyed the outer wall of the nasal fossa and extended into the orbit. I again attacked the tumour twice with caustic points, which caused free bleeding each time. I was still unwilling to resect the superior maxilla on account of the dangers I foresaw both from the operation itself and from the necessity of severing such extensive connections of a very vascular tumour.

Meanwhile, on making my visit one morning in February, 1870, the patient told me that, without having lost consciousness, he had felt when he awoke that morning numbness in his right arm and leg, and we discovered then and on the following days that the upper and lower limbs on the right side were partially, but evidently paralyzed; and as the exophthalmia continued and even increased, I was forced to think that the cribriform plate at the upper wall of the left nasal fossa had been affected similarly to the outer wall, that is, had undergone a destruction and perforation which permitted the tumour to extend towards the cavity of the skull and compress the brain.

However that may be, I at once abandoned all hope, and thought the young man would be soon carried off by meningitis or some other cerebral affection. I regretted that I had not removed and cauterized the tumour at the beginning, after preliminary resection of the superior maxilla, for I now considered such an operation impossible, since there was reason to fear that the removal of the upper

portion of the tumour would open a large communication between
the nasal fossa and the cavity of the cranium; I therefore allowed the
patient to quit the hospital again the 27th of March, 1870.

What was my astonishment to see him return the 16th February,
1871. I had heard nothing of him for a year, and supposed him to
be dead. On the contrary, he came to tell me that since his departure his health had steadily improved in spite of his participation in
the fatigues and privations of the siege of Paris. The weakness of
the right side had disappeared little by little; no cerebral symptom
had occurred; the prominence of the eye existed no longer, and yet
no new treatment had been undertaken. The only incident was
that in September, 1870, more than five months after he had left La
Charité, an abundant epistaxis occurred and obliged him to enter the
Hôtel Dieu, in the wards of M. Laugier, who undertook no surgical
treatment, but contented himself with prescribing some gargles.

By making him breathe through his nostrils, I ascertained that the
air passed freely. Examining him in a good light, I no longer saw
in the nasal fossa the round red bodies which were formerly there.
Opening his mouth, I saw the median division of the soft palate
which I had made, but no tumour above it; I could pass my finger
above the palate throughout the whole upper portion of the pharynx
exactly as in those who have no polyp. The only thing of which
the patient complained was the nasal tone of his voice resulting from
the defective condition of the palate. I proposed staphylorraphy at
once, to which he did not agree, but he promised to return later and
have it performed.

To recapitulate, gentlemen, we have a young man twenty-two
years old, who has just escaped being killed by a suffocating naso-
pharyngeal fibroma. A palliative treatment prevented death, and
afterward kept the tumour from again becoming suffocating. At the
age of twenty-four and a half years, and without any further surgical
treatment, the rest of the tumour disappears spontaneously, being
absorbed, not eliminated. Repair of the orbital and naso-cranial
walls takes place by means which we do not exactly understand. The
symptoms of compression of the eye and brain disappear, and, in
short, the patient appears to be cured.[1]

This fact is certainly favourable to the opinion of M. Legouest, but
we must ask ourselves if, perchance, it is not exceptional. I have
looked for the records of similar cases, but have found none.

M. Legouest said that in the case of the young man eighteen years
old, upon whom he operated in 1865, he intended to make only a
palliative operation by tearing out the tumour through a nasal opening previously established by making an incision in the genio-nasal
fold, dividing the naso-maxillary suture with a Liston's forceps, turning outwards the inner wall of the maxillary sinus, and leaving this

[1] Since this article was put in type, this patient has written to me that he is again
suffering, and has from time to time fresh hemorrhages from the nose. He is far
from Paris, and I have not been able to see him. If it is a relapse, the details I
have given would none the less justify my opinions upon the influence of age, and
authorize me to believe that a new treatment, now that the patient is twenty-five
years old, would yield a definitive success.

abnormal route open so that he might again attack the polyp after the reproduction which he expected, and which indeed took place a few months later. But this time the tumour was attacked by gangrenous inflammation and fell. M. Legouest did not know if the polyp had grown a third time, or if a complementary operation had been performed to close the artificial nasal opening. But if, thus far, surgeons have not been guided, like M. Legouest and myself, in their therapeutical decisions, by the thought of the influence of age, some facts favourable to our opinion have appeared. Thus, in the discussion which took place in the Société de Chirurgie in 1866 upon this subject, Velpeau reported two cases in which the patients, operated upon by the simple method of extraction, one twenty years, the other nine ye r before, had remained perfectly well though retaining upon the basilar process an abnormal prominence which grew no larger. Velpeau indicated the analogy between the behaviour of naso-pharyngeal polyps and that of uterine fibromas at the period of the menopause. We know that often after the cessation of the courses these fibromas or myomas diminish, and even disappear. It may well be the same for the fibromas of the basilar process. On the other hand, it must be admitted that after a certain age naso-pharyngeal fibrous polyps are no longer produced, since to my knowledge no observation has been published of an adult having a polyp of this kind after it had been operated upon during youth. All the published relapses occurred in young people. After the age of twenty-five years we hear nothing of them. The reason is that those upon whom the operation succeeded were permanently cured, or that those in whom a reproduction took place got well spontaneously, like my patient, without undergoing another operation.

Further observation will decide the question, but for the moment I feel justified in repeating to you what I said not long ago about ingrown toe-nail: do not worry too much about relapses; this is a disease of youth; help your patient to become an adult, and, if his tumour does not disappear spontaneously, the chances are great that you will then be able to cure him by a simple operation without relapse.

We must now seek to answer the question which you hear me ask for all the diseases of youth. What is the cause, and how explain the influence of this age upon the development of naso-pharyngeal fibromas?

I shall not spend any time upon this point, because it is impossible for me to give the problem a satisfactory solution. I might indeed tell you that these tumours have their origin in the submucous tissue which is at the same time the peritoneum of the bones of the base of the skull which limit the pharynx above, and that at the period when the development of the skeleton ends, an aberration and an exuberance of nutrition may take place in this periosteal envelope. But I know how hypothetical this explanation is, and prefer to spend no time upon it, but to confine myself to the indication of the fact, as to which there is not the slightest doubt.

I shall be less troubled to draw from what has preceded this therapeutical conclusion, that preliminary operations, intended to give free access to the implantation of these tumours, should be performed only exceptionally. An explanation of this is necessary, for the plan adopted should necessarily vary according to the age of the patient, the size of the tumour, and, above all, the extent of implantation.

1. Suppose first that the patient is still far from the age at which presumably, adolescence being ended, there will be no more tendency to the reproduction of the fibroma; suppose that he is from thirteen to eighteen years old, and suppose at the same time that the tumour is not very large, not larger, for example, than half an egg, and that examinations with the finger and eye have shown that a pedicle exists and is not very large, that the prolongations into the nasal fossæ do not obstruct these cavites entirely, and that there are no appreciable ones on the side of the pterygo-maxillary fossa or of the orbit.

In such a case the surgeon ought to be guided by this thought, that the disease left to itself will increase, and ultimately send out one or another of those prolongations which destroy the bones of the face, and become hemorrhagic, if not so already, and even suffocating. He should therefore consider intervention necessary. But in my opinion, he ought to reject every preliminary operation, and have recourse to one of the simple ones, especially extraction or ligation; and, as extraction through the nostrils is almost impossible, he should attempt it through the mouth, making use of good curved forceps and helping it with a finger. This attempt is rational for two reasons: first, because the pedicle of a fibrous polyp may be small enough to allow of its being torn off; and, second, because certain single nasopharyngeal mucous polyps may, like the example I published,[1] develop in young people, the diagnosis between them and fibrous polyps is almost impossible before removal, and they are very easily torn out.

If the attempt to tear out has failed, recourse must be had to the ligature. Passing through one of the nostrils, the patient being seated before a window, a Belloc sound, the spring of which is projected into the mouth, and fastening to the end of this spring the two ends of a very strong thread of triple silk, or of that kind known as twisted silk; the two ends are brought through the nose by withdrawing the sound, and the loop is carried behind the polyp. This is the difficult part of the operation; if the tumour is not very large it may be done with the fingers; but do not forget that, to render it easier for the patient, it is well to prescribe fifty or sixty grains of the bromide of potassium daily during the four or five preceding days. You know that in many people this drug causes a notable diminution of the sensibility of the palate and pharynx.

If the fingers are not sufficient it will be necessary to use a porteligature. The one which I prefer is that of Felix Hatin. (Fig. 3.) But if you do not possess one, or if you do not succeed with it, you

---

[1] Gosselin, Gazette des Hôpitaux, 1866, p. 453.

may still seize the po   on each side with pronged curved forceps, and while they are held in place by an assistant slide the loop along them.

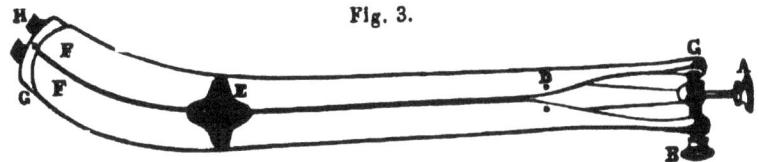

Fig. 3.

After the loop has been put in place, it is well to transfix the tumour above the soft palate with a curved needle carrying a long thread by which the polyp is drawn forward and kept from being swallowed when detached.

The operation is completed by passing the two ends through a Graefe's ligator and gradually tightening the loop.

Here we have to choose between slow section requiring several days, and extemporaneous section in an hour or two. I should now give the preference to the latter, and I should make the intervals between the successive tightenings longer or shorter as the bleeding was more or less abundant; if it was enough to make me expect hemorrhage after the section was completed. I should increase the constriction only once or twice each day—that is, I should make slow, instead of extemporaneous ligature.

Gentlemen, in having recourse to extraction or to ligation without preliminary operation, you offer, it is true, only a palliative remedy. But you give your patient two advantages: you do nothing to endanger his life, you do not mutilate his face or his mouth. Do not forget that division of the soft, and resection of the hard palate, exposes your youthful patient to the chance of having for the rest of his life a nasal tone, and all the discomforts of a permanent communication between the cavities of the mouth and nose. Do not think that you will always be able to remedy this by staphylorraphy, aided, if necessary, by staphyloplasty, for these operations do not always succeed; often they succeed only imperfectly and leave an opening more or less small, the discomforts of which are about as great as those of a large one, and can be remedied only by an obturator. And think for a moment of the discomforts of always wearing an obturator!

On the other hand, resection of the superior maxilla condemns the patient, if he survives, to the deformity of the face, which results from the scars and the loss of teeth. Modern prothesis has made great progress, I know; but, like the obturator, would not artificial teeth be a grievous burden for the long years that follow adolescence?

I much prefer the palliative operations of which I have spoken.

There may be a relapse. Very well! Begin again as often as may be necessary, only advise the patient not to delay too long, not to let the fibroma grow too large. Repeat, as often as may be necessary, those operations which compromise neither the life nor the appearance of the face and mouth, and when your patient reaches the age of twenty-three, twenty-four, or twenty-five years, perhaps even more, reproduction will cease, and you will have rendered him the great service of saving his life without mutilation.

2. But we must now suppose another case, which unfortunately will still present itself too often. The subject, as before, is between thirteen and eighteen years of age; the fibroma has become very large, it sends out many branches, or is suffocating, or is hemorrhagic. Tearing it away can give only imperfect results, and those of short duration; ligation is rendered impossible both by the complete obstruction of the nostrils and the extent of the implantation. I should certainly make one or two atttemps to tear it away, but if they did not succeed we should have no right to hope that, under the supposed unfortunate conditions, life could be preserved until the end of adolescence.

It would then be proper to perform one of the combined operations which we long supposed to be radical, and to give the preference to resection of the superior maxilla as the preliminary operation.

If, as is always to be feared, reproduction should take place, it might be combated successfully until the end of adolescence by partial extractions and cauterizations, as in the case of my patient, practising if necessary a new preliminary operation, division of the soft palate.

You see that here the ideas which we have as to the influence of youth lead us to not despair, and to continue to struggle against the chances of death. But the contest is no longer possible without mutilation; we must accept it, since we can do no better. The important thing is not to inflict these mutilations upon the patients when they can be avoided, and they can be avoided if we remember that simple operations, at first palliative, may by the influence of age become curative.

3. I have now a last supposition to make. The subject is more than eighteen years old, and is nearer the end of adolescence. His constitution is more vigorous, and he is better able to resist the injuries which the polyp may occasion. Moreover he has not to remain exposed so many years to this injurious influence. In this case we should again content ouselves with simple operations, or with palliative cauterization after incision of the soft palate, to which we might add resection of the hard palate as advised by Nélaton. Resection of the maxilla appears to me to be still more exceptionally indicated at this age, and should only be performed if the surgeon, after having long studied his patient, has become convinced that palliative operations will not suffice to keep him alive until the end of adolescence, and if, after the patient has passed this age, when for example he is more than twenty-six years old, the tumour does not diminish by absorption or by spontaneous gangrene.

I do not possess enough facts to be able to tell you what proportion of fibromas disappear spontaneously after the subject has become adult. I certainly believe there will always be found patients in whom this disappearance will not take place without surgical aid. If this intervention is inevitable it is important that it should be deferred until that period of life in which we are almost sure its reproduction *will not* take place.

LECTURE V.

TWO CASES OF SUBACUTE NON-SUPPURATING EPIPHYSARY OSTEITIS.

I. Fall upon the knee—Formation of a painful swelling over the anterior tuberosity of
   the tibia—Absence of fever—Reasons for thinking that the osteitis will not suppurate, and will terminate in a slight hypertrophy after a simple treatment—
   II. Fall upon the great trochanter—Analogous symptoms—Non-suppurating and
   hypertrophic osteitis of youth.

GENTLEMEN: We have at present, in the wards, two young men
affected by the same disease in different regions. One of them is
cured and will soon leave us, the other entered two days ago, and
will doubtless remain for some time with us.

I. The first is seventeen years old and well formed. He told us
when he entered the hospital a fortnight ago, that he had fallen upon
the right knee while running, and that since that time he had not
ceased to feel a pain which was at first slight enough to allow him
to walk and work as usual, but which increased little by little, and
was accompanied by a swelling sufficient to oblige him to stop.

You remember that when we saw him for the first time he was
without fever, and had at the anterior superior portion of the right
tibia, immediately over the anterior tuberosity of this bone, and evidently continuous with it, a hard rounded prominence, slightly painful
when he walked, and very painful when even moderate pressure was
made upon it with one or two fingers. There was no redness of the
skin, no subcutaneous thickening. The temperature of the region
seemed a little higher than that of the opposite side. It was evident
from its situation that the trouble occupied the anterior tuberosity of
the tibia, and that this tuberosity was one-quarter, perhaps one-third,
larger than that of the opposite side. Being carefully questioned
upon this point, the patient assured us explicitly that his two knees
were exactly alike before this last accident, and that the difference in
size between the two anterior tuberosities had existed for only a
week.

I examined the articulation and found in it neither effusion nor
thickening of the synovial, and, as none of the symptoms indicated a
phlegmon, and as the age of the patient, the recent appearance of the
tumour, and its limited extent dismissed the idea of its being an osteo-
sarcoma, I admitted the existence of an osteitis developed almost
exclusively upon the anterior tuberosity of the tibia.

As the pain was moderate, and as the inflammation was not propagated to the connective tissue around the bone, and as there was no
fever, I did not mean by this one of those acute suppurating osteites
which sometimes appear upon the extremities of the long bones while
they are still epiphysary, that is, not united.

Neither did I say that this was an epiphysary exostosis of youth. Its rounded form and hardness certainly recalled exostosis, but its situation dismissed that idea, for exostosis is a bony growth entirely new and generally indolent. This was indeed a bony prominence, but it was not of new formation; it was simply a normal apophysis slightly increased in size.

Dismissing then acute osteitis, osteo-sarcoma, and exostosis, I had to admit a slow plastic osteitis, one that was subacute rather than chronic.

Seeking next the etiological diagnosis, I found none of the general causes which contribute to the development of diseases of the bones. No anterior or hereditary syphilis, no scrofula, no sign of rheumatism. I could find then no other cause than the contusion mentioned by the patient, and as this contusion had been slight, and as, furthermore, I had several times seen a similar swelling develop at the same point upon young people without the intervention of any traumatic cause, I concluded that behind this occasional cause there existed a predisposing one, the age of the patient, and his aptitude to take on, in the neighbourhood of the epiphyses at the time when the nutrition of the bones was working actively to complete ossification, an exaggeration of this movement which thus became an osteitis.

In speaking to you about the prognosis, when the patient was admitted, I said that what preoccupied me most in osteitis was the possibility of its going on to suppuration, and then to purulent infection or caries and necrosis. But I added that in the present case we had but little reason to fear these terminations. I did not expect putrid osteo-myelitis, because the inflammation was not an acute febrile one, and because subacute osteites are rarely followed by these putrid changes which are the sources of poisoning, and of which I shall often have occasion to speak to you.

Nor did I much fear a chronic suppuration which might leave behind it caries or necrosis, or both; for the patient was not lymphatic, and his constitution was not of the kind which predisposes to suppuration of the bones. Furthermore, I had seen several osteites of this kind occupying the anterior tuberosity of the tibia in adolescents, and none of them ended by suppurating.

I therefore told you that, very probably, after a week of rest and care all danger would have disappeared.

All things have gone on as we expected. The treatment consisted simply of poultices and rest in bed. For several days the young man has had no spontaneous pain and suffers very little pressure; I may consider him cured. Still the anterior tuberosity is enlarged, and I think it will remain so. For, indeed, as I shall often have occasion to show you, it is very common to see the hypertrophy which we call hyperostosis follow osteitis, whatever may have been its course, that is to say, whether the termination has or has not been by suppuration, and whether the inflammation of the bone was spontaneous or traumatic. You will scarcely see any disappear without leaving hyperostosis, except the superficial swellings which have chiefly occupied the periosteum, as is the case in syphilitic or rheumatic osteo-periostitis. But in the cases in which the osteitis, whatever may have been its origin, has been interstitial, that is, has occupied the compact and cancellous tissues to a certain depth, and in which the phlegmasia has been accompanied by an increase in size, you may expect to see the hyperostosis persist, and to preserve a tendency towards suppuration when the original osteitis has been suppurative, but, on the other hand, not to have this tendency when the primitive osteitis has not terminated in suppuration. Consequently in the case of this patient, although I see the hyperostosis of the anterior tuberosity of the tibia persist, and though I know that for a certain time and until the completion of ossification he will be exposed to renewals of this pain, especially if there should be another contusion, I do not think he is threatened with suppuration of the bone. If he was going to have it, he would have had it this time.

II. The other patient, who has been here two days, is a young man seventeen years old, who tells us that three months ago he fell upon his left hip, and that since that time, without having been entirely laid up, he has had constant dull pains in the region of the trochanter. These pains have only recently increased, walking finally became so difficult that the patient was obliged to use a cane and enter the hospital.

When I examined him I asked him to indicate the precise seat of his trouble; he placed his hand upon the upper and outer portion of his thigh over the great trochanter, and told us that the pain often extended to the knee. There is almost no pain while he is at rest, it appears especially while he is walking or standing. I pressed with my hand upon all the outer portion of the thigh, and you saw that this pressure caused pain only over the surface of the great trochanter. There we find an ill-defined swelling which at first did not appear very marked, but which is easily recognized when you compare the two trochanteric regions, making the patient lie first upon one side, then upon the other. Trying to discover with the hand the exact position of the swelling, you saw that it was not in the subcutaneous cellular tissue, and was not due to an effusion into one of the two synovial bursæ of the region, for there was no fluctuation. In short, it seemed certain that the part which was swollen and painful on pressure was the great trochanter itself. There is no fever, and the general condition is good.

With what affection have we to deal? The pain, which has already lasted a long time, the lameness which followed it, the diffuse swelling of the upper portion of the thigh, all give at first the idea of a coxalgia. But, the patient lying squarely upon his back, I told him to lift his heel from the bed, to raise his foot well without bending the knee. He made the movement easily, and while he made it I felt with one of my hands placed upon the crest of the ilium that this bone did not budge. If it had been coxalgia the elevation of the heel would have been slower and more difficult, and would have been accompanied by a movement forward of the ilium, a movement due to the fact that, since in this disease the articular surfaces are rendered immovable by muscular contraction, the movements no longer take

3

place in the articulation of the hip, but in those of the pelvis with the spinal column, and in those of the lumbar vertebræ. Then taking hold of the ankle and flexing the leg upon the thigh, and the thigh upon the trunk, I felt that I communicated these movements easily and without experiencing the resistance which is met with in coxalgia, because then the head of the femur and the cotyloid cavity are no longer movable upon one another. Then comparing the height of the spines of the ilium I found that the one on the affected side was not lowered as it would have been in case of coxalgia, and finally, carrying my hand to the lumbar region, I did not find there the bend which is usually found in this latter disease. The result of my examination then authorized me to declare that the affection was not a coxo-femoral arthritis, and before reaching this decision I had made the examination with all the more care because the patient had been sent to me by a physician with a note indicating that he feared the beginning of a coxalgia.

On the other hand, the existence of pains radiating along the thigh might have given rise to the idea of a sciatica. But you saw that these pains were on the outer side, while in sciatica they are especially in the posterior portion of the thigh; that pressure caused them in a region (that of the great trochanter) where they are not found in sciatica, and that finally they were developed while walking, and were not felt when the patient was at rest. Now the principal characteristic of the pains of sciatica is that, although they are sometimes exaggerated during a walk, they appear spontaneously during rest, and even during rest in bed. Consequently there was no reason here to believe in the existence of a sciatica.

You will sometimes hear me speak of a disease, difficult of diagnosis, which occupies the sacro-iliac symphysis, and bears the name of *sacro-coxalgia*. I had also to throw out this disease, because of the localization of the pain in the trochanteric region, and its being awakened by pressure upon this region.

Further, there was no symptom of hygroma, and in addition I knew there was a swelling over the great trochanter.

I recalled the fact that Velpeau had indicated in his lectures osteitis limited to this prominence, and I remembered having met adolescents who had presented symptoms analogous to these.

I thought, then, that we had to deal here with a subacute osteitis of traumatic origin, an osteitis developed, like that of the anterior tuberosity of the tibia of which I have just spoken, upon or in the neighbourhood of an epiphysis. For you know that the great trochanter develops from a special complementary point of ossification, and that it remains until the age of from 20 to 25 years separated from the rest of the bone by a cartilaginous line. There has occurred, then, in my opinion, in this great trochanter, that which occurred in the anterior tuberosity of the other patient. It has been bruised at a period when its nutrition was excited by the needs of ossification, and this contusion has been followed by a phlegmasia which began, perhaps, in the epiphysary cartilage, perhaps in the bone itself. For we cannot determine the starting-point by clinical evidence, the only *evidence which we* have at our disposal.

I do not claim that a similar contusion would never be followed by trochanteritis in an adult; I only say that that is much more rare, and that the affection is seen chiefly in adolescents and in those regions where are found the epiphyses; that is, bony extremities still separated from the rest of the bone by a cartilaginous line.

I now ask myself, gentlemen, what is to be the result of this trochanteric osteitis or subacute trochanteritis. Certainly we may hope that it will behave like the tibial osteitis of which I have spoken; that is to say, that after a rest of a few weeks it will terminate without suppurating, and will leave behind it a slight hyperostosis. But I must say that I fear suppuration more in this than in the preceding case. For the osteitis has already lasted three months, and has steadily grown worse since the beginning. The patient is thinner and paler. Without being distinctly scrofulous, he nevertheless shows us the attributes of the lymphatic temperament, among them a certain aptitude for suppuration. I do not expect the ultimate development of one of those acute and putrid suppurating osteites which may be followed by purulent infection. It is rare for osteitis to take on this acute form in this age, when in the beginning and for a certain length of time it has been subacute.

I shall not fail to show you examples of acute epiphysary osteitis in adolescents, and to point out that they were such in the beginning, and were not preceded by a slow, dull inflammation.

Our present patient is threatened rather by that variety of slow suppuration which leads to caries and necrosis.

He would then find himself in the position of a young man whom I showed you last year, who bore two fistulæ in the trochanteric region. The probe passed through each of them to the bare and roughened surface of the great trochanter, and announced the existence of that variety of suppurating osteitis which ought to end in the elimination of one or more sequestra, and which we call necrosis. I did not feel the probe penetrate deeply enough, breaking its way through the bony lamellæ, to admit the existence of interstitial suppurating osteitis of the cancellous tissue, known generally as caries. But it is probable that this form may also occur in certain subjects after subacute trochanteritis. I cannot give any example; for, since diseases of this kind are not very common, I have not treated a sufficient number of cases to have seen all the forms.

The important thing for our patient is that this osteitis is not so necessarily destined to suppuration as it would be perhaps in childhood, and even during adult life (in case, of course, tertiary syphilis is not involved), and that by reason of his age we may avoid this mode of termination.

What have we to do to obtain that end?

Of course we shall keep him in bed and not allow him to get up under any pretext.

Furthermore, I shall apply compression by means of a layer of cotton batting, kept in place by a figure-of-eight bandage, the loops of which will pass alternately about the upper half of the thigh and the pelvis. This is the bandage which you know by the name of

Spica, but its femoral portion will extend a little lower upon the thigh than in the ordinary spica. I shall renew this dressing every third or fourth day.

At the same time I shall give the patient three or four tablespoonfuls of cod-liver oil daily, and prescribe five ounces of vin de quinquina to be taken before breakfast, and the same quantity before the evening meal, and I shall nourish him as well as possible.

I should like also to protect him from the exhaustion of masturbation; for patients of delicate constitution, in whom we have reason to fear suppuration of the bones, find in excesses of this kind an increase of their debility and its consequences. In private practice I advise the parents not to leave the young man alone, to distract his attention and occupy him as much as possible; in the hospital this care is impossible, but I shall give all the advice necessary.

We shall continue this treatment for a month, and then stop the use of the bandage and allow the patient to get up for a short time each day. If I find that he does not suffer I shall make him walk a little more every day, and if he still does not suffer I shall consider him cured.

If, on the other hand, the attempt shows that a cure has not been obtained, I shall advise him again to remain in bed and shall make use of some revulsive on the skin. For this I shall have to choose between blisters, caustics, and punctate cauterization. I have no absolute preference for any one of these, for thus far my experience has not demonstrated the superiority of one over the other—nevertheless, punctate cauterization is the one which I shall use if after a month's rest in bed this young man still suffers a little on pressure and when walking.

(Punctate cauterization was applied, forty points, with a small iron rod, at white heat, while the patient was anæsthetized with chloroform. Six weeks afterwards all pain had disappeared and the patient was considered cured. He left the hospital, and has not since been seen.)

LECTURE VI.

I. HYPEROSTOSIS OF RIGHT FEMUR. II. NECROSIS OF LEFT TIBIA.

Some considerations upon diseases of the skeleton in the infant and in the adolescent—I. Hyperostosis of the femur and anchylosis of the knee following a non-suppurating epiphysary osteitis—Fresh inflammatory attack, also not terminating in suppuration—II. Necrosis of the tibia following a suppurating epiphysary osteitis—Fresh inflammation—Movable superficial sequestrum, immovable invaginated sequestrum—Long duration of this necrosis probably until adult life.

GENTLEMEN: Chance has recently brought together in our wards two patients suffering from the late consequences of the disease which you often hear me speak of as *acute epiphysary osteitis of youth.*

But first of all, I must make an explanation.

In pointing out to you the diseases of youth I do not mean, and I have never meant to say, that these diseases belong exclusively to youth, and are not seen at other ages; I wished to say that they were more frequent during youth, and that, as a rule, they took on at this age characters different from those which are seen in the same lesion at other periods of life.

I have been criticized upon this subject. Especially with reference to acute epiphysary osteitis, it has been objected that this disease is seen in childhood.

I knew that perfectly well, but I also knew two other things: first, that it is less frequent than in adolescents; second, that it is also less dangerous.

I knew also, in the third place, that osteitis of adults does not take on spontaneously, and without the intervention of solutions of continuity affecting at the same time the bones and the soft parts, those dangerous forms which occur almost spontaneously in the child and in the youth. However, to enable you to decide the question for yourselves I give you the statistics published upon the subject.

Dr. Cullot, author of a very good thesis,[1] gives the following table of the ages at which epiphysary osteitis appears :—

From	1 to 18 months	.	.	2 cases.	
"	2 to 6 years.	.	.	7	"
"	6 to 10 "	.	.	10	"
"	10 to 14 "	.	.	21	..
"	14 to 18 "	.	.	33	"
"	18 to 22 "	.	.	8	" 6 of which were between 18 and 19.
"	22 to 29 "	.	.	1 case.	
"	29 to 30 "	.	.	1	"

M. Sézary,[2] who collected, also, for his graduating thesis, 92 cases, of which 57 were between the ages of 12 and 19, finds an average of 13 years. But the average of 33 cases observed by himself at the Hôtel-Dieu of Lyons was 16 years.

Klose's 13 cases average 13 years.

M. Chassaignac[3] mentions 23 cases, of which 4 were between 9 days and 10 years; 15 from 10 to 18 years; and 4 from 18 to 36 years old.

From all these figures, which have been reproduced in an excellent thesis by Dr. Salès,[4] it results, gentlemen, that the end of childhood and the first years of adolescence, until about the age of 19, are the periods of life during which appear, chiefly, but not exclusively, the diseases which we are about to consider. They are most often met with between the ages of 12 and 18.

And here let me say that in speaking of adolescence, we do not give it perfectly defined limits, sometimes it is considered as beginning at 12, sometimes at 13, sometimes at 14 years, and when we clinicists speak of the diseases of adolescence or youth, and especially of those

[1] Cullot, De l'Inflammation Aiguë primitive de la Moëlle des Os. Paris, 1871.

[2] Sézary, De l'Adolescence. Thèse de Paris, 1871, and Gazette des Hôpitaux, 1871, page 9, et seq.

[3] Chassaignac, Traité de la Suppuration et du Drainage, vol. i. page 413.

[4] Salès, De la Marche et du Traitement de l'Ostéo-périostite dia-épiphysaire suppurée. Thèse de Paris, 1871.

which we attribute to a derangement of nutrition while the bones are
lengthening, and at the moments of that exaggeration of vitality which
prepares the union of the epiphyses, we know that this exaggeration
presents numerous individual varieties. In some patients it occurs at
12 or 13, in others at 16, 17, and 18 years of age, in some the growth
is progressive and slow without any excess of activity more marked
at certain moments; in others, on the contrary, this excess of activity
appears several times and irregularly. In short, a child 11, 12, or 13
years old may be adolescent as to his epiphyses, but not as to the rest
of his body.

At the time when I published my first work upon this subject,[1]
pathologists and clinicists were accustomed to describe diseases of the
skeleton according to the data of pathological anatomy and physiology
without considering age, and without warning practitioners that such
a form of acute osteitis appeared especially at such or such a period
of life. My object was to call attention to this subject, and to show
the relations between the age and growth of the skeleton on the one
side, and the forms of spontaneous osteitis on the other, and I have
seen with pleasure that subsequent works upon this subject have
followed the path which I opened. I made certain reservations
relative to childhood, because, not having practised in the children's
hospitals, I could not know what took place in the first and second
periods of childhood; I insisted particularly upon the frequency with
which I had observed the diseases to occur in adolescents as compared
with adults.

Since then my colleague, M. Giraldès,[2] has well shown that children
may be affected, especially at the end of childhood, or, if you prefer,
at that period of life which is between the end of childhood and the
beginning of adolescence. The excellent works of Messrs. Gamet[3]
and Louvet,[4] and those already quoted of Messrs. Sézary, Cullot, and
Salès confirmed these assertions of M. Giraldès and myself, and
enabled us to draw practical conclusions from this simple fact: the
latter part of childhood and adolescence are exposed to forms of
spontaneous acute osteitis which are seen much more rarely at other
ages.

Let us now turn to the two patients with reference to whom I
thought it necessary to present these preliminary considerations.

I. The first is a young man 19 years old, pale, with chestnut hair,
but with well-developed muscles, showing no scars upon the neck, and
giving no indication, past or present, of tubercular affection. He tells
us that at the age of 13½ years, without appreciable cause, or after a
blow which he does not remember very distinctly, he had severe pain
in the right knee and the lower part of the thigh; that he was very
ill at this time and had much fever; that after a few weeks an abscess
was opened on the inner and lower part of his right thigh, which
suppurated for a long time, and finally closed without the expulsion

[1] Gosselin, Archives générales de Médecine, 1858, tome ii. p. 518.
[2] Giraldès, Leçons cliniques sur les Maladies chirurgicales de l'Enfance, p. 588.
[3] Gamet, Thèses de Paris, 1862.
[4] Louvet, Périostite phlegmoneuse diffuse, Thèses de Paris, 1876.

of any sequestrum or fragments; that at last a cure took place, leaving the knee slightly flexed and immovable, and compelling the patient to use a cane and a shoe with a heel three inches high.

A week ago, without apparent cause, he again began to suffer a little in the lower part of his thigh and knee, and , being no longer able to walk and work at his trade of shoemaking, he applied to us for treatment.

We find the knee completely anchylosed by fusion, the femur and tibia united at an angle of about 40 degrees—what we call angular anchylosis of the knee. There is no notable swelling at this point, and only a little heat.

Above the knee the muscles of the thigh are evidently smaller than those of the opposite side, but yet the lower third of the limb appears a little larger, and on grasping it with the whole hand I feel a very hard circular resistance which gives the idea of a femur much more voluminous than the other or a normal one. I know that one may be deceived by a lesion of the muscles, which I have found in two autopsies, and which has been well described by M. Aug. Ollivier;[1] I refer to atrophy of the muscles, with transformation into a very dense fibrous tissue, which cannot be clearly distinguished from the femur by the hand examining through the skin. But here, as the apparently bony swelling is very large, and as it involves the condyles of the femur themselves in points where there are no muscular fibres of the quadriceps, I infer that the tumefaction occupies, if not the whole, at least part of the lower third of the femur.

Notice also that this swollen portion is painful spontaneously, and upon pressure. As there is no phlegmon which could cause these pains, we may attribute them to the femur; now at this age the bones become more frequently and more easily painful when they are hypertrophied than they do in subjects in whom this condition does not exist.

Furthermore, there is no fever, no notable alteration of health, and the pains, more severe when the patient is standing or walking, have not so far been sufficient to prevent his sleep.

The diagnosis, gentlemen, presents two questions: What is this young man's present disease? and What was the former one which has evidently prepared this one?

As to the present disease, it is composed of combined lesions that are already old, anchylosis of the knee, and hyperostosis of the femur, with concomitant muscular atrophy. These three lesions are irremediable, and they are not what has brought the patient to the hospital. But there is further a recently added pathological condition, a subacute and painful osteitis in the region, and perhaps also in the thickness, of the hyperostosis. If we did not possess the antecedents relative to the acute disease six years ago, we should have to see whether this considerable swelling of the femur were not due to an osteo sarcoma. But with these antecedents, and in presence of the fact that for several years the swelling, instead of increasing, has

[1] Aug. Ollivier, Thèse de Concours pour l'Agrégation, Paris, 1869.

diminished, there is no reason to dwell very long on this diagnosis, and remembering, furthermore, that hyperostosis is often the consequence of osteitis of the long bones, we need not hesitate long; it is subacute osteitis or fresh inflammation in an old hyperostosis.

As to the etiological diagnosis I have nothing in particular to point out.

I shall tell you hereafter that in adults non-suppurating osteo-periostitis is often due to general causes: rheumatism, syphilis, or a feeble state of the constitution similar to the scrofula of children, a sort of acquired or late scrofula.   Here none of these general causes can be accused.   The fresh inflammatory attack appears to have been spontaneous, or if there has been a traumatic cause it has been a slight contusion of which the patient has preserved no recollection. Perhaps the age of the patient and the exaggerated nutrition of the bones have had some influence.   It is true that the union of the inferior epiphysis of the femur was completed long ago, for one of the consequences of these osteites of adolescence is to hasten the union of the epiphysis.   Nevertheless, I think the age has had something to do with the etiology; for you will often see in adults hyperostosis consecutive to simple or compound fractures, and you will notice that the inflammatory attacks, necrosis once ended, seldom occur so late.

Let us now consider the other question: What was the original affection, the traces of which we see here, and of which the present symptoms are a remote consequence?

From the information we have gathered, and from the analogy between what the patient has told us and what we have observed in a certain number of adolescents, there can be no doubt.   This young man was affected at the end of childhood with that disease of which I spoke at the beginning, acute osteitis, ending promptly in suppuration ; and as this osteitis appears to have been spontaneous, or, if traumatic, to have been caused by a slight injury, I feel sure it was one of those osteites which begin in the epiphysary cartilage itself, or in one of the adjoining surfaces of bone, and of which the predisposing cause is the work of ossification.   I cannot say whether the periosteum alone has suppurated, or whether the compact tissue also, and especially the medullary substance, both that of the canal and that of the cancellous tissue, have participated.

I am convinced that in many cases of this kind all the constituent parts of the bone share in the inflammation, and that there is osteo-myelitis at the same time with periostitis.   But when the patient survives, it is very difficult, if not impossible, to show whether the deep portions of the bone have suppurated, as well as the superficial ones, or whether the osteo-myelitis has been non-suppurative, the periosteum, on the contrary, having been attacked and even destroyed by the suppuration.   I shall hereafter have occasion to return to this subject; to-day, I say that there has been suppurative osteitis, at least on the surface, and general osteitis, probably non-suppurative, but presenting the form described by Gerdy as *hypertrophying* or *condensing*. This osteitis does not seem to have been necrotic, as it often is in like cases, and in this respect it is exceptional. But it has got well, leaving behind it the hyperostosis, which is the almost inevitable consequence of hypertrophying osteitis when it occupies the compact tissue of the long bones; and as the peculiarity of this hyperostosis is to preserve, for a certain length of time after its formation, a tendency to sub-acute or chronic inflammation, and as this is more marked during adolescence, we find in it the origin of the recent inflammation which to day torments this young man.

Now, what should be our opinion as to the consequences of this disease? What we have to fear is suppuration. It is true that this may possibly occupy exclusively the cellular tissue, without partici-pation of the bone in the process, and form what Gerdy called a *neighbouring abscess* (abcès de voisinage). Such an abscess would end like a simple one, without ultimate necrosis. But if the hyper-ostosis itself should suppurate, either on the surface, after destruction of the periosteum, or in the interior, that would indicate that a por-tion of the hypertrophied femur was necrosed, and then our patient would be condemned to long suppuration and to the fistulæ which precede the elimination (always very slow) of the sequestra or mortified parts of the bone. Considering all things, I do not much fear this termination, and for the following reasons: the constitution of the patient is not broken down, and as the osteitis escaped necrosis when it was acute, as the present age exposes a little less to it than the one at which the disease of the femur began, and finally, as the inflam-matory symptoms are moderate and subacute, we have the right to hope that the present attack also will end by resolution, and that the patient will continue to escape necrosis, to which he will be so much the less exposed as he grows older.

To favour this fortunate termination we have only a very simple treatment to institute.

We shall keep the patient absolutely quiet, and advise him not to walk so long as there is any pain. We shall cover the affected part with poultices, and prescribe 8 or 10 grains of the iodide of potassium daily. If the disease lasts more than three weeks longer, I shall probably prescribe a blister, perhaps punctate cauterization. But I doubt if these measures are useful; for of two things one: either suppuration is inevitable, and then it is too late to have recourse to them, or resolution is to take place, and then rest and simple means suffice.

II. The other young man is 17 years old, and comes to us for the second time. The first time, two years ago, he was suffering with acute epiphysary osteitis of the right tibia, in its lower portion. We found him very ill, with much fever; and the affection ended with large abscesses, some of which communicated with the lower portion of the denuded bone, and the others seemed to communicate with the tibio-tarsal articulation. In a word, it was one of those serious cases, such as I have described,[1] in which the suppurative

---

[1] Gosselin, Mémoire sur l'Ostéite épiphysaire des Adolescents. (Archives de Méd. 1858.)

inflammation is propagated from the epiphysis and the bone of the
neighbouring articulation. Fearing for the life of the youth, and
seeing him exposed, if perchance he should not die, to a necrosis
which would torment him for many years, I proposed amputation,
but his parents refused absolutely. The suppurating osteo-myelitis
and arthritis did not assume a form sufficiently putrid to cause purulent infection ; the patient also escaped hecticity ; and when he left
the hospital, after six months' stay, he had the tibio-tarsal articulation
anchylosed, without persistent necrosis of the astragalus, and preserved at the lower part of the leg, two fistulæ which suppurated freely,
and through which the probe reached the tibia, which was denuded
over quite a large surface and notably hyperostosed. He walked,
furthermore, with the aid of crutches.

The subsequent course of the disease was such as it is in most of
the young patients who survive acute epiphysary osteitis ending in
suppuration, such, for example, as it was in the case of the young
man whom you saw for a long time in our wards last year with necrosis of the femur consecutive to an osteitis of this kind. Suppuration has continued, and he has not been able to lay aside his crutches.
New pains accompanied by fever appeared twice, and each time a
new abscess formed and a fragment of bone was expelled.

A week ago a new inflammatory attack occurred, which confined
the patient to his bed and forced him to seek admission to the hospital. You saw that the lower part of the leg was swollen, hot, red,
and painful. The tibia is considerably hypertrophied, and the four
fistulæ which lead to it furnish a large quantity of non fetid pus.
The probe passed through these fistulæ reaches a denuded surface, and
I showed you that, placing a probe in contact with the bone through
one of the inner fistulæ, and passing another through the lower one,
and pressing with it upon the corresponding portion of denuded
bone, I transmitted the movement to the first probe. Thence I concluded that a portion of the bone was necrosed and separated from
the rest, that is, that there was a superficial movable sequestrum.
Exploring with the probe upon the other side, I felt upon the
denuded surface an opening through which the instrument penetrated
about half an inch and enabled me to feel another denuded portion,
which was not movable, but which appeared to me destined to
become so, and to form what is called in the description of necrosis
an *invaginated sequestrum.*

The present affection, then, of this young man is a persistent
necrosis of the hyperostosed tibia, with superficial movable sequestrum and invaginated sequestrum not yet movable. You know
that by the name necrosis we designate a mortification of the
bony tissue, that this mortification, affecting more often the compact than the cancellous tissue, is one of the modes of termination
of suppurative osteitis, and coincides quite commonly with hypertrophy and condensation, so that these three things—suppuration,
hypertrophy, and mortification—almost always go together. Undoubtedly Gerdy's condensing or hypertrophying osteitis can occur
in the compact tissue of the long bones without suppuration and

without necrosis. I showed you an example lately in an adolescent, and I shall often show you others in adults. But when this osteitis ends in suppuration, it is at the same time hypertrophying and necrotic; it is what you see distinctly in this case, and what you will also see from time to time in adults;˙ but while in the latter, suppuration, hypertrophy, and necrosis occur, especially after extensive traumatic lesions in which there has been open wound and fracture, or, if you prefer, exposure of the bone to contact with the air, they have occurred in this young man, as is generally the case in adolescents, without external wound, without preliminary exposure, and after an osteitis either purely spontaneous or consecutive to a slight contusion without rupture of the skin.

What will be the ultimate course and what the consequences of this young man's disease? As for the present inflammation, it will cease in a few days, perhaps after formation of another abscess,and the patient's life is not endangered—first, because the fever is moderate, and, according to our experience, is not likely to augment and take on a dangerous character; and secondly, because it is the rule that exacerbated chronic osteitis in an old hyperostosis does not take on the dangerous forms of primitive acute suppurative osteitis.

To what is due this difference in danger between suppurative osteitis preceding hyperostosis, and osteitis consecutive to the latter, when the predisposing cause of age still exists? This is perhaps difficult to explain. I attribute it to differences in structure. Before hypertrophy all the cavities of the bone are filled with fat, the suppuration of which, as I have told you, contributes greatly to give to osteo-myelitis its well-known danger; moreover, there is the epiphysary line in and near which osteitis takes on in the adolescent the intensity and gravity with which you are acquainted. After hyperostosis has occurred the medullary cavity is filled up or greatly diminished, at least in the great majority of cases, and consequently there remains but a small proportion of fat. The cavities of the cancellous tissue and the canaliculi are also diminished and lose most of their fat; hence, as the principal element, suppuration of which causes the danger of osteo-myelitis, is reduced to small proportions, the reappearance of the latter is less dangerous. Furthermore, the epiphysary line has disappeared by ossification, another reason for the mildness of consecutive phlegmasiæ. Notice this, gentlemen: the anatomical result of osteitis is hypertrophy, and with it a certain tendency to relapse; but at the same time it diminishes the number and extent of the bony cavities in which are distributed, amidst the fat, the bloodvessels destined to nourish the bone—hence a certain tendency to mortification in spots, that is, to the necrosis which so often ensues. Consequently, if the favourable result of the anatomical changes caused by the primitive osteitis is to preserve against dangerous relapses, there is yet this other unfortunate result of keeping up prolonged suppuration and necrosis. I say, then, that this young man, in all probability, will not die, and will not even be dangerously ill.

In addition, as his tibio-tarsal articulation is obliterated, we have not to fear a propagation of the suppurative phlegmasia to the synovial membrane; but the necrosis will last for a long time yet, probably for years. Undoubtedly another sequestrum will soon be expelled, but there is still another in course of elimination. There will probably be fresh inflammatory attacks and other portions necrosed which will keep up the suppuration, and that may indeed last until the patient shall have outgrown the age during which the predisposition exists. I know that in this respect there are some varieties, that in certain subjects the new attacks of osteitis cease to occur long before the end of adolescence, notwithstanding the continance of the hyperostosis, and that sometimes these relapses and the continuation of the necrosis are seen in adults. But since we have to form a prognosis we should do it in accordance with the facts furnished most frequently in our practice. Now I noticed long ago that necrosis and persistent suppuration of the large long bones, especially those of the lower limbs, which have been previously hyperostosed by an acute spontaneous osteitis, are seen especially during adolescence, and end with it. The patient having become adult preserves only the articular deformities, the hyperostosis, and the diminution of the muscles caused by the original disease.

Treatment.—We shall make an incision to remove the superficial movable sequestrum which we felt, and at the same time make the explorations necessary to discover if by chance there is another; then we shall keep the patient in bed, apply poultices, and give him tonics. In a few weeks he will leave us, still preserving the fistulæ and the suppuration, and we shall have no other advice to give him than to avoid such fatigue and contusions as might cause another inflammatory attack.

Some one asked me this morning why I did not propose to this young man to relieve him of his present infirmity and his chances of relapse, by amputation of the leg. These are my reasons: first, amputation would endanger his life, which, in my opinion, is not threatened by the present lesions; and second, I have reason to hope, as I have just told you, that the infirmity is temporary and will disappear with adolescence, and that when from 25 to 30 years old he will walk more easily and will have no more pain and suppuration. In short, he will be cured, with a tibia a little large and an anchylosed articulation which will trouble him much less than an artificial limb, and will certainly be more agreeable to him than a mutilation.

LECTURE VII.

ACUTE EPIPHYSARY OSTEITIS OF THE LEFT FEMUR, WITH SUPPURATING ARTHRITIS OF THE KNEE. AMPUTATION OF THE THIGH.

Description of the piece—Difficulty of determining whether the periostenm is stripped off or destroyed—Suppuration and partial disappearance of the epiphysary cartilage—Diffuse suppuration of the cancellous tissue and the medullary canal—Pus in the articulation—Different names given to the disease—Preference for that of acute epiphysary osteitis—Three varieties of this disease: 1st variety, external periostitis without destruction of the periosteum; 2d variety, superficial osteo-periostitis with destruction of the periosteum; 3d variety, general deep osteitis—Difficulties and interest of the diagnosis of these three varieties.

GENTLEMEN: I show you here the specimens coming from an amputation of the thigh, which I performed the day before yesterday, upon a youth 16 years old who entered the hospital for a suppurating osteo-arthritis of the thigh and knee. The patient was taken suddenly, three weeks ago, after a long walk, with high fever which was at first thought by his physicians to be typhoid fever. But soon a painful swelling appeared at the lower end of the right thigh and the corresponding knee; then deep fluctuation was felt, and it was in this condition that the boy was brought to us after he had been ill twelve days.

We at once felt deep fluctuation on the outer and inner sides of the lower part of the thigh, and also very distinctly in the joint itself, which was notably distended.

The day after his admission I made two free incisions, one on the inner, the other on the outer side, and passing through the vastus internus and vastus externus I reached a large purulent collection and evacuated a pint of creamy, thick pus, slightly fetid and mixed with drops of oil. Passing my finger to the bottom of the abcess I felt the femur denuded on both sides. The articulation was not emptied at first, for by pressing upon it I made no pus escape through the incisions. I was not then sure that the arthritis, which was evident, had gone on to suppuration. The patient was a little relieved, but he remained unable to make any movement without suffering a great deal in the knee, which was slightly flexed, the limb resting on its outer side; and the fever continued with 130 pulsations and a temperature of 102° in the morning, and 103° to 104° in the evening.

The third day, by pressing upon the knee, I diminished its size and caused a quantity of pus to escape by the inner incision.

There was then no longer any doubt the abcess was articular as well as ossifluent. Knowing then from my own experience, and especially from *the facts* communicated to the Anatomical Society, in

1858, by my colleague and friend, Dr. Leon Labbé, at that time my
interne at the Hôpital Cochin, that this affection is followed by a
large proportion of deaths, either by pyæmia or by hecticity, and by
long suppuration and necrosis when death does not take place, I proposed amputation to the patient and his parents as a means of
diminishing the chance of a fatal termination.

The operation was performed, and examination of the affected parts
gives us the following details:—

I first show you the cavity in the thigh, which contained the pus;
it surrounded four-fifths of the lower quarter of the femur, not
reaching its posterior part. The vastus externus and internus
muscles were stripped from the bone and formed the outer wall of
the cavity, the inner one being the anterior and lateral faces of the
femur. This bone is, as you see, without periosteum. Whether the
latter was destroyed, or stripped off with the muscles, I cannot say.
You notice, however, that if we seek it on the under surface of the
muscles, near the upper limit of the lesion, we do not find it distinctly.
It appears that its continuity with the rest of the bone is interrupted,
and I do not find on the muscles a fibrous layer resembling the
periosteum. I see only a detritus which appears to belong to the
muscle itself. In a word, I do not find distinctly a simple stripping
off of the per o e m, and I believe rather that this membrane has
disappeared by absorption or by gangrene and prompt elimination.
In almost all cases of suppurating osteitis with denudation you will
have this same difficulty in determining whether the periosteum is
merely stripped off, or whether it has entirely disappeared.

At the surface of the denuded bone we see little else than an
enlargement of the vascular canaliculi, which, on the contrary, would
have been narrowed, and some of them closed, if the patient had
lived and hyperostosis had occurred. We find that the peripheral
portion of the epiphysary cartilage has disappeared, so as to leave a
groove in its place. This groove is filled with pus, and evidently
formed part of the purulent cavity. In order to examine the rest of
the bone we have sawn it vertically and from in front backwards, so
that the section reaches the articular surface between the upper
insertions of the crucial ligaments. You see that the marrow above
the epiphysis is red, infiltrated with blood, pus, and plastic material
in the alveoli of the cancellous tissue and in the lower portion of the
medullary canal, the lesions of which end about an inch below the
point of amputation.

The epiphysary cartilage is destroyed in places and to an extent
greater than was indicated by the groove we saw at the surface.
Reddish, sanious pus is seen at the points where it has been destroyed.
Above and below the cartilage the bony alveoli are infiltrated with
pus, and the surface of section has a red, vinous color.

Finally, the articulation is filled with pus, the diarthrodial cartilage
of the femur is destroyed here and there, and can be easily peeled off,
exposing the compact sub-cartilaginous layer, itself eroded in places.
The pus contained in the articulation communicated with that of the
thigh through an irregular opening in the anterior part of the

synovial membrane near the edge of the cartilage of incrustation, up to which, furthermore, the periosteum is destroyed. It seems that the synovial membrane adjoining the cartilage, and at the point where it covers the periosteum of the groove above the condyles, has also shared the destruction, so difficult to explain, of the periosteum. The diarthrodial cartilage of the tibia and the semilunar inter-articular cartilages are not affected.

In presence of these lesions you can understand the different names which have been given to the disease of which they are the expression. These names are not recent, and the difficulty about establishing one definitively was due to the fact that our predecessors had not studied the disease, and had confounded its description with those of deep phlegmon and necrosis.

I heard, at the beginning of my studies, Professor Roux indicate these deep abscesses about the long bones of the lower limb, and point out the fact of their appearance, especially in young people, and the denudation of the bone which ensues. I have even heard him express his regret at not having found in the authors any particular account of these abscesses.

But it appears to me that attention was only called seriously to this subject by two works of M. Chassaignac, one upon osteo-myelitis,[1] the other upon acute subperiosteal abscesses.[2] In creating the word osteo myelitis, and causing its adoption, M. Chassaignac described lesions of the marrow of the bone which had been first published by Dr. Raynaud in a remarkable work.[3] But while this latter author had spoken only of traumatic osteo-myelitis following amputation, the former pointed out spontaneous or primitive osteo-myelitis and its coincidence with deep abscesses external to the bone, and with the disappearance or loosening of the periosteum.

Furthermore, M. Chassaignac has the credit of having indicated the frequency of these abscesses during early life, their development with intense febrile symptoms, and the concomitant and consecutive necrosis. He recognized that this affection has close relations with osteo-myelitis, that the latter differs from it especially by its coincidence with articular suppurations which do not accompany sub-periosteal abscesses.

Still later, Klose[4] (of Breslau) published, under the title *Separations of the Epiphysis*, a suppurative inflammation of the extremities of long bones which causes a separation between the epiphysis and the diaphysis, and of which the anatomical and clinical description has much analogy with those of the osteo-myelitis and acute subperiosteal abscesses of M. Chassaignac.

Then similar lesions were described under the name of *juxta-epiphysary osteitis* by Dr. Gamet, of Lyons, and under that of phleg-monous periostitis by Dr. Louvet and M. Giraldès.

[1] Chassaignac, Gazette Médicale, 1854, p. 505.

[2] Chassaignac, Abcès sous-périostiques Aigus. (Mémoires de la Société de Chirurgie, tome iv. p. 281.)

[3] Raynaud, Sur l'Inflammation du Tissu médullaire des Os longs. (Archives Générales de Médecine, 1831, tome xxvi. p. 161.)

[4] Klose, Archives Générales de Médecine, Aug. 1858.

Referring to these different descriptions and to the specimens which I have just shown you, you see that we might really employ any one of these names. There is no doubt, for example, that we have here M. Chassaignac's spontaneous osteo-myelitis, since the medullary substance is inflamed and suppurating, as is likewise the neighbouring articulation. In like manner the presence of a purulent collection in the position which this author assigned to acute subperiosteal abscesses would permit us to choose this appellation, just as the presence of the same collection at the point of union between the diaphysis and epiphysis, and for a certain distance along the femur, would justify the expressions "juxta-epiphysary osteitis" and "phlegmonous periostitis." And, finally, do you not see that the epiphysary cartilage is beginning to be destroyed, and that if this destruction had continued the epiphysis would have separated from the diaphysis and given us Klose's spontaneous separation of the epiphysis?

It seemed to me necessary to choose a name which should not localize the inflammation so much as others have sought to do in such or such part of the bone, which should indicate the origin of the affection in the exaggeration of the nutritive process, at the junction of the epiphysis and diaphysis, while the bone is lengthening, and which should at the same time indicate the period of life at which this exaggeration takes place. Therefore I used and continue to use the expression *acute epiphysary osteitis of youth*.[1]

Look at these specimens.

Here is an osteitis which is general and complex, since it occupies all the constituent portions of the bone, periosteum, bony tissue, medullary substance; and there is no more reason for calling it exclusively osteo-myelitis than periostitis or osteo-periostitis. It was acute, for it ended promptly in suppuration. It is very intense in and about the epiphysis; and, finally, it was developed in an adolescent. If the affection appears in a child I will willingly call it acute epiphysary osteitis of childhood, but it will remain none the less true that we shall be in the presence of lesions which are rarely seen in the adult, and for the development of which the incompletion of the ossification of the skeleton is the capital predisposing condition.

Now, to make the present case accord with those which you have already met, and those which you may hereafter meet, it is necessary to add that this epiphysary osteitis of youth appears clinically under several different forms.

First, there are the differences of location. The disease may develop in the upper or in the lower limbs, but it is much more common in the latter. You will find it especially at the lower portion of the femur, and lower extremity of the tibia; more rarely at the upper end of this bone. In one case which I have published[2] the suppurating osteitis appeared at the upper end of the femur, at the junction of its neck with the shaft, and of the upper with the lower portion of the great trochanter.

[1] Gosselin, Ostéites épiphysaires des Adolescents. (Archives Gén. de Méd., 1858, vol. ii. p. 513.)
[2] *Gosselin, loc. cit.*, 1858.

Then there are varieties of intensity. I think I may say that there exists a subacute form without fever and with moderate pains, which does not end in suppuration, but nevertheless leaves behind it hyperostosis and sometimes incomplete anchylosis. This form is rare. I cannot, at this moment, show you any examples; but I remember to have seen, in 1864, at the Hôpital de la Pitié, a boy 18 or 19 years old, who had incomplete angular anchylosis of the left knee, with a swelling of the lower portion of the femur, which, a few days before, had again become painful after a fall. This patient told us that he had been taken, three years before, without appreciable cause, with swelling and pains which had kept him in bed for two months; that his physician had expected abscesses, but that they had not formed, and that he had been left with an enlarged femur, and unable to extend his knee completely. According to all the appearances he had had a subacute, non-suppurating epiphysary osteitis.

The acute form advancing rapidly towards suppuration, like that of the patient from whom these anatomical specimens come, is the one you will most often see, and the principal characteristics of the disease will then be that it is accompanied by intense fever, that it causes great pain, and that it occupies a sufficient length of the affected bone to deserve the name of diffuse suppurating osteitis. But this acute form itself presents three varieties which depend upon the location and the abundance of the suppuration.

In the first variety, of which the patient described on page 38 offered an example, the suppurative inflammation appears to occupy only the external face of the periosteum. The osteitis is none the less complicated by it; but it is suppurative neither in the compact tissue nor in the medullary substance, but only between the periosteum and the muscles. The abscess heals without leaving either fistulæ or necrosis; but hyperostosis results, thus demonstrating that the entire thickness of the bone has been affected. It is in such a case that I should consent to use the term phlegmonous periostitis; and yet I should wish to add external, plegmonous, and suppurative external periostitis. It is certainly the least dangerous of all the suppurating varieties of epiphysary osteitis; but it is also the rarest.

In the second variety, such as was seen in the tibia of the young man of whom I have heretofore spoken (page 41), there was suppuration of the surface of the bone after destruction of the periosteum, and also in the peripheral or superficial layers of the epiphysary cartilage. The compact tissue and the marrow—that is, all the rest of the long bone—share in the phlegmasia; but they do not suppurate as the surface of the bone does; nor, if the neighbouring articulation takes part in the inflammation, does the arthritis become suppurative, probably because the intensity of the disease is not sufficiently great to propagate the suppurative form of the phlegmasia as far as the synovial membrane. This is the variety which M. Chassaignac described under the title of *acute sub-periosteal abscesses*. I should call it *diffuse phlegmonous osteo-periostitis*. But I call your attention once more to the fact that in these cases the disease is not limited to the superficial part of the bone, it occupies the whole thickness; but the

4

other parts do not suppurate ; in them the osteitis remains plastic, and causes the hypertrophy of which I have so often spoken.

Finally, in the third variety, of which we have an example before us, all the constituent parts of the bone are not only affected, but suppurate, and the suppurative inflammation is propagated, either along the periosteum or along the parenchyma of the epiphysis, and through the eroded diarthrodial cartilage to the neighbouring synovial membrane. This is undeniably the most dangerous form, the one which I call osteo-arthritis. It ends very often in death, or, if the patient survives, in an interminable necrosis.

It remains now to decide whether the diagnosis between these different forms can be easily made. It is easy for the subacute form, and for that one of the acute ones in which the outer surface of the periosteum suppurates without destruction of the membrane, and without deep suppuration of the bone. It can be established especially by the aid of the general symptoms, which are moderate in these cases, and by exploration of the cavity when the abscess has been opened. If the periosteum has not been destroyed, there is no denudation of the bone; if it has been, there is. The only real difficulty is to distinguish between superficial suppurating osteitis and general suppurating osteitis; that is, at the same time superficial and deep, or osteo-myelitis. These two forms differ, perhaps, in the intensity of the general symptoms, which is greater in the second than in the first. But this difference is scarcely appreciable when you have only one patient before you. In short, in both cases the fever and all the resultant functional troubles are very marked, and the differences of intensity are too slight to furnish a means of diagnosis. The pus has no distinctive characteristics; the oily drops mentioned by M. Chassaignac are found in both forms, as is easily understood, since these drops come from the fat of the bone, and in both cases the pus is supplied by the bone, of which both the outer and inner portions contain this medullary fat, which exists as well in the external vascular canaliculi as in the alveoli of the cancellous tissue, or in the central medullary canal of the compact tissue. The diagnosis, and especially the diagnosis which is important for the treatment, is completely established only by the presence of pus in the articulation, or the appearance through the opening of the abscess of the bare dislocated extremity of the diaphysis. When one or the other of these has been discovered (and the former is the more common), there is no doubt of the existence of deep complex osteitis, such as M. Chassaignac had in view in his description of osteo-myelitis.

The interest of this diagnosis is due to the following reasons : So long as the suppuration is superficial, and the articulation is not affected, the preservation of the limb is the rule, and the surgical treatment consists chiefly of free incisions, to open the purulent cavity and allow it to be washed. It is true that death by purulent infection or hecticity may occur; but it is much less probable than when the suppurating osteitis is deep, because, as I have often had occasion to explain to you, pyæmia is chiefly due to suppuration of the marrow in osteo-myelitis.

The chances are, then, that the patient will get well when the disease is superficial. It is true that this will only be after a long-lasting neurosis, which will generally end with adolescence. On the other hand, when there are at the same time suppurative arthritis, suppurative osteo-myelitis, and osteo-periostitis, the chances of purulent infection and hecticity are so great that amputation gives the patient a better chance to escape with his life.

LECTURE VIII.

TARSALGIA OF ADOLESCENTS.—(FIRST, SECOND, AND THIRD DEGREES.)

1st degree, tarsalgia with contraction of the peroneal muscles disappearing after rest, reappearing after walking—Methods of examination in this disease—Treatment by rest and the immovable apparatus. 2d degree, tarsalgia with contraction which disappears only by the aid of anæsthesia, treated by straightening the foot during anæsthetic sleep. 3d degree, tarsalgia with retraction—Treated by section of the tendons of the lateral peronei—Examination and discussion of the theories of MM. J. Guérin, Bonnet (de Lyon), Nélaton, Duchenne (de Boulogne) concerning *painful valgus.*

GENTLEMEN: We have before us two young men suffering from that affection to which I have given the name *tarsalgia of adolescents.*

I. The first has been in the wards for more than two months, and will soon leave us. Let me describe briefly his condition at the time of admission.

He is 17½ years old. Two months before his admission into the hospital he felt pains in his left foot. When questioned as to their probable cause, he replied that he knew of none. He had never had rheumatism; he had not sprained his foot; he enjoys general good health, and nothing about him indicates a scrofulous constitution. We learned only that he had grown rapidly during the last year, that six months ago he commenced work as a grocer's boy, and that this work compelled him to remain on his feet all day, and to take long walks. At first the pain was slight, it began at the end of the day, disappeared during the night, and did not reappear at all during the morning; then about three weeks later the pain became sharper, was accompanied during the day by a slight swelling, and became at times severe enough to force him to rest for half an hour or an hour, after which he was again able to walk and attend to his work. Then for about a fortnight before admission the pain during the afternoon was so severe that he limped, and was obliged to rest, and even to lie down two or three times toward the end of the day.

The day he presented himself at our consultation, I called your attention to the fact that his foot was turned outwards in the position which characterizes that vice of conformation known as *valgus*, and that it was kept in this position by persistent contraction of the extensors and lateral peronei.

The next morning, after he had been in bed for nearly twenty-four hours, we no longer found the valgus and contraction observed the day before; the foot possessed all its movements, those of laterality as well as those of flexion and extension.

Questioning him about the pain, he replied that, for the moment, he did not suffer at all. Still, by pressing with one finger on the outer side of the foot a little in front of the external malleolus, in a rather circumscribed point corresponding to the junction of the calcaneum with the cuboid, I awakened some pain. Pressure on the inner side, a little behind the tubercle of the scaphoid, caused a similar pain, and the patient told us that those were the points where he suffered after standing and walking all day.

You then saw me extend forcibly the great toe with one hand, place the thumb of the other against the under portion of the head of the first metatarsal bone, and ask the patient to press back my thumb. He did it as easily as with the other foot, which showed that the peroneus longus, which, as you know, is designed to form and maintain the arch of the foot, was at that moment neither paralyzed nor inert.

It was evident that to understand the affection thoroughly we should have to examine the patient again after he had walked for an hour or two; so I told him to get up the next morning at six o'clock and walk about the wards until the hour of my arrival (eight o'clock).

When we came to his bed the next day, you saw that the left foot had again taken the position of valgus, which we noticed the first day at the consultation, that is to say, the outer border of the foot was raised and the toes slightly turned outwards, and on the inner side the head of the astragalus was notably more prominent under the skin, and hence apparently larger, than on the other foot. But this was only an appearance, for the day before, when the foot was in its natural position, there was no difference in size between the two. We could also see under the skin the tendons of the extensor longus, extensor proprius pollicis, and tibialis anticus; and we could both see and feel above the external malleolus the rigid prominence of the contracted peronei. Finally, we could feel and follow with the finger along the outer side of the foot the prominent cord formed by the tendon of the peroneus brevis. When asked to let his foot go, to relax the contracted muscles, the patient was entirely unable, in spite of his good will, to meet our wishes. Grasping the leg firmly with both hands above the ankle, and raising it from the bed, I shook it sharply from side to side, but was not able to give any lateral movement to the foot, while by the same manœuvre on the right side I produced marked lateral movement. Then fixing with one hand the lower part of the left leg, and grasping the sole of the foot with the other, I tried in vain to turn the latter outwards or inwards. All my efforts were transmitted to the leg, and the foot executed no lateral movement, that is, none of those which take place in the medio-tarsal and calcaneo-astragalian articulations.

On the other hand, I could easily give the foot the movements of flexion and extension, those which take place chiefly in the tibio-tarsal articulation.

Examining then the sole of the foot, I found exactly the same arch as on the other side, so that if I had wished to use the name so often employed by our predecessors, I should have had to say "painful arched valgus." Furthermore the skin behind the inferior projection of the heads of the metatarsal bones presented the normal folds which go with the existence and proper conformation of the plantar arch.

Of what disease were these the symptoms? Of a singular disease, the nature and anatomical lesions of which are still imperfectly known, and which has three dominant clinical characteristics: pain, provoked especially by prolonged walking; outward deviation of the foot, or valgus; and prolonged contraction or contracture of the anterior and exterior muscles of the leg, or, if you prefer, of all the muscles supplied by the peroneal nerve. It is evident that in this case the valgus was not congenital, that it was accidental, and even temporary, since it disappeared completely after rest.

The question then to be answered was this: was the pain caused by and closely connected with the contraction, or was the contraction only the consequence of the pain which was itself the primitive phenomenon?

To answer this question in the case of our patient, I turned to his clinical examination, and to the remembrance of a similar case in which I was enabled to make an anatomical examination.

In our clinical investigation I called your attention to two things: first, according to the commemoratives pain was the initial symptom, not only of the disease, but of all the attacks which occurred at the end of the day. During two or three weeks the young man suffered without noticing any deviation of the foot; the latter only appeared later, and, in every painful attack of an evening, the valgus appeared only some time after the pain. Moreover, the first day, when, after twenty-four hours' rest, the muscles were relaxed and the valgus had disappeared, pressure caused pain, not along the course of the muscles of which I have spoken, but over the posterior bones and articulations of the tarsus. For me then in this case there is no doubt, the pain was primordial, was increased by walking, and caused, by reflex action, the muscular contraction and deviation of the foot outwards.

But then what was the origin and seat of this pain?

Here, I invoke the result furnished by pressure with my fingers. The pain which that caused could have no other origin than the bones or the articulations.

But I prefer to refer to the case, unique, I think, in science,[1] in which I was enabled to make an autopsy.

It was a young girl, 18 years old, who presented the same symp-

[1] I should add that M. Leroux, of Versailles, communicated to the Société de Chirurgie (*Gaz. des Hopitaux*, 1865) a case in which dissection of the foot showed articular lesions similar to those which I now mention. These lesions belonged to a case of tarsalgia of adolescents. But the foot was turned inwards, in varus, instead of being in valgus, as it was in all the cases which I have observed.

toms as this young man does, and who died suddenly of cholera a few days after admission to the Hôpital de la Pitié.   The anatomical examination, the details of which I communicated to the Académie de Médecine,[1] showed us that the astragalo-scaphoid and calcaneo-cuboid articulations were affected with dry synovitis, that in several points the diarthrodial cartilages were destroyed by a process of erosion or ulceration, and that below these points the corresponding cancellous tissue was red and infiltrated with blood as in osteitis of the first degree.   These lesions, similar in several respects to those of chronic dry arthritis, and to the principal of which Brodie gave the name of *ulceration of the cartilages*, left me no doubt of their connection with the clinical symptoms in this young girl.   The ulceration mentioned, the subjacent partial osteitis, and the dry synovitis had become painful during exercise, and the pain had brought about contraction of the muscles and valgus.

In my opinion, the same things have occurred in this young man, and in the three or four other examples which we see every year in these wards of different degrees of the same disease.

Let us now see, gentlemen, what there is that is strange or uncommon about this affection, and how far we can explain it.

The first thing that strikes us is that we are in presence of a variety of articular disease, chronic dry arthritis, which is found in the other articulations only at the end of adult life and the beginning of old age, and in these the tarsal articulation appears to be confined exclusively to adolescence.   For it is found in subjects who, while they are growing rapidly, are exposed to fatiguing toil, and compelled to take long walks, often with the addition of a more or less heavy burden.

What connection is there between the growth of the skeleton and this arthritis, or rather arthro-osteitis with ulceration of the cartilages? I cannot say.   To explain the osteitis of adolescents, I referred to the exaggeration of nutritive work going on about the epiphyses.   But here in the astragalus there is no epiphysis, and the one on the posterior portion of the calcaneum is far from the articular surface on which the lesions appear; in my autopsy it was already united, and no lesion existed in it.   We must then admit that completion of growth predisposes, without accompanying union of the epiphyses, to the lesion which now occupies our attention, and I invoke the process of growth because this is another of the diseases of youth.   I do not deny its existence in children, although I have never seen an example, but you will not meet with it in the adult.   You will see adults affected with irremediable valgus, but they will tell you their deformity began at the age of 16, 17, or 18 years.

But is the contraction of the muscles equally uncommon?   No, and yes.   I say no, for the clinic often shows us spasmodic contractions in connection with articular lesions.   Think of coxalgia, at the beginning of which you find the joint fixed, often in extension, sometimes in very marked flexion, by all the peri-articular muscles, and especially by the psoas.   Then remember the arthrites of the knee

---

[1] *Gosselin, Tarsalgie des Adolescents* (valgus douloureux), Lésions anatomiques de cette Maladie.   (*Bull. de l'Académie de Médecine*, 1865, tome xxx. p. 144.

with permanent flexion due to contraction of the biceps, semi tendi-nosus, and semi-membranosus. Finally, does not temporary torticollis, which is also a disease of childhood and adolescence, appear in many cases to be caused by a contraction due to rheumatic arthritis of the cervical articulations?

But let us remain in the region of the foot. I have sometimes seen in adults, and I have shown in my clinic two patients who, whilst suf-fering from gonorrhœal tibio-tarsal arthritis, had a deviation of the foot inwards, which was clearly due to contracture of the tibialis pos-ticus. These were not the muscles of which we are speaking to-day, but the contractures were due to an articular affection.

That which is unusual and very difficult to explain, is the constancy of the contracture of the anterior and outer muscles in adolescents affected with tarsal osteo-arthritis. This constancy is such that I can understand perfectly how eminent clinicists should have considered the disease as located in the muscles. When MM. Jules Guérin and Amédée Bonnet[1] (de Lyon) described painful splay-footed valgus, and advised as principal treatment tenotomy of the lateral peronei, it is incontestable that they believed in a deformity produced by contrac-tion, and then retraction of these muscles.

When Nélaton compared this disease to writers' cramp, he thought it was a contraction, becoming painful, of the peronei and the exten-sors, just as in writers' cramp there is painful contraction of the flexors and extensors of the thumb.

This same idea of a lesion primarily muscular, led M. Duchenne (de Boulogne) to an analogous theory, according to which the origin of that variety of valgus in which the foot remains arched is an ex-aggerated contraction or contracture of the peroneus longus. Beyond the fact that it is impossible to prove this theory, it has the inconve-nience of taking into account neither the initial pain, which is much more marked over the tarsal bones than along the course of that muscle, nor the articular lesions which I pointed out, nor the ten-dency to anchylosis which is one of the possible terminations of the affection. It offers also this singular contradiction that, according to it, as I shall soon tell you when speaking about another patient, con-traction of the peroneus longus would give, with the exception of the hollow instep, exactly the same physical and functional symptoms as would incomplete paralysis of the same muscle, which latter, accord-ing to M. Duchenne, would produce the flat-footed valgus.

Furthermore, it was because in my opinion there were, together with an origin in the skeleton, consecutive effects, singular and im-portant lesions of the muscles, in this strange disease of youth, that I proposed for it, in 1865, the name, which prejudges nothing of this nature, of *tarsalgia of adolescents*.

I add that in this patient we have to deal with what I have called the first degree of tarsalgia, that in which the pain, and especially the contracture and the valgus disappear after a few hours' rest, to reap-pear when walking has been renewed and kept up for a certain time.

[1] Bonnet, Thérapeutique des Maladies articulaires, Paris, 1853.

What would have become of it if we had done nothing?

Perhaps a cure would have taken place spontaneously: but that doubtless would have been only in case the young man had given up for a time the fatiguing occupations which had been the occasional cause of his trouble.

I have met several patients who, from the information furnished by them, appeared to me to have had tarsalgia of the first degree, and to have been cured without surgical treatment by refraining from long walks. I treated in my private practice a young girl, sixteen years old, who had been affected with valgus for a week, after having felt pain for a fortnight when walking. She was relieved by keeping the bed for a week, and by avoiding for some time thereafter prolonged standing and walking.

But as, in our young man, the tarsalgia was very marked, and had already lasted several weeks, and as the necessity of working for his living would have led him to endure the pain after obtaining a slight diminution by temporary rest, I had every reason to suppose that the tarsalgia would have passed first to the second degree, that in which the contracture and valgus no longer disappear by rest, but only during anæsthetic sleep; then to the third, that in which the muscles no longer relax, even during sleep, and may be considered as having passed to the condition of permanent shortening, which you know by the name of retraction; perhaps finally to the fourth, that in which the medio-tarsal articulations, or at least one of them, and especially the astragalo-scaphoid, are anchylosed by fusion. For one of the consequences of the slight arthritis, of which you have seen the first degree in this patient, is the formation of one or more anchyloses. A few years ago I showed, at the Hôpital de la Pitié, a man fifty years old, in whose left foot there was, together with an old valgus, a union of the astragalus and calcaneum; and he told us that at the age of eighteen he had had a sprain, which he did not think it necessary to have treated by a surgeon, and in consequence of which this deformity was produced. I should add that this anchylosis, after having troubled him for a long time, and having rendered long walks impossible, had ended by becoming indolent, and causing no further functional trouble.

You see, gentlemen, that in speaking to you of the course of this affection when abandoned to itself, I made no mention of suppuration. I should fear it, perhaps, if I had found at some points of the tarsal region a diffused swelling and doughiness with semi-fluctuation, such as we find in fungous synovitis or white swelling. Not only were these signs absent, but moreover the existence of valgus and contracture led us to dismiss the idea of an articular affection which might terminate some day in suppuration. For it is a remarkable fact, and one abundantly proven by clinical observation, that arthritis tending to suppuration is not accompanied by these symptoms (contracture and valgus), and when we see these latter appear, especially in a patient who shows no signs of scrofula, we know that the affection will end neither in articular suppuration nor in caries.

In this respect the prognosis was favourable; but it had this inconvenience, in case the disease had been abandoned to itself, it would undoubtedly have lasted several years, during which the young man would have been constantly disturbed in his occupations, and it might perhaps have ended in definitive retraction and anchylosis, which are always the cause of great trouble in walking until adult life has fairly begun.

Treatment.—It results from all that I have told you, that the chief indication in this case was to keep the foot motionless. In that way we could cause the pain to disappear, and with it the muscular contracture which was its reflex effect. It was also the means by which to obtain the cure of the articular lesions, the existence of which we had the right to assume; notably that of the osteitis and the ulceration of the cartilages. I am unable to tell you if this ulceration is capable of cicatrizing purely and simply, without restoration of the cartilage; or if the latter can be reproduced, which does not seem to me impossible at this early period of life. But I have had no anatomical demonstration on these points. I only know, from the results which I have obtained in a dozen patients whom I have been able to follow, that all the clinical phenomena of tarsalgia of the first degree may disappear after a rest of two or three months.

I therefore applied an immovable apparatus whilst the muscles were well relaxed. While the foot was kept turned inwards, I wrapped about it a thick layer of cotton batting, which I carried nearly half way up the leg; over this I rolled tightly a dry bandage, then another soaked in plaster mixed with a solution of one part of gelatine in a thousand parts of hot water. The plaster dried in a few hours. The patient remained in bed for six weeks without having the bandage removed; at the end of this time I let him sit up, and a fortnight later—that is, at the end of two months—I removed the bandage, and let him walk as much as he chose.

To-day, a week later, all appears to be in good condition. No pain, no contraction has reappeared. I hope the young man is cured, and I shall let him leave the hospital in a few days. I shall advise him to wear an elastic stocking and snugly-fitting shoes, so as not to turn or sprain the foot, and thus bring back the tarsalgia; also to come and see us from time to time; and if I notice that his foot has any tendency to turn outwards again, I shall make him wear a laced shoe, the sole of which will be nearly half an inch thicker on the inner than on the outer side, so that he will have to walk with his foot turned inwards.

Unfortunately, I am not certain that the cure is final and definitive. I have seen, in several patients who had been treated in this way, the pains, contractions, and valgus reappear a few weeks after they had again begun to walk, so that it was necessary to repeat the treatment. The reason doubtless was that the articular lesions were not completely healed; for you understand that in certain cases the ulceration of the cartilage is not cicatrized or repaired in two months, and it is to be regretted that there is no sign by which we can determine the persistency of the lesion after it has been sufficiently diminished by treatment to no longer occasion functional disorders, the reappearance of which is afterwards caused by walking and standing.

II. The other patient whom I mentioned at the beginning is eighteen years old. He thinks he sprained his left foot three months ago; he suffered but little from it, and kept at his work as house servant, remaining on his feet most of the day. For a few weeks he had moderate pains, which, like those of the preceding patient, were notably greater at night. Then he noticed that his foot turned outwards when he suffered most. This deviation disappeared by rest; but a fortnight ago it ceased to disappear, the pain became greater, and a week later the patient was obliged to enter the hospital.

The first and second days, after twenty-four and forty-eight hours' rest, we found that the left foot was flat, almost without any plantar arch. But this conformation is not connected with the present affection; it is old, perhaps congenital, although the young man cannot give us any categorical information on this point. In any case, it is as marked upon the right foot, which is the seat of no disorder, as it is upon the left, which has been lame for some time. Further, we find the same physical and functional symptoms as in the preceding patient; that is, deviation of the foot outwards. apparent enlargement of the astragalus, suppression of the lateral movements of the foot, pain upon pressure on the outer side over the calcaneo-cuboid articulation, and prominence of the tendons of the extensors and lateral peronei.

It was necessary to know if the shortening of the muscles, which was betrayed by the prominence of the tendons and the deviation outwards of the foot, was definitive and irremediable, or if it could disappear and be replaced by relaxation. You saw that the shortening persisted in spite of the repose. In order to ascertain if it could cease, I subjected the young man to the influence of chloroform, and after he had become well anæsthetized you saw that all the muscles were relaxed, and that I profited by it to turn the foot inwards, and fix it with a plaster apparatus.

In this case then, as in the preceding one, we had to deal with tarsalgia of adolescents, but it was tarsalgia with splay-footed instead of arched valgus. The succession of the phenomena—first, pain without contracture, then pain with temporary contracture, finally pain with prolonged contracture and valgus without intermittence—authorized me to believe that this was again a disease, the origin of which was in a lesion of the tarsal articulations, but in which the contracture, a secondary reflex effect, was liable to become of chief importance, because prolonged contracture might become retraction, that is, the muscles would be unable to relax, and as this retraction would be inevitably accompanied by immobility of the joints, the latter would be so much the more disposed to anchylosis. If I have obtained by means of the anæsthesia a permanent relaxation, if, the articular lesions disappearing under the influence of rest, the pains are not reproduced and no longer cause reflex muscular contraction, the articulations will be able to renew their functions, and the foot to reestablish itself in a normal condition. It was with this hope that I *applied the plaster* apparatus upon the foot placed in varus after *anæsthesia.*

I must now ask again if the explanation which I repeated here of the lesion which now occupies us is a sound one, and if we ought not to invoke the theory of M. Duchenne (de Boulogne). This theory is as follows: Splay-footed valgus presumes insufficient action on the part of the peroneus longus, since the action of this muscle, by its simple tonicity, is to maintain the hollow of the instep by drawing the first metatarsal bone downwards and outwards. The origin of the affection might then be in this muscle, which would contract too feebly, or, as the author says, might be the seat of an impotence. In consequence of this impotence the foot would flatten: the plantar nerves, having become painful by the increased pressure, would provoke by reflex action a painful contraction of the peronei and extensors; perhaps, even, the flattening of the foot might subject certain points of the articular cartilages to an unaccustomed pressure which would cause their ulceration.

I ought to say, however, that M. Duchenne, in his last article upon this subject,[1] does not say much about the articular lesions, or the origin of the pains. I do not clearly understand whether, in his opinion, these latter have their origin or their principal seat in the impotent muscle, in the muscles contracted consecutively, or in the nerves, or even in the bones and the articulations.

This is, furthermore, the objection which I address to all those who attribute valgus to a functional lesion of the muscles. Why this radiating pain? Why, above all, this pain on pressure when the muscles are relaxed and the patient at rest; this pain which, moreover, in most cases, is the initial phenomenon and precedes contraction for quite a long time?

In the present case I cannot admit the impotence, always very problematical, of which M. Duchenne speaks. My chief reasons are that the flat-foot far antedates the pain, and that it exists upon the right side where there is no pain, as well as upon the affected left side; that the pain, as I have just said, was the initial phenomenon, and that finally before using anæsthesia we found the peroneus longus contracted as well as the peroneus brevis. Perhaps they will claim that this muscle, at first impotent, became afterwards contracted. I will grant it if they wish; but I ask how then will they prove this impotence to have been the cause of the trouble? Suppose the theory correct, it cannot be demonstrated by clinical study in cases like this one, where the foot was flat long before the appearance of painful symptoms.

I recognize, too, that M. Duchenne rests his theory of impotence upon a powerful argument; the cure of certain patients affected with splay-footed valgus by faradization of the peroneus longus. But this argument should not have too much weight. Whatever we may think of the theory, there will always be a singular functional lesion of the muscles in tarsalgia, and I understand how the passage of

---

[1] Duchenne, De la Crampe du Pied, ou de l'Impotence fonctionnelle du long péronier et de la Contraction fonctionnelle de ce Muscle. Union Médicale, tome xxxviii p. 599, 1868. It will be noticed that the case of splay-foot reported in this article was that of a woman forty years old, and not of an adolescent.

electric currents might advantageously modify this lesion and the trouble of innervation which causes it.

I do not accept then the theory of impotence, because clinical and anatomical study of the disease does not confirm it. But if necessary, I shall make use of the therapeutical resource offered us by M. Duchenne. If, after two months of immobility in a good posture, the pain and contraction return, I shall try electrization of the peronei and the anterior muscles of the leg. You may have seen last year a youth affected with flat-footed tarsalgia, who improved and seemed to be cured by twenty applications of electricity; but I still think, that, by reason of the presumed beginning of the disease with articular lesions, we shall do well to first combat these lesions by immobility, and to address ourselves to the muscular element only when it shall have taken a marked predominance, and an importance which it had not at the beginning.

III. Tarsalgia of the 3d degree with retraction of the lateral peronei; treatment by tenotomy.

Here is a new case of tarsalgia in a subject 19 years old. The foot is arched and in valgus. The extensor muscles relax by rest, but it is not the same with the lateral peronei; they remain tense and prominent under the skin. I anæsthetized the patient, but did not get them to relax. I am then justified in thinking that these muscles are definitively shortened by the production, consecutive to prolonged contraction, of the condition which we call retraction. The commemoratives are also favourable to the opinion that there was first pain in the articulations and bones, and that the contracture occurred afterwards. Now that the retraction exists, the muscular lesion has become the most important. For, even if the articular lesions should diminish, the foot would still remain deviated outwards, a condition which would make walking difficult and at times painful. I know that after a time this difficulty and this pain would cease, but still they would exist for a certain number of years. Moreover, instead of diminishing, the articular lesions might extend and terminate in the anchylosis characteristic of the 4th degree of tarsalgia, anchylosis which would still cause functional disorders for a certain number of years.

It is in cases of this kind that tenotomy of the lateral peronei is indicated. I consider it useless when the contracture can be overcome by rest or anæsthesia.

You saw me perform it yesterday on this patient. It consisted of a first time, in which I made a fold in the skin, and pricked its base with a pointed tenotome three finger-breadths above the external malleolus. In a second time I introduced through this opening, between the skin and the posterior face of the tendons, the blade of a pointed tenotome lying on the flat. I then turned the blade towards the tendons and divided them, one after the other. I was at once able to turn the foot inwards and fix it there with a simple roller bandage, and in four or five days, when the slight cut in the skin is healed, and we are sure there will be no suppuration, I shall apply a plaster apparatus to fix the foot and keep it slightly turned inwards. I have *already performed* this operation twice for tarsalgia of the 3d degree (with retraction of the peronei). The patients met with no accidents, and left the hospital apparently cured. As they have not come back to me, I have reason to hope that the cure has been maintained.

If from the results of clinical investigation we had reason to think that the peroneus longus did not share in the retraction, and that the peroneus brevis alone was affected, we might spare the first, and divide the second only on the dorsal surface of the foot. I know that M. Duchenne (de Boulogne) has recommended this modification for those cases which he attributes to the impotence of the peroneus longus. Thus far I have met with no cases of this kind. If I should meet with any I should not hesitate to divide the peroneus brevis alone.

PART II.

FRACTURES OF THE LIMBS.

LECTURE IX.

ANATOMICAL AND CLINICAL PHENOMENA OF CONSOLIDATION AFTER FRAC-
TURE OF LONG, FLAT, AND SHORT BONES.

Necessity of studying consolidation in long bones, flat bones, and short bones.
§ 1. Consolidation of the shaft of long bones:—1st period, when the fragments
are end to end—when they have overridden—Study of the process in a guinea-
pig—Repair of the periosteum; 2d period, musculo-periosteal capsule—Its successive transformations into fibrous and fibro-cartilaginous substance—New differences according as the fragments are end to end or overridden; 3d period,
completion of ossification—Interpretation of the provisional callus and the definitive callus; 4th period, obliteration of veins—Synovitis of neighbouring ten
dons and articulations—Muscular atrophy. § 2. Consolidation of the extremities
of long bones. § 3. Consolidation in flat bones and short bones.

GENTLEMEN : You will find in your books rather lengthy descriptions of the consolidation of fractures, descriptions in which mention
is made of experiments upon animals, and of the authors of these experiments. It is undeniable that this subject is one of those in which
experimentation has been most useful, for it is seldom that we have
occasion to study upon man the anatomical character of consolidation,
death happening very rarely during its course. But there are some
parts of the skeleton upon which experiments are difficult to make,
and, in consequence, have not been made; these are the spongy ends
of the long bones and the spongy short and flat ones. In the first
two the force cannot be concentrated with sufficient exactitude upon
the parts which we wish to study to produce the fracture at the desired
point; in the last we are liable to injure at the same time the organs
contained in the cavity which the flat bone contributes to form, and
to cause death before the time necessary for the study of the consolidation has elapsed. The result is, that fracture of the shaft of long
bones has been well studied, for these experiments are easily made,
and that the ideas thus acquired have been a little too freely applied
to fracture of the extremities of these bones, and to the short and flat
ones.

It is true that in his thesis, so justly esteemed, Dr. Lambron[1] has
indicated perfectly the differences presented in the formation of the

---

[1] Lambron, Thèses de Paris, 1842.

callus at different points of the skeleton. But as this distinction is made only at the end of his work, and after a great display of erudition which calls attention only to the authors of experiments upon the diaphyses, and as it is not made sufficiently prominent, I think, perhaps, proper attention has not been paid to it. It therefore seems to me indispensable, in order to leave no false ideas in your minds upon this subject, to describe separately consolidation in the shaft of long bones, in their extremities, in the short bones, and in the flat ones.

§ 1. Consolidation in the Shaft of Long Bones.

I show you here twelve femurs of guinea-pigs, the shafts of which present different periods of consolidation after fracture. The shortest of these periods is forty-eight hours, the longest ninety days. I do not claim to apply to man all the results which we find here. I wish you to remark especially that in these animals the work of consolidation advances more rapidly than it does in our femurs, and in most of the bones in the human race. For, besides the varieties in the aptitude of each kind of animal, there is a rapidity which depends upon the size of the bones. The smaller they are, the more rapidly do they consolidate, and as the bones of guinea-pigs are much smaller than those of men, this is the principal reason why the fractures which I now show you have advanced so much more rapidly towards a cure.

Leaving this rapidity out of account, we find the work of repair is accomplished in these animals, as in us, in three periods, of which you here see specimens sufficiently well marked.

1st period.—Clinically, we have a first period which I seldom fail to point out to you in fractures of the large long bones. It is characterized by three principal symptoms : ecchymosis, and its progressive extension to a certain distance from the fracture ; swelling of the limb ; spontaneous pain, and especially pain increased by pressure and motion. The first of these symptoms is sometimes absent, the other two almost never. We call this first period *inflammatory*, because the swelling and the pain, accompanied sometimes by a little redness and heat, the febrile movement which is added in certain cases, can hardly be explained otherwise than by an inflammation. This period lasts, in the human race, for from six to fifteen days, more or less, according to the size of the bone, the degree of the contusion, and the idiosyncrasies.

In the guinea-pig this period is shorter, but the anatomical and physiological phenomena which occur during it are the same as in man. They differ a little if the fragments are end to end or if they have overridden.

There is one point, however, which is common to all cases, and which we find in these specimens of recent fracture: it is the effusion of blood between the fragments, in the thickness of the periosteum, between the periosteum and the bone, in the medullary canal, and in the muscular interstices, to a certain distance above and below the solution of continuity. In the most recent fracture of these four, the blood is the most abundant, most coagulated, and purest. In the oldest, a week, the blood is less abundant, less coagulated, and more liquid. Why this last circumstance? Is it because the solid part of the blood, the corpuscles and the fibrine, have been in part absorbed, and the serum has remained? But this is not what usually happens. The serum is the first to be absorbed, and there remains a thick paste formed by the clots. When, instead of a paste, the collection becomes more liquid, as is sometimes seen in subcutaneous effusions of blood, we attribute it to the effusion of a new liquid, the serosity, into the collection, and its mixture with the blood. Is it not probable that the same thing has taken place here, and that the blood has become a little more fluid by the addition of a certain quantity of serosity? And, as this has occurred under the influence of the inflammatory process, we may consider it as the plastic or coagulable lymph pointed out by Hunter, as the blastema of contemporary histologists, that is to say, as a product analogous to that which is furnished by all solutions of continuity, and which is capable of undergoing the transformations necessary to ultimately reconstitute the divided tissues. In this serosity you find also the substance which the ancient authors, and, in the eighteenth century, Haller called the bony or glutinous juice poured out at the beginning of consolidation.

The effusion and infiltration of blood are about the only lesions which I shall show you in the most recent fractures, those of the second, third, and fourth days.

I. But here is one a week old, in which the fragments are nearly end to end. There is still some of the sero-sanguinolent liquid, but you see that continuity is re-established on the outside of the bone by a quite thick, fibrous-looking substance, forming about the fragments a casing or capsule, which is not sufficiently stiff to prevent their moving upon one another. By its outer surface, this capsule is in relation with, and even very closely adherent to, the deep muscular layer, and is continuous above and below with the periosteum. Its inner surface looks towards the fragments, and is in contact with the sero-sanguinolent and glutinous liquid interposed between them. In this capsule you find what Duhamel, Dupuytren, Breschet, and Villermé, described under the name *virole externe*, external ferrule. What is this ferrule? How, and by what has it been formed? If we were sure that the periosteum had not been torn when I broke the bone, we should say that it had been formed by this membrane which had become inflamed and thickened in consequence of the accident. But as I took care, after having made the fracture, to press the fragments several times outwards and inwards, I presume that the periosteum was torn, if not all around the bone, at least over a great portion of its circumference. If, then, we find to-day the continuity re-established, it is because repair or cicatrization has taken place by the thickening and rapid transformation into connective tissue of the plastic lymph exuded and mixed with blood, of which I have just spoken. That does not prevent the periosteum from being thickened above and below the solution of continuity. But I *want you to notice* that in addition to this thickening, there has been formation of a new periosteum all along the solution of continuity of the primitive periosteum; and it is probable that the materials for this repair have been supplied not only by the periosteum itself, but also by the muscular layer which has participated, more or less, in the solution of continuity, and which, at all events, participates in the consecutive phlegmasia. You will thus appreciate what there was of truth and what of exaggeration in the celebrated opinion of Duhamel, an opinion shared by many experimenters, and notably by Dupuytren, Breschet and Villermé, Flourens, Lebert, that the periphery of the callus, what they called the external ferrule, was formed by the thickened periosteum. This is true for the portions of this membrane which lie above and below the solution of continuity, but at this latter point the capsular ferrule is completed by a tissue of new formation which is a periosteum, if you choose, but a new or cicatricial periosteum which is the result of a prompt transformation of the lymph or blastema exuded after the accident. There was evidently exaggeration on the part of Duhamel and his successors, when they attributed the whole ferrule to a thickening of the normal and primitive periosteum.

As for the marrow and the space between the fragments, you see there nothing more than the infiltration of blood, and thus you determine a first period characterized at once by effusion of blood, effusion of lymph, repair by means of the latter of the periosteum, and its thickening, which seems to me to be undeniable, and as to the existence of which, I am surprised to see doubts expressed in some works, particularly in that of Billroth.

II. Here now are two guinea-pig femurs broken eight and nine days ago, in which the fragments, instead of remaining end to end, have overlapped. You still find liquid blood at the extremity of the fragments and between the surfaces where they correspond to one another. But you notice that the periosteal casing is not so complete as before. It is interrupted at two points, those which correspond to the greatest prominence of the overlapping fragments, and its continuity exists only over part of the circumference of the fracture. The repair of the periosteum has been incomplete. It is lacking at those points where the separation between the edges of this torn membrane was too great, or where there was interposition between these edges of one of the fragments. You understand from this how inexact it was to say, with Duhamel, that in every case there was a complete periosteal ferrule which, by its ulterior transformations and its interfragmentary prolongations, formed the whole callus. The truth is that the periosteum contributes to a certain extent to the formation of the callus, to a very great extent when it has not been torn at all, or when, having been torn, the edges of the tear have been brought together by the exact setting of the fragments, but to a much less extent when the torn edges have been separated by a great interval, or by the interposition of overlapping fragments. I am now going to show you that nature has other resources than the periosteum, and that the repair of broken bones must not be attributed to this membrane alone.

5

2d period.—Look at these four femurs (still those of guinea-pigs), which were fractured ten, twelve, fifteen, and twenty days ago.

I. Of not one of them have the fragments remained end to end, as happens when the experiment is made upon a dog, and when immobility has been obtained by means of some apparatus. Here I was not able to keep on any apparatus, on account of the disposition and smallness of the limbs, and the vivacity of the animals. Therefore, in order to describe to you that which takes place when the fragments are brought end to end, I am forced to refer to what I have observed upon dogs in which I have obtained this result, and to the reports of other experimenters who have observed facts of this kind.

In such cases, we find at this period, quite a thick capsule, adherent to, and enveloping the two fragments. This capsule appears to be formed by the periosteum; but it is doubled externally by a muscular layer which adheres closely to it, and which you will soon verify upon our overlapping fragments. The union is so close, that we may believe that the deep muscular layer has taken part in the formation of this external callus. This capsule, which we shall therefore name *musculo-periosteal*, is much more dense than the former ones; it adheres closely to the fragments, has a grayish appearance on section, and when examined under the microscope, shows cartilaginous cells. In the earlier cases it was the fibro-cellular callus, now it is the fibro-cartilaginous callus. On section, we see a certain number of orifices, through which the blood oozes, and which belong, some to the natural vessels of the membrane, others to vessels of new formation. Here and there can be already seen a few calcareous spots scattered through the thickness of the fibro-cartilage, and which are the first points of ossification of the latter.

I do not wish to dwell too long upon the intimate mechanism of the transformations which have taken place; that of the plastic lymph into a cellular, or connective substance for the new portion of periosteum; that which brings about the thickening of the old periosteum; then the invasion of the fibrous tissue by the fibro-cartilage, and the bony deposits in the latter. Nor do I wish to discuss the question whether, instead of a transformation of the primitive elements into others, there has not rather been a substitution, that is, a successive replacement of elements and tissues by others. For these questions are still under discussion, on account of the difficulty of settling them by histological examination, and, furthermore, these studies have no very direct clinical application. I will remind you only, in order to enable you to understand these controversies, and their degree of utility, that, at the beginning of the repair, and thickening of the periosteum, we find in the· organic gangue, rounded nucleated cells, similar to those which precede the formation of our normal tissues. For the French school, represented by M. Chas. Robin, these primitive cells are formed in the exuded lymph, which we compared to a blastema. For the German school, represented by Virchow, they come by proliferation from the cells of the torn tissue. It makes but little difference to me whether you adopt the one or the *other of these* theories, I have no unanswerable arguments for either;

but I believe that the French opinion is better supported by observation than is the German.

A little later we find fibres of connective tissue, then cartilaginous cells, and here again I am unable to say if these are transformed primordial cells, or if, as M. Robin[1] claims, the fibres have grown beside and in the place of the latter, that is, by a substitution instead of a transformation. As to the deposits of calcareous molecules, soon supplied with thin bone, corpuscules, and vessels analogous to those of Clopton Havers, no one is able to say how they are formed; quite recently they have advanced the theory, without, however, being able to prove it, that the corpuscules, or osteoplastes, were the result of a calcareous infiltration of the primitive cells which I have just mentioned. As for myself, I can suggest nothing else by way of explanation, than a tendency, a nisus, analogous to that which must be admitted for the primitive formation of the bones. This nisus exists in the points of our organism where the skeleton is to form, and it still exists in those where, a longer or shorter time after its formation, a solution of continuity occurs.

But, thus far, I have spoken to you only of the periosteum; let us now see what has taken place (when the fragments are end to end), in the other parts of the fracture, in the medullary substance, and the compact tissue of the fragments themselves.

As for the medullary substance, as it is not well marked in these small animals, I can show you only the anatomical modifications which have been observed in the large animals, and even in the human race. However, after separation of the fragments, and comparing the interior of the canal with that of the other side which is healthy, you see in the centre of the bone a gray coloration, a greater density of the contained substance, and a diminution of the fatty aspect. It is evident that the marrow has been modified in its texture, and I do not think that I overstep the limits of permissible hypothesis in telling you that this marrow has been inflamed like the periosteum. There has been medullitis at the same time with periostitis. This inflammation has likewise given birth to plastic lymph, and this has been replaced by a fibro-cellular substance at the same time that the fat has been absorbed. It is even possible that cartilaginous cells have already appeared here. Thus far, I have not found any; but, as every one admits that the medullary substance becomes cartilaginous, and then bony in the process of consolidation, I suppose that the cartilage would soon have been developed, if it is not so already. We have then here what the authors have named the internal ferrule, or the beginning of that part of the process of repair which is performed by the medullary substance. But, the work is not so far advanced as it is on the side of the periosteum.

Now look at the end of the fragments. In the inter-fragmentary space there is no appearance of consolidation; we find there only a little blood, or, rather, sanguinolent serosity, and if it were not for the thickened periosteum and marrow, we could easily separate them

[1] Dictionnaire de Médecine et de Chirurgie, par Littré et Robin (13th edition), Art. Cal.

from one another. Still the compact tissue of the extremity of the fragments is red; if we detach the periosteum for a certain distance above and below, we find the compact tissue pink and its vascular canaliculi enlarged. We have then here the anatomical character-istics of non-suppurating osteitis of the compact tissue. I give the name *plastic* to that osteitis under the influence of which the exu-dation destined to repair is poured out, by opposition to the osteitis in which there is formation of pus with or without a concomitant reparatory process.

The anatomical modifications of this period in a fracture set end to end may then be resumed in this: periosteum thick, fibro-carti-laginous, with beginning of ossification; marrow dense, fibro-cellular, soon becoming cartilaginous, but without bony deposit; no sign of interfragmentary callus; osteitis on the surface and in the thickness of the compact tissue of the fragments. In a word, repair by means of the periosteum and the muscles more advanced than repair by the other tissues.

II. We have now to see what has taken place in this second period (from the eighth to the fifteenth day) in overriding fractures. You still find here the fibro-cartilaginous condition of the periosteum and the deep muscular layer, with beginning of ossification. But as the periosteal capsule is incomplete that part of the work of repair which is performed by this capsule is necessarily less solid than in the preceding case. As to the marrow, it is grayish and thick as when the fragments are end to end; but that of the upper and that of the lower fragments no longer correspond on account of the over-riding; consequently this thickening of the medullary substance does not help the consolidation. But between the fragments there is a fibro-cellular, partly cartilaginous substance which aids in keeping them together. This is the beginning of an interfragmentary callus. But it is furnished exclusively neither by the marrow nor by the compact tissue; it evidently has its origin in all the surfaces which are brought into contact with one another by the overlapping. Such are the outer face of the periosteum and a part of the compact edge of the fragments. There, in a word, we must not seek circular repair in the periosteum nor in the interfragmentary compact tissue, still less in the marrow which contributes nothing to it since its two divided surfaces are removed from one another. A mixed lateral interfragmentary callus is produced, the materials of which are formed by the muscles and by the outer surface of the periosteum, without its being possible to prove that this latter is thickened and trans-formed, and without our being able to admit anything else than the effusion from it, as well as from the surrounding cellular and mus-cular tissues, of plastic juices which are ultimately transformed. But we must not expect to find regularity of the phenomena which we observed in the end-to-end fractures, and which the authors have erroneously indicated as occurring indiscriminately in all fractures.

3d period.—During the third period, which lasts from the fortieth to the sixtieth day, new anatomical modifications ensue in the fibro-cartilaginous substance which was formed during the second. The most important is the formation of the bony substance, that is, the deposit of calcareous matter, and the more abundant deposit of osteoplastes or bone corpuscles. As for these latter, we may again ask ourselves if they are the result of a transformation of the cartilaginous cells or of a substitution. This is a point which histological observation has not been able to clear up, and upon which only suppositions are permissible. You know that I lean toward the theory of substitution.

Let us see what observation has taught us concerning the succession of the phenomena in the different portions of the fracture; and here let us distinguish again between an end-to-end and an overlapping fracture. The observations have always been made upon the end-to-end fracture only. They have formed what I show you here upon this guinea-pig's femur, the lesion of which has reached the sixtieth day; a very large external bony ferrule; a bony mass, a sort of internal ferrule, within the medullary canal, but an intermediate substance between the fragments which is not yet quite ossified, and the greater part of which remains fibro-cartilaginous. In other words, you see here what Dupuytren described under the name *provisional callus*, and Miescher under the name *primitive callus*. By these names these authors wished to indicate that the periosteal and medullary portions of the bony callus were destined in great part to disappear by absorption, and that the true callus was formed by what was left of these and by the bony substance which ultimately formed between the fragments. But there was an exaggeration on the part of these surgeons in the expression of their thought in this way, first, that all is not provisional in the periosteal and medullary calluses, since a part is to remain; and secondly that, as I shall presently explain, the theory given by them as a general one, is not applicable to overriding fractures.

I ask you to notice, in passing, upon this human tibia, in which chance has permitted us to study a callus at the sixty-fifth day, that at the level of, above, and below the fracture, which is not an overlapping one, the compact tissue has become very vascular, very dense, and enlarged; that it offers, in short, the characteristics ascribed by Gerdy to condensing osteitis. When I shall study the clinical phenomena of fractures in detail I shall recur to this habitual intervention of hyperostosis after fractures of the long bones. But here, while studying the question anatomically, I am justified in telling you that the work of consolidation of fractures is dependent upon a modification of the vitality of the fragments which we can ascribe to nothing else than osteitis, and that the variety of osteitis which here intervenes is that which Gerdy named *condensing osteitis*. I go even further. In diaphysary fractures of long bones the intervention of this condensing form of osteitis seems to be necessary. When there is lack of consolidation and pseudarthrosis, rarefying osteitis has intervened. Fortunately that is much more rare, and that is why we so rarely see pseudarthrosis follow simple fracture of the shaft of long bones.

Now let us look at overlapping fractures. We have here an

example in the femur of a guinea-pig. I have sawn it longitudinally, and you can see that the new ossification, or, if you prefer, the calcification and production of osteoplastes, have taken place between the two bony surfaces in contact, there where the fibro-cartilaginous callus already existed, but that there is no mention to be made here of a medullary bony callus. It is true that the marrow at the line of the fracture is in great part ossified. But you see that this ossification is of no use to the callus and does not contribute to the consolidation, since that of the upper and that of the lower fragment are not in continuity as they were in the end-to-end fracture.

Nor is there any question of an interfragmentary callus formed by the compact tissue. Consequently, we have no longer to speak of provisional callus and definitive callus. Say, if you please, that the lateral interfragmentary callus is perhaps larger to day than it would have been six or eight months hence. But do not think that Dupuytren's and Miescher's ideas are applicable to cases of this kind, which are the most frequent in man. I have also to point out the same hyperostosis consecutive to the condensing osteitis, as that of which I spoke in end-to-end fractures.

4th period.—For the fourth period, which extends from the sixtieth to the one hundred and twentieth day, and sometimes beyond, I have but few anatomical details to point out: the callus becomes denser and diminishes in size, the medullary canal generally remains filled by the interior ossification, and the shaft of the bone remains a little larger than is normal.

I have further to mention lesions which I can show you only imperfectly in animals, and of which I have at this moment no specimen belonging to man. But we often notice the consequences in the living. I refer to—

1st. Obliteration of the veins;
2d. Synovitis of neighbouring tendons and articulations;
3d. Muscular atrophy.

1st. Obliteration of the large veins near the fracture is quite a common lesion. Are we to explain it by a phlebitis due to the propagation to the interior of the veins of the phlegmasia which arises at the point of fracture, or is it due to simple coagulation of the blood without preceding inflammation of the internal membrane of the vens? The pathological anatomists are still discussing these two theories. As for myself, I hold the first opinion. In most cases, and especially in those in which this lesion occurs in the course of a fracture, I attribute the coagulation of the blood in the veins to a phlebitis by propagation. I even ask myself (but I shall never be able to answer the question by positive facts) if this phlebitis is not due to the passage into the large veins of irritating materials coming from the inflamed marrow or osteomyelitis. But, leaving aside the theoretical question, I point out to you this spontaneous coagulation and the resultant obliteration as the cause of a complication which is not dangerous, but is troublesome and lasts a long time, œdema of the limb about and below the point of fracture.

2d. Synovitis of the tendons and joints is not so frequent in fractures of the shaft as in those of the extremities of the long bones. Nevertheless, after one of the former you often see one of the neighbouring joints inflame and preserve for a long time a more or less painful rigidity, which is explained by the loss of extensibility and of suppleness of the synovial membrane and the connective tissue which lines it. This is particularly common in the knee after fracture of the shaft of the femur, and in the ankle-joint after fracture of the leg.

3d. The muscular atrophy consecutive to fractures which I have studied for several years, and which I made known in a thesis of Dr. Lejeune[1] based upon my lectures at the Hôpital Cochin, and a little later in my work upon *irreductibility and the consecutive deformities of long bones*,[2] is a phenomenon, if not constant, at least very frequent. We often see examples in living patients. The diminution in size of the limbs, the diminution of strength, are easily recognized. In three guinea-pigs whose muscles I here show you, this lesion is very evident. The muscles of the thigh which was broken a few months ago are a little paler and smaller than those of the opposite side. I weighed the muscles of the thighs of one of the animals and found on the healthy side 142 grains, and on the fractured one 117.

Dr. Lejeune weighed separately the muscles of both limbs of a patient who died at the Hôpital Cochin, and found a notable difference in each one.

According to these results, you may consider it an incontestable fact that the muscles diminish in size after a fracture, and I have ascertained that this diminution is permanent, and not temporary.

I have sought[3] for what might be the cause of this slight atrophy, and reached this conclusion, that it should be attributed neither to the compression nor to the immobility, and that it was doubtless due to a change in the distribution of the nutritive materials which is the consequence of the process of consolidation. Not only does the fracture draw towards itself a greater quantity of these materials, but the callus itself, when once formed, and after its completion the hyperostosis, require a greater proportion for their nourishment. This seems to me to be proved by the difference in weight between the fractured and the opposite healthy bone of the same subject. For example, look at these two femurs of a guinea-pig. The right, which was broken forty-three days ago and which is consolidated, weighs 19.8 grains, the left, 15.75 grains. Is it not probable that the right has taken, and would have continued to take, if the animal had lived, more material from the blood, and that consequently there would have been less left for the muscles?

Whatever may be the explanation, the anatomical fact exists and accounts for the persistent weakness so long complained of by patients in limbs which have been broken. I admit that in many patients the diminution of strength is not great, and is scarcely

[1] Lejeune, Thèses de Paris, 1853.
[2] Gosselin, Mémoire sur l'Irréductibilité et les Déformations consecutives des Os longs. (Gaz. Hebdomadaire de Méd. et de Chirurgie, Paris 1859.)
[3] Gosselin, loc. cit.

appreciable. That is because the innervation is not affected, and the muscles receive from the nerves a stimulus sufficient to diminish the physiological results of the atrophy. It is no longer the same when the nerves have been wounded at the same time as the bone. There may then be paralysis as well as atrophy, and the functional troubles are much more marked.

§ 2. PHENOMENA OF CONSOLIDATION IN THE EXTREMITIES OF LONG BONES.

In the extremities of long bones, as in their shafts, we have a first period, called inflammatory, during which the blood and the plastic lymph are effused between the fragments, and at the same time the adjoining connective tissue is swollen for a certain distance above and below the solution of continuity. The beginning of consolidation has not been so well studied here as upon the shaft, for the fractures are so difficult to produce, that experimental study has not been possible, and on the other hand, occasions upon men are rare. We know, however, that the fragments are almost never entirely separated from each other, and that consequently we have not to make a separate study for the end-to-end and for the overlapping fractures. They are almost always end to end, with a more or less marked displacement according to thickness and sometimes according to direction. On the other hand, there is no medullary cavity, and consequently no internal ferrule. The repair is periosteal and interfragmentary, and in this first period, the solution of continuity of the periosteum begins its repair at all the points where its borders are a little separated. But in general the periosteum does not thicken as much as it does on the shaft, and does not form from the beginning this thick ferrule of which we have spoken. No consolidation yet takes place between the fragments; we find there only extravasated blood.

During the second period the new periosteal portion becomes fibro-cartilaginous. At the same time the interfragmentary consolidation commences by the production, probably through the transformation of the exuded lymph, of a fibro-cartilaginous substance. But here several varieties must be pointed out.

In the first, the fragments, composed almost exclusively of cancellous tissue, have not been crushed; they offer neither the reciprocal penetration so well described by M. Voillemier[1] for fracture of the lower extremity of the radius, nor the reduction into small fragments, sometimes into dust, of a portion of this bony tissue which is broken by the mechanism of crushing. In such cases the blood is absorbed, and the fibro-cartilaginous substance, the beginning of the interfragmentary callus, is formed.

In a second variety, which is often found in fractures of the lower extremity of the radius the pieces are in contact, but are reduced by crushing into a certain number of fragments, some of which are very small, almost pulverized. In such cases, especially when there is penetration, the work of consolidation is preceded by the absorption

---

[1] Voillemier, Clinique Chirurgicale, Paris, 1861.

of a part or of the whole of the fragmentary portions. Nothing in the clinical symptoms indicates this absorption, but as, after fractures long consolidated, we find a shortening which cannot be explained by overriding, and which we can attribute only to this absorption, I presume that it takes place during the first few days at the same time as that of the blood infiltrated between the fragments.

In a third variety, of which the intra-capsular fractures of the neck of the femur and of the humerus give us quite frequent examples, the fragments are in contact but do not penetrate one another; the interposed blood is reabsorbed, and so too is the bone dust. But no intermediate fibro-cartilage is produced, and this absence of the first rudiments of a callus is the indication of non-consolidation which has been pointed out by all the modern authors as frequent in fractures of this kind.

To what cause must we attribute this unfortunate result? It has been claimed to be due to the shortness of the upper fragment, the insufficiency of vessels, and therefore of nutritive materials, in this fragment, and consequently the necessity for the lower fragment to do the whole work of repair, a task which it is unable to perform properly.

I would here say that if this were the only cause, or even the principal one, all fractures of the extremities would be exposed to non-consolidation. Now some of these, those of the lower extremity of the radius for example, consolidate very well.

In those which consolidate rarely I see the intervention of a condition which ought in great part to explain it; I refer to the free communication between the seat of the lesion and the articular cavity, such as exists in intra-capsular fractures of the neck of the femur. I suppose that, as it has been claimed for fractures of the patella, the blood and plastic lymph flow into the articulation, and not enough of the latter remains between the fragments to ultimately produce the fibro-cartilaginous substance.

In the third period, absorption of the pieces goes on if the conditions of the fracture are favourable thereto; the periosteal callus ossifies without becoming thick enough to form a ferrule comparable to that of fracture of the shaft. The interfragmentary callus is completed and assumes a greater and greater importance through the ossification of the fibro-cartilaginous substance, according to the same mechanism, and in the same mysterious conditions which I indicated above. This intermediary callus is often very thick and very resisting, especially at the lower extremity of the radius; but sometimes, and in particular at the neck of the femur, it remains fibrous and more or less dense, almost always dense enough to allow the patient to walk with crutches without inflection or rupture of the callus.

In any case, the capital difference to which I wish to call attention between the callus of the shaft and that of the extremities is that, at the beginning, the former is much more peripheral than interfragmentary; that if it is interfragmentary in overlapping fractures, it is at the same time lateral and periosteal; while the second is interfragmentary in the most rigorous sense of the word, that is, it is formed

in great part or in totality by the spongy tissue through which the
solution of continuity was made.   And the result of this comparative
study is to show that all the constituent parts of the bone, spongy
tissue, compact tissue, periosteum, contribute to repair fractures of
the bone, that even the layers of muscular tissue and the surrounding
cellular tissue contribute also to it, and that, finally, the authors
erroneously attributed a much too large part to the periosteum in this
reparatory function   Furthermore, the same conclusion will be drawn
from the study of the consolidation of simple fractures of flat bones
and short bones.

In the fourth period, the patients are tormented by the consequences of articular and tendinous synovites, and so much the more
so because these fractures being near a joint or synovial grooves, and
often even in communication with them, the inflammation has spread
to the latter and left behind it the dryness and stiffness which in the
joints, characterize plastic chronic arthritis and dry arthritis.   These
consequences are so much the more marked and rebellious because
the patients affected with these lesions of the extremities are almost
always advanced in age, for the predisposing cause of fracture with
crushing is rarefaction of the cancellous tissue, rarefaction which, in
consequence of inexplicable modifications of nutrition, is a very
common consequence of age.   Now it is also the case that in old
people traumatic arthritis and synovitis, although they do not go on
to suppuration, are very slow to end and often pass to that condition
of incurability which causes dry arthritis.   Finally, muscular atrophy
occurs after these fractures as well as after those of the shaft.

§ 3. ANATOMICAL PHENOMENA IN FRACTURES OF THE FLAT
BONES AND SHORT BONES.

I have not much to say on this subject; nature uses the same
resources in the consolidation of these two kinds of bone as in that
of long bones.   The muscles, the periosteum, and the whole fractured
surface furnish the materials, and the same ulterior modifications of
these materials cause the formation of the callus.   But in the flat
bones, and especially in those which. have no diploë, or only a very
thin one, the periosteum is the chief agent where it has been preserved, and it must not be forgotten that if it has been divided, which
very commonly happens, it begins by repairing itself, and the material
which it supplies to the callus comes as much from its cicatricial
portion as from that which remained intact about the fracture.
Further, no matter how thin the bone may be at the place of fracture,
it can still furnish the materials needed for repair.   I had occasion,
in 1871, to trepan for intra-cranial suppuration following gunshot
fracture of the right parietal bone, a young man twenty-four years
old, who was employed in the museum of natural history, and had
been brought to the ambulance of that establishment after the battle
of Buzenval, where he had been wounded.   Not only did he survive
the operation, but a bony growth formed all around the opening and
advanced towards the centre, so that this sort of flattened callus

closed entirely the hole made by the crown of the trepan. Larrey has reported similar cases, in which, as in mine, the calluses were formed during suppurative osteitis, but I wish to mention them here in order to show you once more the power and the multiplicity of means which the organism possesses to repair not only solutions of continuity but also losses of substance in the bone.

LECTURE X.

PHENOMENA OF CONSOLIDATION AFTER COMPOUND SUPPURATING FRACTURES.

1st Variety: Consolidation after benign and superficial suppurating osteitis. 2d Variety: Consolidation after deep osteitis or non-putrid suppurative osteo-myelitis. 3d Variety: Death before consolidation by putrid osteo-myelitis and purulent infection.

GENTLEMEN: Do not lose sight of a first point which is capital in the history of fractures complicated by wounds; they may get well, exactly like simple fractures, but on one condition, which you should always bear in mind when you are called upon to treat such a case, on condition, I repeat, that the bone does not suppurate.

When the broken bone suppurates, and unfortunately all the efforts which you have made and should have made to prevent it do not always succeed, the clinical and anatomical phenomena of consolidation are peculiarly modified, sometimes hindered by this new complication which I shall study especially in the long bones.

Moreover, we have differences depending upon whether the suppurating osteitis occupies the superficies or the entire thickness of the bone, and according to its greater or less intensity. Let me explain these two points.

1. In a first variety, which I call *benign and superficial suppurating osteitis*, the patient has no general symptoms and consequently no fever. The swelling of the limb is moderate, suppuration is established the fourth or the fifth day in the wound itself. The eschars begin to be eliminated, and if you probe the wound gently, you feel the bone denuded superficially. Suppuration becomes a little more abundant after the eighth or ninth day, but the pus is laudable, not fetid, and the apyrexia continues. Things go on in this way for twenty or thirty days; the suppuration continues rather scanty, with no burrowing of the pus, no indication of a deep collection. Mobility of the fragments begins to diminish; in short, except for the superficial suppuration and denudation, the fracture resembles a simple one that has reached this period. But the denudation continues and the *fracture goes on* to the sixtieth, sixty-fifth day; about the seventieth

day we find it consolidated. Increase of volume can be felt above and below, showing that the osteitis on both sides of the fracture has taken on the condensing form with which we are acquainted. But the fistula persists and the suppuration which it supplies only ends twenty, thirty, or forty days later, after elimination of a splinter or mortified piece comprising a more or less considerable portion of the thickness of the bone. To use the ordinary terms, there has been superficial necrosis, and, after expulsion of the necrosed part, the callus and cicatrix have been completed. The osteitis, instead of remaining plastic over the whole fracture, became suppurative and necrotic in one place, hence the anatomical phenomena which have taken place. In the deep parts of the bone, that is to say, between the fragments, in the medullary canal, and at that portion of the circumference of the bone which is opposite that with which the wound communicates, the osteitis has been plastic, that is, non-suppurative, and the' callus has been formed, as in ordinary cases, by effusion and ultimate transformation of the lymph. Adjoining the wound the periosteum has been destroyed by absorption or by mortification; part of the bone has necrosed. Suppuration has taken place about the necrosis without extending to the interfragmentary space. After expulsion of the sequestrum, the suppurating granulations have covered the surface of the bone, and it is in them that have taken place the ulterior transformations, that is, into fibro-cartilage, and then into bone, which have brought about both the reproduction of the periosteum at this point, and the reproduction, sometimes excessive, of the subjacent layer of bone. Here then you see a new element intervene in the formation of the callus, an element which is itself a product of the consecutive inflammation; the granulations, which whilst they suppurate on the surface, ossify below and are transformed into a bone cicatrix, just as they are transformed upon the skin and subjacent tissues, when there is suppuration, into nodular fibrous tissue. The intervention of this new element shows you once more how many assistants the periosteum needs in order that the callus may form under all the conditions where its production becomes necessary.

2. In a second variety, suppuration invades the surface and the depths of the bone, that is to say, the interfragmentary space, the medullary canal, and that portion of the circumference which is furthest from the wound. The osteitis, in a word, has become a general suppurative one, and is no longer partially suppurative as in the other variety. This is the form which we call suppurative osteo-myelitis, so as to indicate also the participation of the marrow.

At first the clinical phenomena vary according to the intensity of this osteo-myelitis. If this is moderate, if the osteitis is subacute, the primitive or traumatic fever is not very violent; the pulse does not go beyond 100, 110, nor the temperature in the axilla above 101° to 102°; you do not see the subicteric tint, the delirium, the dryness of the tongue, the tympanism of the abdomen, which announces the dangerous form of traumatic fever. Suppuration begins on the fifth *or sixth day in the* wound; the pus burrows in the neighbouring tissues. Through the wound and the new openings made by the suppuration, the probe, and sometimes the finger, show that the bone is denuded to a considerable extent above and below the fracture, both about the wound and on the opposite side. The probe penetrates deeply between the fragments and brings out pus. If in order to dress it, you are obliged to move the limb, you see at each movement the liquid escape from the deep parts; furthermore, the suppuration is very abundant. These are so many indications of the presence of suppuration in the depths of the bone, and consequently in the medullary canal.

The case goes on thus for weeks and months unless complications, particularly erysipelas or purulent infection, should intervene. Suppuration continues to be abundant, from time to time slivers of bone are eliminated, the fragments remain movable, repair does not go on, and yet the tumefaction of the bone above and below the fracture indicates that there the osteitis has become condensing, a circumstance which generally augurs well, because, in cases of this kind, the osteitis is reparatory at the same time that it is condensing, that is, the nisus which increases the size of the bone above and below the fracture tends also to repair it.

Finally after a length of time which varies from three to six months, a large callus exists at the seat of the original lesion of the bone. There are still superficial slivers of bone, others, surrounded by new bone, are invaginated; more or less numerous fistulæ lead to these sequestra. In short, the suppurating osteitis has at the same time been hypertrophying and necrotic, as is generally the case in acute suppurating osteitis of youth, and finally, the fracture is really replaced by necrosis consecutive to this osteitis.

How is this callus produced? Very probably by the two mechanisms which we already know; in spite of the intensity and abundance of the suppuration there are perhaps here and there a few points where it has not taken place, and where the plastic exudation has been deposited either by the muscles or by the portions of bone furthest removed from the wound. But in addition, at those points where suppuration takes place without necrosis and elimination, the callus is formed by the granulations themselves, as Sabatier formerly pointed out, and as well by those of the medullary canal and compact tissue as by those of the periosteum. Another proof in support of the opinion that the periosteum is far from being the only agent in the formation of the callus.

3. In a third variety, the osteo-myelitis becomes as intense as possible; it is hyperacute, gives rise to traumatic fever of the most dangerous kind, and is followed, if life is prolonged, by putrefaction of the marrow and periosteum which becomes the point of departure of that other fever which we call purulent infection. But I do not wish to treat to day of putrid osteo-myelitis. I only wish to point it out to you, placing it beside the other forms of suppurating osteitis and the mode of consolidation after their appearance.

LECTURE XI.

FRACTURES OF THE LEG.

GENTLEMEN: I. You have just seen in No. 5, a man 82 years old, of habitually good health, who fell yesterday evening in the street, was unable to rise, and was brought to the hospital on a stretcher. He was put to bed and his left leg placed in a wire trough extending a little above the knee. The patient suffered during most of the night, and has slept but little; this morning we find him in the following condition:—

The left leg, compared with the right, is notably larger, without showing either phlyctenæ or redness. Pressing with one finger upon the inner face of the tibia we feel only a little thickening; there is neither ecchymosis nor phlyctenæ. The finger passed along the anterior border and inner face of the bone, finds nowhere any inequality which could be attributed to a displaced fragment. Pressure with this finger causes pain only at the junction of the middle with the lower third of the leg. This pain on pressure in a fixed point, the suffering experienced during the night, the extensive though moderate swelling, taken together with the difficulty of moving the limb, and the patient's inability to get up and walk, are the rational signs of fracture. But you saw that by raising the limb with my two hands, one of which embraced its middle, the other its lower third, and by trying to move the lower part of the limb alternately outwards and inwards with the hand which held it, while the other held the upper two-thirds firmly, I produced an abnormal movement, the centre of which was at the lower part of the shaft of the tibia. I thus demonstrated mobility, and during the same manœuvre I also felt crepitation. We have then no doubt upon the first point of the diagnosis. The patient has a fracture.

But is it only a fracture of the tibia, or are both the bones broken? It is again the mobility which enables us to answer this question. If the tibia alone had been fractured, I should have been able to impress only very obscure movements which would have left me in doubt; *to establish my diagnosis* I should have had to insist upon the pain on pressure, and to renew the examination for several successive days. I should undoubtedly, after several days, when the swelling and the muscular contractions had diminished, have ended by finding a sufficiently appreciable mobility ; perhaps also one day or another, during these examinations, I might have found crepitation. But when the very first day you find a mobility so marked that the hands of the surgeon appreciate it very easily, and that even the assistants can see it, there is no hesitation ; it is a simultaneous fracture of the tibia and fibula.

Can I now tell you what is the direction of this fracture, if not in both bones, at least in the more accessible one, and to what anatomo-pathological conditions the absence of displacement is due? Upon these points I am obliged to maintain the greatest reserve. Before Malgaigne's publications we might have thought that it was a transverse fracture; but since Malgaigne[1] has shown positively that fractures of this kind, especially in adults, do not exist, and that the cases which were supposed to be such were toothed fractures, we may believe that we are in presence of a fracture of this kind, and that the non-displacement is explained by the preservation and interlocking of these irregularities. It is probable at the same time that the periosteum and attachments of the muscles are preserved upon a part of the contour of the solution of continuity, and aid to keep the fragments together.

However that may be, you are in presence of the most favourable clinical variety. The patient will get well without deformity, and in all probability will get well rapidly. At least we foresee no circumstance which would retard consolidation.

II. Not far from this patient is another, at No. 15, who was admitted three days ago, and who presents an example of the second clinical variety of fracture of the leg.

He fell, like the preceding one, and was not able to get up or walk. It was the left leg which was injured. The functional and physical symptoms are the same. But in addition, by passing the finger along the anterior border of the tibia we felt at the lower part of the inferior third an abnormal projection which raised and distended the skin and was painful on pressure. Furthermore, there were two quite large phlyctenæ, one of which was filled with yellowish serosity, and the other with sanguinolent serosity, and a few smaller ones. Let us consider for a moment these two particularities.

1st. What is this abnormal projection? It is evidently formed by the upper fragment of the tibia, and is due to the fact that this fragment, pushed forward by the impulsion which was communicated to it at the moment of the accident, is at the same time drawn up and held by the traction of the quadriceps femoris upon the point where the ligamentum patella is attached. This displacement, the most frequent of those which you will see in fractures of the leg, belongs to the category of transverse displacements. When you meet with it, you will ask yourselves two questions : one theoretical, To what is it due? the other essentially practical, Is it reducible?

[1] Malgaigne, Traité des Fractures, p 66.

To what is it due? I told you a moment ago that it was due to an impulsion forwards by the cause of the injury, and to the action of the quadriceps femoris. But the anatomical condition which really explains it is the principal direction of the line of fracture. This direction, instead of being nearly horizontal as in the preceding case, represents an oblique direction downwards and forwards, a section so disposed that the upper fragment terminates in a more or less pointed extremity. This disposition has received the name of oblique fracture, and you understand that it is very favourable for the displacement which we see here. It is sufficient that at the time of the accident an impulsion be communicated to this fragment, so that, drawn up by the action of the quadriceps, it forms the projection which you saw.

Are there not, also, in the manner in which the fracture is produced, in its mechanism, as they say, reasons which explain the displacement? I do not think so, or at least if the reasons exist, they escape us entirely. For I learn from the information given by the patient that, as in the preceding case, the fracture was produced without the intervention of any more or less heavy vulnerant body. It is not then a fracture by direct action, but by indirect action. But in fractures of this kind which we are unable, on account of the resistance of the tibia, to reproduce upon the cadaver, the solution of continuity is the result both of irregular muscular actions, some of which tend to give the bone an unusual curve, and the others to twist it, and the pressure of the weight of the body upon this bone, already a little bent and twisted. But it is impossible for us to analyze strictly the muscular phenomena which are produced at the moment of the fall; and as it is also impossible to study them by experiments upon the cadaver and upon living animals, I am unable to tell you how and why, in consequence of this complex intervention of muscular action and the weight of the body, there is obliquity of the fracture and propulsion forwards of the upper fragment of the tibia.

Content yourselves, then, with knowing and remembering this capital fact; the most frequent displacement in fractures of the leg is the one you see here, a transverse displacement in which the extremity of the upper fragment projects forwards.

Let us now consider the practical question: Can this displacement be reduced, and will it be possible for us to keep it reduced, so that the patient may get well without a deformity due to the persistence of a transverse displacement? This problem is in great part solved for this patient. For yesterday I reduced the displacement in the following manner: I raised the leg from the wire splint in which it had been placed the evening before. With one hand I held the upper fragment; with the other, grasping the two malleoli, I drew them downwards, exerting what, in classical language, is called extension. As I felt a little resistance I asked an assistant standing at the end of the bed to help me make extension, grasping the instep with one hand, with the fingers upon the dorsum and the thumb upon the sole of the foot, and the calcaneum with the other. I asked him to draw on the foot while I myself exerted traction with the left hand and made counter extension with the right. The projection having disappeared, we replaced the limb in the trough well lined with cotton; I satisfied myself that the coaptation continued; and, fearing lest in the manœuvre an angular displacement might have been substituted for the transverse one which we had just corrected, I looked to see if the foot was in a good position, drawing an imaginary line from the middle of the first metatarsal bone to the inner border of the patella. When the foot is in a proper position, this line is parallel to the axis of the leg.

As this condition existed, I concluded from it that the reduction had been well made. I asked the patient if he felt any painful pressure on the heel; he said he did not. For greater security I placed a supplementary pad of cotton behind the tendo Achillis above the posterior projection of the calcaneum, so as to diminish pressure on the latter—pressure which is the cause of the severe pain so much complained of by many patients with fracture of the leg. I completed the dressing with a bag filled with oat chaff placed upon the front of the leg, an anterior splint, and some straps with buckles. I examined the leg yesterday and this morning, and found, by passing my finger along the inner face and the anterior border of the tibia, that the fragments were kept in place. I have now no doubt that they will remain so until the end of the treatment. You will then have seen upon this patient one of the most frequent forms of fracture of the leg, that is, fracture with transverse displacement, reducible and easily kept reduced.

3d. What are we to think of the phlyctenæ and of the influence which they may have upon the course of the disease?

In themselves they indicate nothing bad. They are due to a singular modification of nutrition which follows traumatic perturbations. More frequent perhaps when the fracture is direct, they occur also, as you see in this patient, after the intervention of indirect causes. They accompany fractures of the leg much more frequently than those of other parts of the body. Why? It is absolutely impossible for me to tell you.

As to the influence which these phlyctenæ will have upon the course of the disease, I consider it very simple. I cut them open with the scissors, let out the serosity, and placed upon each of them a small piece of perforated linen; and, as the surface of the derm is neither very much bruised nor sloughy, I presume that they will dry promptly, without suppurating, and that in a few days they will be healed.

You will sometimes see phlyctenæ of the leg followed by suppuration of the derm for ten or fifteen days. You may also find under the raised epidermis an eschar, not comprising the whole thickness of the derm, but which nevertheless will have to be eliminated; hence a suppuration which may last long enough to necessitate a special dressing every morning and to oppose the application of the immovable apparatus. This suppuration of phlyctenæ, with or without eschar, is

6

seldom seen except in cases where there has been intervention of a direct cause and more or less violent contusion of the skin.

In short, the prognosis in this patient, as in the other, is favourable in this sense, that the cure will take place without persistent deformity. But it has this disadvantage, that, whatever we may do, the patient will be obliged to keep the bed for about sixty days, walk with crutches for from four to eight weeks, and then with a cane, slowly and limping, for a certain time. The most favoured adults, after a fracture of the leg, do not walk in a perfectly satisfactory manner before the end of four months.[1] Perhaps ours will not be such. Many conditions which we cannot foresee, but which nevertheless may easily intervene, may perhaps ultimately appear. Thus I advance the opinion that the callus will be solid and that mobility will have disappeared after 45 days. But who knows whether in them, as happens from time to time, and without our being able to know very well or foresee the reasons, 60, 75, and even 80 days, instead of 45, may not be necessary to obtain this result? Who knows also whether the tibio-tarsal and tarsal articulations will not remain painful and stiff for many months? I do not think so, because the patients are still young, and are neither gouty nor rheumatic, and because I have no reason to suppose the existence of a fissure extending into the articulation; but, whatever may be the favourable presumptions, you should know that in many cases fracture of the lower third of the leg is followed by an arthritis ending in a semi-anchylosis which long remains rebellious and painful during walking.

You have seen in what the *treatment* has thus far consisted. The leg is kept quiet in the wire trough by means of three canvas bands which are properly tightened and buckled in front over a splint, behind which is a chaff-bag. The foot is also fixed to the sole of the frame by a figure-of-eight bandage, the loops of which surround the apparatus, one opposite the lower part of the leg, the other opposite the foot.

Immobility is assured by means of the mechanical bed which we use for all fractures of the leg and thigh, and even for all painful diseases of the lower limb. The one which we use in the hospital is more simple but a little less convenient than those which we make use of in private practice, and it has the advantage of being easily arranged everywhere, even in the country. It is composed of a rectangular oak frame, the length and breadth of which are the same as those of the mattress. At about 18 inches from the upper end is fastened, by means of a hinge on each side, another smaller frame, intended to hold the pillow, and capable of being fixed at any angle. This smaller frame has but three sides, the one between the two hinges is lacking, and is covered with a stout piece of canvas. The corners of the large frame are furnished with stout hooks, and smaller ones are placed at intervals along the sides, by means of which sheets or strong sail-cloth bands, 6 to 8 inches wide, can be fastened upon the frame. Two

---

[1] In children consolidation takes place more rapidly. The muscles and articulations resume their functions sooner, so that they have scarcely any need of crutches, and at the end of two months walk quite easily.

cords, the four ends of which are attached to the corners of the frame, and a pulley, whose hook receives their loops, complete the apparatus. The upper pulley is attached to the ceiling, or to the frame of the bed in our hospitals.

Fig. 4.

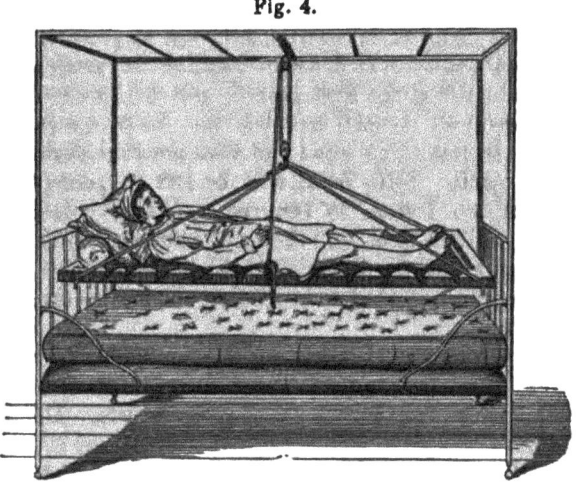

Hospital Bed.

The patient is placed in the middle of the frame, which has previously been arranged with five or six bands. By means of the small frame his head can be raised for the purpose of eating or drinking, without causing the least sudden movement. If the bands are not properly placed, new ones can be easily substituted by raising the frame a little or by passing them under the patient as he lies, and attaching them to the hooks. By raising the frame with the cord and pulley, the wants of nature can be attended to, proper cleanliness observed, and the bed and bedclothes changed, all without giving the slightest injurious movement to the limb.

As our patients are young and healthy enough to endure without pain the prolonged pressure of the sacrum upon the bed, I do not use the water-bed, which, however, I should make haste to employ if, after a little while, they should complain of pain and sores in that region. I should have recourse to it at once if the patients were weakened by age or by anterior diseases.

The beds occupied by these two patients are in a well-lighted part of the ward. That is a point which should always be seen to. Light is necessary to the maintenance of good health, and good health favours the formation of the callus.

I saw at the Hôtel-Dieu, in 1847 and 1849, two patients who had been lying for six weeks in the darkest part of ward Sainte Marthe, and in whom a fracture of the leg was not at all consolidated. I had these two men placed in better lighted beds in the centre of the ward, and consolidation took place at once.

It is unnecessary to say that the patients will be nourished as well as possible, and that the limb will be examined from time to time to make sure that no displacement has occurred, and, for the one which has the phlyctenæ, to renew the cerate dressing which is applied to them.

In fifteen or twenty days, when the inflammatory period is ended and there is no more swelling, and when the second phase of the affection has begun, during which we have fibro-cartilaginous transformation and the beginning of calcareous deposits in the soft, sanguinolent, and glutinous substance which forms outside the bone and inside the medullary canal during the first period, you will undoubtedly see me change the apparatus: I shall envelop the limb in a layer of cotton, and wrap about it first a dry band and then another soaked in dextrine or silicate of potash. This band will be left in place for twenty or thirty days. When I wish to remove it, I shall place the limb in warm water for half an hour, and then, the bandage being thus softened, take it off carefully, while the leg is held by two assistants, so that no shock may be communicated to it in case consolidation should not be sufficiently advanced.

The bandage removed, I shall see if any mobility remains; it is probable that I shall find none. The rule is that it does not last until the forty-fifth day in fracture of the leg in adults. Does that mean that the callus is complete and perfect at that period? By no means, it only means that it is solid enough to resist the lateral impulsion which one hand gives the lower fragment while the other one holds the upper one immovable. But a few anatomical studies which I have had occasion to make upon fractures at this period in man, and the analogy with that which we find in the bones of animals subjected to experiment, oblige me to admit that, notwithstanding the disappearance of abnormal mobility, the callus is still in part fibro-cartilaginous, and is not so exclusively bony as it will become. These same studies have also taught us that it is only the peripheral periosteal callus which has become solid and partly ossified; but that the interfragmentary callus, so well demonstrated by M. Lambron,[1] is still soft and without admixture of calcareous molecules and bone corpuscles.

Finally, clinical experience has taught us that if the patients now begin to walk, the callus may bend, yield, and an iterative fracture be produced. In a word, the callus will be so solid on the forty-fifth day in both patients that mobility will no longer be felt; but not sufficiently solid to allow us, without danger, to subject it to the trials of walking or even standing. Therefore we shall advise them to remain a fortnight longer in bed, and not to begin to walk with crutches until the sixtieth day. By that time the peripheral callus will have completed its ossification, and the interfragmentary one will have commenced and will be able to continue and complete its own notwithstanding the movements and exercise of the patients. As its ossification advances, the volume of the exterior callus will diminish.

But let us return a moment to the treatment which I have begun and which I propose to continue in both patients. I want you to understand that I might employ many others and obtain an equally

---

[1] Lambron, Etudes sur les Formations du Cal, Paris, 1842.

good result. You will find in your text-books the description of a certain number of apparatuses for fractures of the leg, and you may even, by consulting a masterly thesis written by Malgaigne,[1] make yourselves acquainted with all the inventions bearing upon this point which have been produced since the days of Hippocrates. They are very numerous; and indeed any one of them might do for our present patients. For when we find ourselves in presence of a fracture with a displacement which it is easy to reduce and keep reduced, all apparatuses are good if they are sufficiently restrictive and if the patient will keep as quiet as possible. You will then be able, in your practice, to employ, instead of this wire trough, one made of tin, gutta-percha, or wood. Above all, you will be able to use the system of short separate bands, called Scultet's apparatus. Its advantage is that it can be constructed everywhere out of materials which are almost always at hand, and which, if necessary, can be replaced by others quite as easily found. Before applying it, it is to be prepared in the following way : —

Arrange upon a table three or four cords parallel to one another, or, better, three or four bands of stout duck or elastic webbing furnished with buckles. Over these place a large napkin or towel; upon this towel you place small bands, three inches in width, whose length is double the circumference of the limb; each band overlaps three-quarters of the breadth of the preceding one. They are to be placed perpendicularly to the axis of the limb, beginning at what is to be the upper end of the apparatus and continuing until you have obtained a length equal to that of the injured limb. Upon these bands, and beginning at the same end, you place doubled compresses five inches wide, each of which covers half the breadth of the preceding one. A splint, as long as the limb, is then placed along each side, and the towel, bands, and compresses rolled over them until they meet in the centre. Thus arranged, the apparatus can be easily transported.

To apply it, the assistant, who makes the extension, raises the foot, drawing it towards himself, while the surgeon, seizing the leg with his left hand (if it is the right leg) above the fracture and with his right hand below, maintains the reduction. Another assistant places the bandage under the limb, and, unrolling the splints, spreads out the apparatus. The limb is then placed carefully in the centre, and, while the assistants keep up extension and counter-extension, the compresses and bands are freely wet with a mixture of two parts of water and one part of camphorated alcohol. The surgeon then takes the lowest compress by one end, while an assistant holds the other, rolls it smoothly over and engages its end under the limb on the opposite side; he then brings over the other end and tucks it under on his own side. He does the same for each compress, one after the other, and then applies the bands in the same way. He then rolls up the outer splint in the towel and places a chaff-bag, an inch thick, between it and the leg; an assistant does the same on the opposite side, and the apparatus is completed by means of an anterior bag upon which is a shorter splint.

[1] Malgaigne, Sur les Appareils contentifs des Fractures en général (concours de professorat, Paris, 1841), and Gaujet, Arsenal de la Chirurgie contemporaine, Paris, 1867, tome I.

The assistant then holds the three splints in place while the surgeon ties or buckles the straps. He takes care that the heel does not press upon the bed, so as to avoid those intolerable pains which are sometimes caused by continuous pressure of the calcaneum. If this pain occurs the surgeon places a small square cushion under the lower part of the leg so as to raise the heel from the bed. A hoop or cradle protects the leg from the weight of the bedclothes.

Sometimes the point of the foot has a tendency to incline to the right or left. I then fix it in a good position by means of a long compress wrapped about it and fastened on each side to the bed. The foot is in a good position when a line drawn from the patella to the great toe is parallel to the axis of the leg.

I advise you to familiarize yourselves with the construction and application of Scultel's apparatus; for in private practice you will often employ it. But, when you make use of it, do not forget one principal precaution, that of not making it too tight at first. It has been often discussed whether it is better, for fractures in general, to reduce them and apply at once the restrictive apparatus, or to wait until the inflammatory period is ended. That is a question which should not be examined generally ; its answer varies according to the regions.

As for fractures of the leg, it is incontestable that the patients feel better and suffer less when the limb is kept in a good position. I advise you then to apply the first day the restrictive apparatus which you may select. But do not forget that the limb will swell, on account of the distant infiltration of the blood which continues to be poured out by the fractured surfaces, and of the serosity exuded during the inflammatory process. Consequently it must not be tightly applied at first, for a slight constriction might be turned into a strangulation by this inevitable increase of volume. Of course, in a limb so well supplied with muscles and whose arteries are so well protected, gangrene is not to be feared, at least in an adult, but the constriction might cause new phlyctenæ, and, above all, it would have the disadvantage of causing the patient to suffer, of preventing sleep. Now, our duty is to avoid causing useless suffering, and, moreover, suffering affects the health.

I told you that to have a regular and prompt consolidation it was necessary that the general health should be troubled as little as possible. With troughs and straps we can easily avoid too much constriction, and if by chance it should be too great, any one can loosen the straps without disarranging the apparatus. With Scultel's apparatus this is not so ; when the constriction is painful, it is necessary to await the arrival of the surgeon, and consequently long suffering is needlessly inflicted upon the patient. You will avoid this by not tightening at first, and by renewing the application every day so as to proportion the compression to the increase or diminution of volume.

I have sometimes used Malgaigne's box, or Jules Roux's *planchette polydactyle.*[1] The latter is very convenient, especially if you take care

---

[1] A trough pierced with holes through which pegs are passed to press upon the fragments and keep them in position.—TRANS.

to pad it well with cotton or with a sheet, and if the holes through which the pins are to pass, are numerous enough to furnish, on each side of the foot and leg, sufficient support for the limb.

These apparatuses have the advantage of allowing the surgeon to easily uncover the fractured limb to see what is going on, treat the phlyctenæ, arrange the degree of constriction according to the change in size, and make, if necessary, a new reduction. Among these apparatuses, I may even establish a distinction between those which leave the anterior part of the limb uncovered, and those which allow the fractured point to be seen only after they have been entirely, or in part, removed.

The first, which I also call *open apparatuses*, are the troughs, when they are not closed by means of the anterior splint and strips, Roux's planchette polydactyle, the simple cushion-trough which I have sometimes used, and which consists of a large square cushion, filled with chaff, upon which the leg is placed, and then its sides are turned up and fastened with straps, taking care to leave an open space in front through which the leg can be seen and felt. I might add, as forming part of this category, Maisonneuve's plaster splints. They are made of two pieces of linen, folded in eight thicknesses, and long enough for one of them to pass along the back of the leg and sole of the foot to the ends of the toes, and for the other to encircle the sole of the foot like a stirrup, and pass up each side of the leg as far as the knee. These pieces of linen, dipped in plaster, and folded so as to be two and a half inches wide, are applied to the leg, and kept in place by a roller bandage until they become dry, when the bandage is removed, and three strips of diachylon substituted, one about the foot, the other two about the leg, leaving a part of the anterior face of the leg, and particularly that which corresponds to the fracture, uncovered. This apparatus is very restrictive, but after having used it for more than a year I have given it up, for two reasons: first, because upon patients with a fine and delicate skin, especially women, the diachylon causes an erythema and unpleasant itchings; and secondly, because I have twice seen an eschar produced on the heel, on the most prominent part of the calcaneum.

The second, the *enveloping apparatuses*, are all those which hide the fractured limb from the sight of the surgeon, and allow him to examine it only by removing them in whole or in part. The Scultet apparatus and the roller bandage are types of this variety. The first is much to be preferred, because the limb can be uncovered without raising it, and consequently without giving it any movements which might be painful or might disarrange the position of the fragments or the work of consolidation. The trough, with straps, bag, and anterior splint, belongs to the same category. If I have given it the preference, it is simply because, without spending too much time, I can unbuckle it, remove the splint and the bag, examine the limb, and put everything in place again. But I repeat that if you are willing to give it a little more time, the indication is met as well with the Scultet or any other apparatus, as with that which I now use upon our two patients.

I have already told you that in about three weeks I shall change the apparatus, and substitute an immovable roller bandage, made with a very concentrated solution of silicate of potash. Why this change? It is certainly not that the consolidation may take place more regularly or rapidly. You know what are the anatomo-physiological pheno-mena which accompany the formation of the callus; you are acquainted with the first period, that which is characterized by the effusion of blood and plastic lymph about and between the fragments, that which almost always, passing beyond the simple needs of repair, gives us, clinically, the inflammatory phase. You know the second period, that which begins between the eighth and thirteenth days, and during which the plastic matter, and perhaps the blood, are transformed into a cellulo-fibrous substance about the fragments and the periosteum. Finally, you know the third period which, beginning from the twelfth to the fifteenth day, and continuing until the end of consolidation, is characterized by the deposit of phosphate of lime and the formation of bone corpuscles in the fibro- cartilaginous substance. Well, these phenomena go on independently of our apparatuses ; we apply the latter that the former may follow one another while the limb is fixed in a good position, and that the callus may be as little of a deformity as possible. If we should put on no apparatus, the consolidation would, none the less, take place, provided that the limb was kept nearly immovable, but it would be irregular.

If then we have recourse afterwards to an immovable bandage, it is not to accelerate nor to regulate the callus; in this respect the trough, continued until the forty-fifth day, the Scultet's apparatus, if we had used it, would give exactly the same results. We have no other in-tention in thus modifying the treatment than to make the patient a little more comfortable. You have often heard me ask patients with broken legs a day or two after the application of an immovable appa-ratus if they felt more or less comfortable than with the one that had been first applied, and you have heard almost all of them reply that they felt easier because it was lighter, and because the limb, especially the foot, being better immobilized, they can turn and move a little in the bed without causing any pain. It is then because the immovable apparatus is more convenient and more agreeable to the patients that we use it. As for any preference for the silicate of potash, it is not absolute, and nothing would prevent us from using dextrine, simple plaster, or plaster mixed with gelatine, or starch upon linen or paper. It is quite indifferent. The important thing is to know how to well utilize these different substances.

A few years ago I used a good deal, and even now sometimes use plaster or dextrine, which I applied in the following way : —

With the plaster we first make a clear paste by mixing it with water, and then roll a dry band about the limb, previously covered with a thick layer of cotton, while the leg is held by three assistants, two of whom make extension and counter-extension, and the third supports it at the point of fracture. I then roll a band of coarse tarlatan about the limb, beginning at the foot, soaking it in and covering it, as I ad-vance, with the clear plaster paste placed in a basin under the leg. I apply the plaster thus in three superposed layers of tarlatan so as to have a sufficient thickness.

I much prefer this method to that of first applying the plaster to an ordinary band and then rolling it about the limb.

Dextrine is applied as follows: it is not easy to dissolve this substance rapidly in water, and it would require too much time to make a homogeneous glue. In order to obtain it immediately we first mix the dextrine with alcohol, which does not dissolve it, but which gives it the appearance of a fine moist sand, then we slowly add hot water. As the water has a great affinity for the alcohol, it penetrates into all the interstices and dissolves the dextrine at once. The alcohol has the additional advantage of making the solution dry more rapidly.

When the solution is brought to the consistency of a thick syrup, a bandage is unrolled and rolled up again in it so as to be thoroughly impregnated with it. The bands thus prepared may be kept for some time.

The limb is covered with a layer of cotton kept in place by a dry band over which the dextrinated one is applied. When this application is ended, a little of the solution is spread over the outside to fasten the edges down. Bottles of hot water are placed about the leg to hasten the drying, and yet, notwithstanding that, it does not become perfectly solid in less than forty-eight hours.

That is the disadvantage of dextrine: plaster dries too quickly, dextrine too slowly. We possess now an intermediate substance, of which I have spoken—the silicate of potash. The prepared solution is kept for sale. It is obtained by heating to red heat a mixture of one part of powdered quartz with four parts of carbonate of potash. The substance thus obtained is dissolved in water, and. evaporated to the consistency of a thick syrup.

It is applied exactly like dextrine, and has the advantage of drying much more rapidly, but the impure article which we sometimes receive dries quite as slowly. At present I use the silicate because it is good, but you would see me return to the dextrine in case I found that the silicate furnished by the administration did not dry rapidly enough.

You might also use plaster with the addition of gelatine, in the proportion of two parts in a thousand of water, as recommended by Prof. Richet. The mixture, which is quite convenient, has, like the silicate of potash, the advantage of drying less rapidly than ordinary plaster, and more rapidly than dextrine.

When you wrap the band soaked in a solidifying mixture about the limb, it is necessary : 1st. To have the limb supported above and below the fracture by two aids, who will make extension and counterextension; 2d. To make sure that displacement is not produced, an accident which is not probable, since we have reached a period in which the consolidation is sufficiently advanced to prevent the fragments from separating with so much ease ; 3d. To see that the foot is so placed that a line drawn from the centre of the inner border of the first metatarsal bone to the inner border of the patella, is parallel to the axis of the leg ; 4th. To surround the limb with a layer of cotton, so as to protect it from too much pressure upon certain points; 5th. To tighten it only moderately; the effects of too great constriction would undoubtedly not be so bad as during the first period of the fracture, but yet this excess of constriction might cause pain and oblige the surgeon to remove the apparatus the next day or the day after. Of course it ought to be examined after it has become dry, to see if it threatens to cause excoriation or gangrene of the skin at any point, and to prevent this complication, either by putting some more cotton between that part of the skin and the apparatus, or by cutting away the offending part. These precautions are especially necessary in persons, such as women and children, whose skin is thin and easily irritated or broken.

LECTURE XII.

FRACTURES OF THE LEG—Continued.

Fractures of the leg in the lower third, continued—" V" fractures with displacement which is reducible, but difficult to maintain reduced, and fractures with irreducible displacement (3d and 4th clinical varieties)—Fractures with incomplete perforation of the skin (5th clinical variety).

Gentlemen.: I. At No. 26, Ward Sainte-Vierge, is a man 35 years old, of habitual good health, who was brought to us ten days ago with fracture of the lower third of the right leg, caused by a fall down a staircase, but which still seems to have been indirect.

I shall not occupy your time with the question of diagnosis. As in the other cases of which I have had occasion to speak, the diagnosis was easy; inability to walk, pain, swelling during the first few days, mobility, crepitation, left us no doubt of the existence of a fracture of the two bones.

I showed you, from the first, that there was an angular displacement, for the leg described a curve the concavity of which was directed upwards, and a rotatory displacement, for the foot rested on its outer portion, and had turned outwards with the lower fragment. I told you that we had easily corrected these two displacements. But in addition we had the most common variety of transverse displacement, that in which the upper fragment projects in front. You were able to feel the first day, when as yet there was no swelling, that this projection of the upper fragment, instead of terminating in a sharp point corresponding to the crest of the tibia, as is the case in oblique fractures, had its point placed upon the antero-internal face, and at the extremity of two lines of equal length, so that the edge of the upper fragment had the form of a projecting V.

I reduced this displacement, as I did the other two, the first day by the classical manœuvre of reduction, then placed the limb in a wire trough, and completed the dressing with the bag, the anterior splint, and the straps with which you are already acquainted. But when I examined the leg the following morning, I found, that, although the angular and rotatory displacements were not reproduced, the transverse one had reappeared, and that the point of the projecting V exerted quite a strong pressure upon the under surface of the skin. I reduced it again, and then, replacing the limb in the trough without completing the apparatus, I observed what took place. We saw the upper fragment resume almost immediately its vicious position and project under the skin. Again reducing it, I tried to maintain the reduction by means of a layer of cotton and two longitudinal graduated compresses, which I placed along the whole length of the upper fragment from two finger-breadths above the point of the V, so as not to make compression over the point itself. My intention was to distribute a moderate compression all along the upper fragment. Above the graduated compress I placed the bag and anterior splint, which I bound down with three straps about the upper fragment, and one about the lower one. The foot was also fastened to the sole of the trough with a band.

The next morning, by slipping my finger underneath, I felt that the point did not again project, and thence inferred that the displacement had not been reproduced.

But the following morning it was not the same. The projection had again become very notable. I again reduced it, and renewed the compression all along the upper fragment by means of a triple graduated compress and a layer of cotton.

The apparatus has now been five days in place, and the displacement has not reappeared; I therefore hope that it will remain reduced. Of course, if it should reappear after a few days, I should again reduce it, and try to make a more efficacious compression along the upper fragment.

Two peculiarities here require attention: 1st, the V-shape of the upper fragment; 2d, the difficulty of maintaining the reduction.

1st. The V shape of the upper fragment has not in itself a very great importance. But it has the advantage of indicating some anatomo-pathological details of a certain clinical value, which without it we could not suspect.

I have made several autopsies of fractures of this kind while they were quite recent, and found that when the upper fragment showed this projecting V in front, its posterior surface was very irregularly divided, and showed also two lines of fracture forming a re-entrant V with its point directed upwards, that at the same time the inferior fragment presented in front a hollow V corresponding to the projecting one of the upper fragment, and on the posterior surface a point fitting into the re-entrant V of this latter. Hence an irregularity in the main line of fracture, which cannot be included in the anatomo-pathological divisions, heretofore admitted, of transverse and oblique fractures, and which was better described by Gerdy under the name of *toothed or pointed fractures*. It is a curious and inexplicable thing, this irregular and complex direction of the line of fracture in a bone so voluminous as the tibia, and under the influence of the indirect causes which I have had occasion to explain (page 80). But this is not all: when the fragments present this alternation of large V-shaped

Fig. 5.   Fig. 6.   Fig. 7.

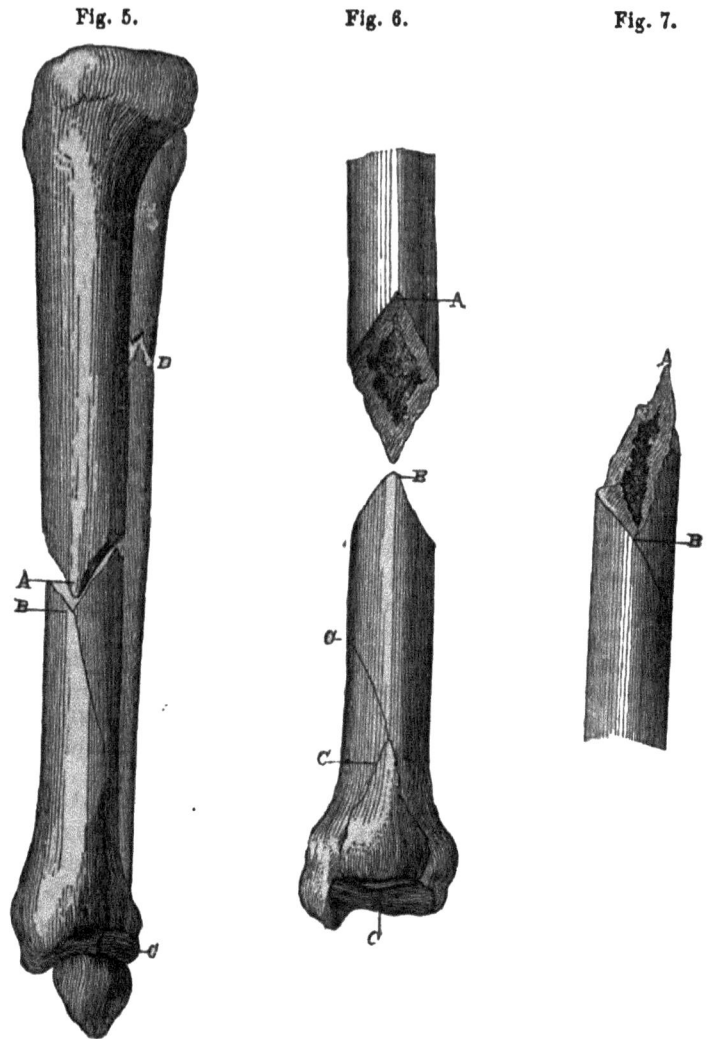

Fig. 5. V-shaped fracture of the right leg, with spiral fissure of the tibia, inner face. A, projecting V of the upper fragment, inner face ; B, re-entrant V of the lower fragment and beginning of the fissure ; C, articular portion of the fissure ; D, concomitant fracture of the fibula.

Fig. 6. V-shaped fracture of the right leg, tibia, posterior face. A, re-entrant V of the upper fragment, seen from behind ; B, projecting V of the lower fragment, seen from behind ; C C C, fissure, extending to the articulation.

Fig. 7. V-shaped fracture of the right leg, inferior fragment, with its anterior re-entrant and its posterior projecting V ; B, origin of the fissure at the angle of the re-entrant V.

points and indentations, we find also the marrow considerably bruised, and in the lower fragment a fissure which, starting from the point of the re-entrant V, winds in a spiral about the inner face of the tibia, then the posterior face to the tibio-tarsal articulation, traverses this articulation near its posterior border, and rises again along the posterior face, thus circumscribing upon it a lamellary fragment.

The first time I saw this long fissural prolongation, causing the seat of the fracture to communicate with the ankle-joint (it was in 1854, at the Hôpital Cochin), I supposed it to be a very uncommon lesion, and although I had occasion to see successively two examples (Figs. 5, 6, 7, 8, 9), which were described in a note[1] and in the thesis of Dr. Bourcy,[2] I could not believe that a fact so curious could, if often met with, have escaped the investigation of surgeons so completely that no author, up to that time, should have spoken of it.

Fig. 8.   Fig. 9.

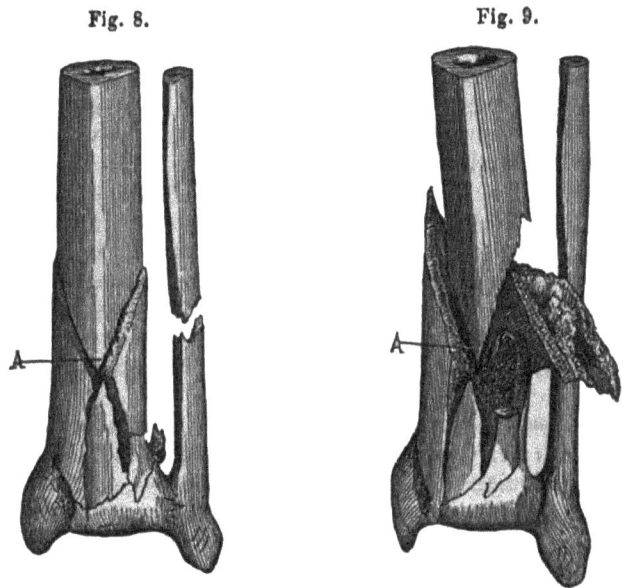

Fig. 8. V-shaped fracture of the leg, with splitting of the inferior fragment of the tibia-pieces in place ; A, the V of the upper fragment.
Fig. 9. Same fracture, with the upper fragment replaced in the medullary canal.

But soon new observations collected by my colleagues, especially by MM. Chassaignac, Houel, and H. Larrey, and myself, showed us that indirect fractures of the lower third of the leg very often presented this irregular main line in form of a V, and the long accessory line in form of a fissure, extending to the articulation of the foot, and that consequently it was necessary to admit three principal anatomical varieties of fracture of the leg in the lower third, corresponding to as many clinical varieties : *toothed fracture* (*transverse* of the old authors), *oblique fracture*, and *V fracture*.

I see among our contemporaries a certain tendency to suppress this latter denomination, and to replace it by that of spiroid fracture given by Gerdy to some which, though analogous, differed in many respects,

[1] Gosselin, Leçon clinique faite à l'Hôpital Cochin sur les Fractures en V du Tibia, Gaz. des Hôpitaux, 1855, p. 218.
[2] Bourcy, Thèses de Paris, 23 June, 1855.

and which he had described for the thigh. For my part, I reject the name spiroid, because it indicates only the secondary lesion, the fissure which cannot be discovered in the living patient by physical signs, while the denomination *V)fracture* is based upon the direction of the principal line of the fracture, and indicates a distinction which can be recognized, at least in part, through the skin. We should, however, remember that this name indicates not only a particular form of the principal line of fracture, but also a spiroid fissural prolongation extending to the articulation. It is unfortunate that a single word cannot express these two facts.

Before going any further, let us see what relation exists between the V shape and the fissure on the one side, and the V shape and bruising of the marrow, which I have already mentioned, on the other. I believe that I gave, in my earlier publications upon this subject,[1] the only possible explanation, in saying that, in consequence of the absolutely inexplicable direction of the principal line of fracture, the upper fragment exerted, at the very moment of the accident, a pressure like that of a wedge upon the lower fragment, causing it to burst into pieces, and that this same pressure crushed the marrow. I thus extended to fractures of the lower third of the leg, the study of the results of the reciprocal pressure of the fragments immediately after the production of the main line of the fracture, a study which, in other fractures, and notably in those of the lower extremity of the radius and those of the neck of the femur, has given us penetrating fractures.

Let us now return to our patient: he has a V fracture, that is to say, a fracture with crushing of the marrow and fissural prolongation towards the articulation. Now these latter lesions, and even the form of the lower fragment, are not indicated by physical signs, but only by the projection of the upper fragment which we feel through the skin when the swelling has not yet become very great or when it has sufficiently diminished, and by our anatomo-pathological studies which have taught us (the pieces in the Musée Dupuytren prove it) that, in those cases where the upper fragment presented this form, the other lesions mentioned were not lacking. What conclusions should we draw from these notions with reference to the ultimate course and prognosis of the fracture? The patient will have a tibio-tarsal arthritis, and this arthritis will leave behind it for a longer or shorter time a semi-anchylosis or stiffness. Unquestionably this is not a coincidence which belongs exclusively to V fractures, for we often see the articulation inflame by simple proximity, but that which is possible in other cases is almost inevitable in those where the fracture extends to the articulation. As to the subsequent stiffness and difficulty in walking which it occasions, I should fear its long duration if the patient was a little older or subject to rheumatism or gout, for, as I have often told you, the duration of this painful stiffness and loss

[1] Gosselin, Mémoires de la Société de Chirurgie, tome v. 1855 ; and Bulletin de la Société de Chirurgie, tome vi. p. 262, 1855 ; tome ix. p. 148.

of function following spontaneous arthritis and long immobility depends upon the age. The older the patient, the longer the duration.

We draw from the above-mentioned notions this other conclusion, that the patient is a little more exposed than others to suppurating osteo-myelitis.

Upon this point I was led into an error by a singular chance at the beginning of my labours upon this subject. My first two patients affected with V fracture had, the one a compound fracture, the other a simple one, and both died of purulent infection following suppurative osteo-myelitis. I did not infer that all those who should have V fractures without communicating wounds would have suppurative osteo-myelitis, but I concluded that they were exposed to it in a certain measure.

Since then I, as well as others, have often seen simple fractures of this kind which were not complicated either by suppuration of the marrow or by purulent infection.

I say to you then, our patient, because he has a V fracture, and with it a crushing of the marrow, is more predisposed than others to an osteo-myelitis. But as there is no external wound, the suppuration of which might extend to the fracture, it is more than probable that he will escape this dangerous complication and will get well.

2d. I now come to this displacement, which is reducible and difficult to keep reduced. To what is it due? To this, that at the moment of the accident and of the wedge-like action by vertical pressure and rotation of the upper fragment upon the lower one, extensive ruptures were caused about the first. Not only was the periosteum divided, but the muscles were extensively torn at the moment of the great muscular effort during which the bone was broken and acted like a wedge upon the lower fragment. Freed from all its connections, this upper fragment is easily drawn upwards by the action of the quadriceps femoris, and it is only by means of a considerable and constant pressure that we can keep it in place.

But what disadvantage would there be if we paid no attention to this displacement and did not correct it? First, its point might perforate the skin immediately or after the formation of a small eschar by its pressure, which would change the simple fracture into a compound one, and would expose the patient to the tedium and dangers of a consolidation after suppuration. Secondly, supposing that this unfortunate complication should be avoided, the patient would get well more slowly because the callus would be made by only a part of the contour of the fragments, that by which they touched one another, and all the materials poured out by the rest of the contour or between the fragments would not be utilized. Finally, the callus would be irregular in two ways, because an abnormal projection would persist indefinitely, and because the persistence of the transverse displacement would cause longitudinal displacement and a permanent shortening of the leg.

I know that in such cases it is more important to attend to the function than to the shape, and that notwithstanding the irregularities of which I speak, the limb would recover its usefulness in walking and standing. Nevertheless, patients, especially women, are always dissatisfied with being deformed, and if we do not wish to be accused of negligence or incapacity, we should make every effort to obtain a cure of fracture of the leg with a callus as little irregular as possible.

What means are at our disposal to correct this tendency to displacement? It is evident that ordinary restriction by the apparatuses with which you are acquainted is insufficient, and that it is necessary to add something to them.

I told you what I did for our patient: compression all along the upper fragment except at the point where it might cause an eschar. Take care not to yield to the idea which at first presents itself of compressing the extremity itself of this displaced fragment by means of a cushion and a small splint. If you should do that you would run great risk of causing mortification. For the skin would be compressed at this point between the fragment which tends constantly to be drawn outwards, and the accessory apparatus which would press it backwards. It would be better, as I said, to distribute the compression above the point of the V, than to concentrate it at that point. It is, furthermore, necessary to tighten it a little more than usual, and relax it if the patient suffers. You remember that the limb has been attentively watched, and that I have renewed the reduction whenever the displacement has been reproduced. I do not advise you to have recourse in cases of this kind to the Scultet apparatus, because in order to make compression efficaciously along the whole length of the upper fragment it is well that the limb should rest upon a hard plane, and because it is indispensable to examine the fracture once or twice every day, and to repeat the reduction if necessary. Now it is not easy to make up your mind to open so often a complicated Scultet dressing; it is much easier with the trough, or Malgaigne's box, or Roux's polydactylic box. You understand, also, how necessary it is in such cases not to withdraw the limb from observation by enveloping it in an immovable bandage. The fracture should be constantly examined until at least the 25th day, that is to say, until the time when consolidation is so far advanced that, even if it should seem necessary, reduction could no longer be made.

Compression, such as you see me apply, is not the only means which we possess. We might use in this case Malgaigne's point, which consists of a metal rod attached to a steel hoop through which it can be raised and lowered by means of a screw.

I have twice used Malgaigne's point for fractures similar to this one. In one of them the final result was very good, but was obtained at the price of quite severe pain. In the second, the patient complained of violent pains which obliged him constantly to loosen the screw, and finally he had an erysipelas, of which he got well, but which caused the treatment to be suspended. In short, I find that compression is preferable because it is less painful and can produce the desired result without any lesion of the skin, and I should use Malgaigne's method only in case this compression did not prevent displacement.

I advise you also to accustom yourselves to do without these special apparatuses. The fractures for which they can be used are not frequent, and when they are met with, these apparatuses are not always at hand or are in bad condition, as are always those instru-

Fig. 10.

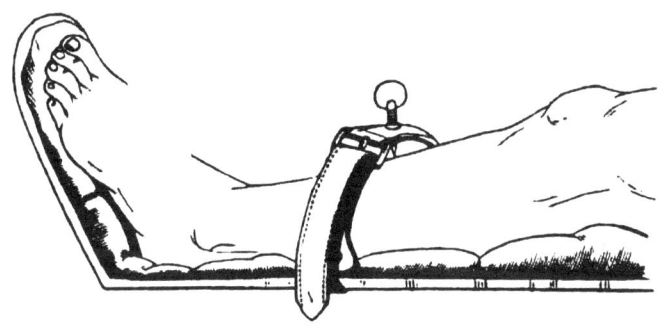

ments of which we do not make daily use. Keep them, if you choose, for hospital practice and the large cities, but in ordinary practice use the means which are always at hand, such as cotton wadding, oakum if you have no cotton, or pieces of linen folded into long and narrow compresses.

II. *Fracture with irreducible transverse displacement.*—At No. 45, there is another variety of fracture in the lower third of the left leg, which we have had under observation for a fortnight. It is in a rather young and vigorous man who fell while running, and in whom we have no reason to believe in the intervention of a direct cause.

Since the first day we have recognized the projection of the upper fragment and its V shape; but it was in vain that I tried to make it disappear by executing the manœuvres of extension, counter-extension, and coaptation; I did not succeed; I applied poultices for three days, gave opium, and left the limb untouched, hoping that perhaps reduction was prevented by spasmodic muscular contraction, and that this contraction would disappear with time. The fourth, fifth, and sixth days I failed as on the first. I succeeded in diminishing the projection by means of the compression mentioned in the preceding case, without causing an eschar; but I did not get complete reduction, and I am obliged to recognize that I am in the presence of one of those irreducible displacements which our predecessors did not describe. For in all the books which preceded Malgaigne's, reduction of fractures is spoken of as a very simple thing, which is always easy and never meets with obstacles. Now the case before us, the examples of which, fortunately, are not very frequent, shows you that it is not always so.

Can we at least explain this irreducibility? I might be permitted to attribute it to muscular action which, the transverse displacement once produced, had caused the over riding, and had been too strong to yield to the attempts at reduction. But it is very rarely and with

7

much difficulty that the upper fragment entirely abandons the lower one. On account of the breadth of the bone and the irregularity of the fracture, the fragments always touch at some points, and muscular action does not produce so much overlapping that our efforts at extension cannot overcome it. Moreover, experience has shown us that in fractures of the leg longitudinal displacement, which is always the result of muscular contraction, can most often be easily corrected.

In these exceptional cases where reduction cannot be obtained, I think it ought to be attributed to some obstacle offered either by a strip of muscle or by a splinter or piece of bone, which has slipped into the place of the upper fragment.

We can never demonstrate materially either in our present patient or in those of the same kind which we meet from time to time, the interposition of a foreign body between the fragments; but as autopsies of recent fractures have demonstrated it sometimes, we have a right to believe in its existence in irreducible cases. I have in my collection a specimen which came from a woman in the Hôpital de la Pitié, who had a compound fracture, the upper fragment of which I was unable to bring into place. This was due to a large muscular bundle of the tibialis posticus which had caught upon the end of the lower fragment and occupied the place of the upper one.

I have often met also with splinters of bone placed crosswise in the inter-fragmentary space, and I have found them especially in V fractures. For the result of the splitting and rotating action of the upper fragment upon the lower is sometimes that one of the sides of the lower or hollow V breaks, and the fragment, drawn by the muscular fibres attached to it, or in consequence of an impulsion communicated to it by the lower fragment, or of some outside pressure, leans towards the inter-fragmentary space and is caught in it so as to oppose reduction. What happens with one of the sides of the hollow V may also happen with some detached point or with several, and thus, instead of one, we have several obstacles to reduction.

I repeat that I do not know what is the obstacle in this case; but I presume, from what I have seen in the cadaver, and from the full V shape of the upper fragment, that reduction is prevented by a cause of this kind, and that it would be impossible to reduce it completely.

We shall then expect to see this patient get well slowly and with a deformed callus, which will, however, in no way affect the functions of the limb. I shall forewarn the patient of this result.

Let us also meet the indication of pushing back this fragment as far as possible towards its proper place, so as to avoid an eschar over the point, and render the deformity as slight as possible.

For that purpose we apply graduated compresses all along the upper fragment. This would be a suitable case for Malgaigne's point[1] if we preferred it. But although this eminent surgeon claimed that his apparatus was almost infallible, you may be sure, that in a case of this kind, it would not have succeeded in removing the deformity entirely.

In any case, remember this fact, that although our classical authors

---

[1] Malgaigne, Traité des fractures et luxations, Paris, 1847–1854.

have represented fractures of the leg as always susceptible of reduction, it must be admitted that some are irreducible, and that the consecutive deformities are due to the circumstances of the fracture and not to the carelessness of the surgeons. I treated this subject fully in 1859.[1]

III. *Fracture of the lower third of the leg with transverse displacement and projection forwards of the lower fragment.*— I do not wish, gentlemen, to describe fully all the varieties of fracture of the leg; but let me tell you, in passing, that if displacement of the upper fragment is the one which is the most often observed, you will also see in some rarer cases transverse displacement of the lower fragment forwards.

We have an example in the woman who occupies No. 10. At the time of her admission there was a notable projection of the lower fragment which I was able to reduce and keep reduced.

But you will also meet with patients in whom reduction and retention are difficult. That may be explained in the same way as the irreducibility of the upper fragment, by a peculiar interlocking, or by the interposition of a splinter or piece of muscle. But we must also attribute it in part to the action of the gastrocnemius and soleus, which, drawing the calcaneum and lower fragment upwards, keep the broken end of the latter in front of the upper fragment.

I do not know what causes this kind of displacement; in any case, it does not coincide with a V fracture, and is found in certain toothed and oblique ones. The prognosis and treatment present no peculiarity.

IV. *Fracture with very prominent angular displacement forwards.*— Notice also the patient in No. 26, in whom, on the day of his admission, we found a fracture in the lower third of the two bones of the left leg with a very prominent angular projection in front (angular displacement). Lateral angular projection is not very rare, it is easily corrected, and rarely reproduced. But the same is not true of angular displacement with prominence in front; it is easily corrected, but has a great tendency to reappear, and the surgeon should struggle against this tendency so long as the callus is not sufficiently strong to oppose its reproduction.

I make the reduction in this case very easily every morning, and compress with a cushion and anterior splint as well as possible. The next morning I find a little of the projection which I had effaced so well the day before, and I am obliged to make a new reduction.

This is another of those cases in which it is necessary to examine the limb every day, and to correct the deformity as often as possible. Be careful in such circumstances not to apply the immovable apparatus too soon, for if the callus has not already acquired a certain solidity when you inclose the limb, the angular projection will be reproduced little by little under the apparatus without your perceiving it, and when you remove the bandage you will find the leg solid but very irregular, with an angular callus which will shorten it very much, and compel the patient to walk upon his toes and to wear a shoe with a very high heel.

[1] Gosselin. Sur l'Irréductibilité et les Déformations consécutives dans les Fractures des Os longs. (Gazette hebdomadaire, t. vi. p. 130.)

I shall undoubtedly not apply the silicated apparatus before the thirtieth day, and even if I then find marked mobility I shall not apply it at all, and shall continue to use the ordinary apparatus, examining it often, until the end of the treatment.

I have not thus far spoken of section of the tendo Achillis as part of the treatment of fractures of the leg with displacement difficult to correct, because this operation, proposed long ago by Laugier, seems to me useless in the transverse displacements to which I have called your attention. For of two things, one: either these displacements can be reduced and maintained by the aid of the measures which I have mentioned, in which case tenotomy would only add to the consecutive muscular weakness of the limb; or the displacement cannot be corrected, which is due, as I have told you, rather to certain peculiarities of the fracture than to contraction of the gastrocnemius; tenotomy, therefore, would be useless.

But in angular displacements forward which are so easily reproduced, it is allowable to think that the contraction of this muscle has a great influence, and that consequently division of the tendo Achillis by temporarily suppressing the cause would also suppress the effect. But I can support by no personal experience the advantages of this operation, for I have had no occasion to perform it, and the examples published by Laugier, who, according to Malgaigne, introduced this modification of the treatment, and by M. Meynier d'Ornans, are not numerous enough to bring conviction.

In a word, the procedure is not generalized in practice; is it because it has not been considered good, or because the particular class of cases to which it is appropriate, the one which now occupies us, has not been clearly indicated? I do not know; but it is for this reason, and also because I expect to succeed without it, that I have not had recourse to it. On one occasion, however, I keenly regretted not having employed it, for, notwithstanding all my care, my patient got well with an infirmity and a shortening which tenotomy would undoubtedly have avoided.

V: *Fracture with engagement of the point of the fragment in the thickness of the skin.*—Finally, gentlemen, I wish you to notice, in passing, the patient in No. 7, who presents a singular fracture of the tibia.

The point of the upper fragment is implanted in front in the under portion of the skin, that is to say, has *spitted* it without traversing its entire thickness. This case establishes the transition between fractures without wound and fractures with wound. You saw that I tried at once to withdraw the bony point from the skin, and in this case I succeeded quite easily with my hands alone and by the ordinary manœuvres of reduction.

It is not always so, and once I had to draw the skin downwards with a double hook implanted on the sides of the point.

In another case all my efforts to disengage the point were unsuccessful. I then treated the fracture without occupying myself any further with this incident, and had the satisfaction of seeing that little by little the depression of the skin diminished; at the end of the treatment it was no longer adherent, the point had been reduced spon-

taneously.   Remember this peculiarity if ever you have to treat a case
of this kind.   Try to disengage the point, and if you do not succeed,
treat your patient as for an ordinary fracture.

LECTURE XIII.

COMPOUND FRACTURES OF THE LOWER THIRD OF THE LEG.

I. Small wound.   Diagnosis completed by the flow of blood and drops of oil.   Possible termination without suppuration.   After mild suppurating osteitis, and
necrosis.   After putrid and infecting osteo-myelitis.   Importance of occlusion.
Methods of practising it.   Imbricated strips of diachylon plaster.   Bands dipped
in collodion.   II. Large wound.   Suppuration more difficult to avoid.

GENTLEMEN : We visited this morning, at No. 41, a man about 40
years old, who broke his left leg by a fall upon the ice.   When he was
picked up his stocking was found to be wet with blood; and after we
had undressed him, and cut off this stocking, we found at the anterior
portion of the leg, near the junction of the lower and middle thirds,
a wound nearly half an inch long, through which a bony point projected slightly.   Blood, mixed with drops of oil, flowed from the
wound.   There is also an abnormal mobility which leaves no doubt
as to the existence of a fracture of both bones.   But this fracture is
complicated by a small wound with issue of the upper fragment.

This patient reminds you of two others whom we have seen during
the year, and in whom you did not have the opportunity of seeing
the projection of the upper fragment.   In one of them the reduction
had been made by the interne on duty the evening before our first
visit.   In the other the dressing was also made in the evening.   The
interne had not found the bone projecting, but as he saw a considerable quantity of blood escaping, and as by passing a probe carefully
into the wound, he felt the denuded extremity of the fragment, he
was convinced, and I shared the conviction, that the wound communicated with the fracture.   But had this wound been made, like the
two preceding ones, from within outwards by the fragment itself, or,
on the contrary, from without inwards by some external vulnerant
body?   There we had to deal only with probabilities, and it is so in
most cases of this kind; certainty almost never exists.   The probability that the bone was the vulnerant body is based upon the narrowness of the wound, and the absence of a severe contusion, such as
would have been produced by a blow.   Still, this question is not of
capital importance.   The wound was not quite half an inch long, its
edges were not bruised, and its condition was favourable for immediate
union, which is the essential point.   Let us here recall the case of
another patient.

Toward the end of last year I called your attention to a patient, who, with a fracture, probably toothed, at the junction of the middle and lower thirds of the leg, had on the anterior and outer portion of the limb a wound through which no one had seen a fragment project, and through which a probe, passed with all the precautions indicated in such a case, had not reached the fragments or the intervals between them. Was the wound in communication with the fracture, or was it independent? We had two reasons to think that it communicated: the first was that from the information furnished us, and from the quantity of blood that had soaked into the dressing during the fifteen hours that had elapsed between the patient's admission to the hospital and our visit, we saw that the wound, although small, had bled a great deal, but without the interrupted spirt and the bright colour which characterize arterial hemorrhage. Wounds occupying the soft parts do not bleed so freely and for so long a time, unless an artery is wounded, and that, I repeat, is not the case here. On the other hand, when the wounds communicate with a fracture the fragments always furnish a large quantity of blood which comes from the capillaries of the periosteum, from the bone itself, from the marrow, and from the nutrient arteries. It is this abundance of blood which causes the effusions and infiltrations of the first days, the extensive ecchymoses which you see increase during the first two or three weeks, and which disappear so slowly.

The second reason for believing in the communication was the presence of drops of oil in the blood which flowed the first day. I admit that this is not a pathognomonic sign; I know, and I should warn you that the fat of the subcutaneous cellular tissue can supply drops of oil to the blood of a recent wound interesting only the soft parts; but these drops appear only in small quantity and for a short time, especially when the wound is small. On the other hand, the marrow of the bone, the fat of which is more liquid, furnishes more and for a longer time when it has been torn. That is why the appearance of oily drops in the blood of small wounds coinciding with a fracture, ten, twelve, or fifteen hours after the accident, is a strong presumption in favor of the opinion that the fracture is compound, that the wound communicates with it. When the flow of blood is moderate, and the oily drops are not found, we have to remain in doubt, and incline towards the opinion which involves the treatment most favourable to the patient. Admit, in such a case, communication, rather than not. There is no disadvantage, if the wound is independent, in treating it as if it communicated, and there are very great ones in treating it as independent if by chance it communicates.

But to return to our patient: I reduced the fracture very easily, and was able to replace the point of the upper fragment which is on the anterior border, and does not indicate a V fracture. Here, then, is a patient with a nearly transverse wound one-quarter of an inch long, about which the skin is probably loosened for a certain distance, and which communicates with the seat of the fracture, a sort of accidental cavity limited by the fragments, and filled with liquid and coagulated blood. What would happen if we should leave the wound in the state in which it now is, and occupy ourselves only with the ordinary treatment of the fracture? One of the four following things:—

Either the wound, being narrow and but slightly bruised, would heal promptly and without suppuration. In three or four days the fracture would be no longer *exposed*, and would advance to a cure like any other simple fracture.

Or the wound would not heal by first intention; it would suppurate, but the suppuration would be limited to its edges and would not extend inwards to the seat of the fracture, the deeper layers of the soft parts having united immediately and opposed a barrier to the extension of the suppuration towards the deep parts. In this case the fracture would also heal like a simple one.

Or the suppurative inflammation starting from the wound, immediate union of which had not taken place, would extend further and further towards the seat of the fracture, that is to say, to the bones, and especially the tibia, whose greater size renders its suppuration more important and more dangerous; the suppurative inflammation would invade, in all probability, all the constituent parts of the bone; periosteum, compact substance, and medullary substance. In a word, osteitis would supervene, or rather—uncomplicated, mild, suppurating osteo-myelitis of acute or subacute form; we should have as local symptoms of this disease:—

1st. During the first few days a diffuse and painful swelling of the limb, and the development of a more or less intense fever which we have called, since Dupuytren,[1] *traumatic fever.*

2d. A little later, and for a long time, an abundant suppuration following subcutaneous or intermuscular diffuse phlegmons, a necrosis keeping up fistulæ until elimination of the mortified parts has taken place, and finally cure with one of those more or less considerable hyperostoses, of which I shall have occasion to show you examples.

Or finally, the suppurative inflammation extending to the bones would there take on the form which I call putrid or infecting osteomyelitis, which differs from the preceding one by two capital characteristics:—

1st. By the formation of eschars and the putrid decomposition of the blood upon the soft parts of the wound, and especially by the gangrene and the decomposition of the medullary substance and the extravasated blood in the medullary canal, and in all the canaliculi which have been opened by the solution of continuity.

2d. By the coincidence, with this putrid decomposition, of an intense fever during the first few days, with a pulse of 120 or 130, and an axillary temperature of 104°, headache, thirst, sometimes delirium, and, later, purulent infection.

Do not forget, gentlemen, that by the very fact that a patient is exposed to suppuration of the bone, he is exposed to this putrid and

---

[1] Dupuytren, Leçons orales, tome vi.

malignant variety of acute osteitis and the consequences I mentioned, especially to death by purulent infection, which happens more often than death by traumatic fever, the latter being really primitive putrid infection, while the other is consecutive or secondary putrid infection, and the hecticity, which sometimes occurs still later, may be considered as a tertiary putrid or septic infection.

But perhaps you would ask me the following question: If this man is threatened with an acute suppuration of the bones, have you any reasons for hoping that this suppuration will take on the mild rather than the malignant form, or for believing rather in the development of the latter, and of one of the varieties of dangerous septicæmia which you attribute to it? I can reply only with presumptions.

If the patient was in the country, if he was not in a hospital, if I was sure that he was not given to drink, I would reply: Yes, his wound, in itself, exposes him to acute suppurating osteo-myelitis, but there are, in the circumstances mentioned, reasons for hoping that this suppuration will not take place, or that, if it does, it will remain simple and mild, or, if you prefer, non-putrid and non-infecting. But, on the one hand, the atmospherical conditions in which he now finds himself, and on the other, his previous life in a great city, his exhaustion by fatiguing labour, his alcoholic habits, his present position in a ward charged with nosocomial emanations, are so many unfavourable circumstances which predispose him to suppuration of the bone and to the putrid and gangrenous form of this suppuration. It is true, that this predisposition exists only in a certain measure, and I cannot tell you just what that measure is. For above all these causes one other is needed which is purely individual, and which is inherent to the constitution and to its aptitudes. Multiple as are the causes of which I have spoken, it may be, nevertheless, that the constitution does not favour suppuration of the bone and especially putrid suppuration. On the other hand, moderate as may be all the occasional causes, the constitution may be one of those which engender pus and putridity easily, notwithstanding all that is done to prevent, and it is because we are in the most absolute ignorance upon these individual aptitudes which annihilate or fortify the action of all the other causes, that I cannot say what will happen. I tell you what is possible, but I cannot tell you in what degree it is possible.

The only thing which I wish to fix in your minds is that a wound, even a small one, which complicates a fracture of the leg, exposes it to suppuration and all its possible consequences; dangerous traumatic fever, suppurative, acute osteo-myelitis, purulent infection, hecticity, or necrosis, and slow cure with a deformed and painful callus.

But there is one circumstance which diminishes the gravity of the prognosis in the case of our patient. All that I have just said is under the inexact supposition that we should not try to do anything for the wound. But, on the contrary, we shall treat it with great care, and I hope that our efforts will meet with success, and that we shall prevent suppuration of the bones and its consequences. I have the more reason to expect this result because the wound is small, its edges are not bruised, and there are no eschars to be eliminated. Under such conditions I have every reason to hope for immediate union and a cure without suppuration.

The means by which to obtain it are very simple, and yet it is only within the last twenty years that they have been well understood, formulated, and applied.

The surgeons of the seventeenth and eighteenth centuries advised, it is true, that the wound should be closed by means of agglutinatives, but they devoted themselves above all to the reduction of the fracture, as Boyer's article on compound fractures[1] will show you. They thought little about the wound, they indicated neither the mode of application nor the length of time during which the agglutinatives should be kept on, and, furthermore, they possessed only insufficient ones which softened in contact with the blood and became loose the first or second day after their application, and did not keep the edges together long enough to prevent suppuration. Consequently the surgeons of the beginning of the nineteenth century did not comprehend the precept sufficiently to apply it vigorously. Led away by the ideas which ruled at that time about inflammation, they tried to moderate it by various topical applications, hoping thereby to prevent it from becoming suppurative. Poultices, leeches upon the injured limb, systemic bleeding, diet, in a word all that constituted antiphlogistic treatment, was recommended, and the dressing of the wound was made of secondary importance, consisting in the application of a piece of diachylon or court-plaster, which met only temporarily and incompletely the main indication, that of keeping the edges of the solution of continuity together, and protecting them as long as possible from contact with the air.

It was still with the hope of moderating the inflammation that A. Bérard, Breschet, and many others after them, had recourse to continuous irrigations of cold water, and Baudens to refrigeration by means of ice. Undoubtedly they sometimes succeeded with these means when the wound was a small one; but they often failed, while, on the contrary, with the dressings which we have at our disposal to-day, success, that is to say, non-suppuration, is the rule, and failure the exception.

To M. Chassaignac[2] belongs the merit of distinctly formulating this surgical point under the name of *occludent dressing*. This dressing consisted, when its author recommended it, of small strips of diachylon overlapping and crossing one another over the wound, the edges of which had previously been brought as well together as possible. He placed several layers, one over the other, so as to form a sort of cuirass, and left it all in place for ten or twelve days.

But the occludent dressing has been singularly improved by the use of collodion. With this substance we make an apparatus which dries rapidly and remains firmly attached to the skin without becoming soft or wet by contact with organic liquids. The pieces may

---

[1] Boyer, tome iii., 1st edition, p. 68.
[2] Chassaignac. Des Opérations applicables aux Fractures compliquées de Plaie. Thèse de Concours pour la Chaire d'Opérations et Appareils, Paris, 1850, and Traité de la Suppuration et du Drainage, tome i. p. 514.

easily be left in place for the necessary time, six, eight, and even ten days.

By its exact application and adhesion collodion gives a first and very important result. It protects the wound and the rest of the fracture from contact with the air, the presence of which leads so easily to decomposition of the blood and exuded products, an alteration which inevitably causes suppuration. It satisfies two other capital conditions, that of keeping the edges as exactly together as possible, and that of immobilizing them by preventing any slipping or folding of the skin.

For we have to obtain permanent reunion as well as occlusion, in order to reach the great result which we seek.

We have to choose between two methods of applying the collodion.

The first consists in cutting a certain number of strips of linen, half an inch wide and from two to three inches long, and in dipping each one successively in a mixture of collodion and castor oil, the so-called elastic collodion, which is less irritating than the ordinary collodion. The leg being well placed in the trough or fracture-box where it is to remain, an assistant brings with two fingers the edges of the wound together, and while he holds them in contact the surgeon applies the first collodionized strip. He places a second over the first in the form of an X, then a third parallel to and covering about two-thirds of the first, a fourth parallel to the second, and so on, so as to cover the wound itself and about an inch of the surrounding parts with a sort of collodionized cuirass. When the dressing is completed the strips are very tightly applied, close the wound, and confine the skin all around it.

The second method consists in covering a piece of goldbeater's skin about an inch and a half in diameter with collodion, sticking it upon the wound, and placing a second over the first.

I have used both methods and prefer the first. The separate bands are better than the goldbeater's skin, for the latter sometimes leaves a gap which might favour the displacement of the edges of the wound, and it compels the use of a larger quantity of collodion, which sometimes causes phlyctenæ.

I applied upon our patient the collodionized and imbricated strips of linen, after having satisfied myself again that reunion had been well made, and I completed the dressing with the anterior splint, cushion, and straps. I placed him upon the mechanical bed, and I advised him, even more strongly than usual, to avoid every kind of movement. During the following days I shall examine the leg, press upon the cuirass to see if this pressure causes a pain which might indicate inflammation, or if it causes the issue of a few drops of sanguinolent or purulent serosity. If, as is very probable, I find neither pain nor oozing, I shall leave the dressing in place for ten days; at the end of that time I shall remove it, and I can tell you beforehand that the little wound will be cicatrized, and that the fracture, transformed into a simple one, will heal after the usual lapse of time. During the last four years I have used this dressing a dozen times in cases where, as in this one, the wound was not very much contused and was not half an inch long, and in no case did suppuration of the bone ensue.

Consider it then as certain that this mode of treatment is superior to any other, and relieves you from having to make use of antiphlogistics, continuous irrigation, and ice, the success of which is much less probable.

While speaking of these recent small wounds which heal under the occludent dressing, I wish to remind you of a patient whom you saw a few months ago in our wards. He was a man 30 years old, who, in consequence of a fall from some high place, had a fracture with irreducible displacement. We made every effort to reduce the fracture, but without success, and the upper fragment pressed strongly from within against the skin. In spite of all our efforts to prevent it, the skin, although not compressed by any part of the apparatus, was at last perforated. Fortunately, this took place twenty days after the accident; consolidation had already begun, and this late wound had no unfortunate consequence. The seat of the fracture, undoubtedly protected by the callus, did not suppurate, but the skin and the superficial part of the denuded bone did suppurate, and left a cicatrice slightly adherent to the bone.

II. *Compound fracture with a large wound.*—We have in No. 5 a man 40 years old, who offers an example of compound fracture. This lesion also is below the middle of the leg, and nearly at the place of election. It was caused by a fall from a height of two or three yards, in consequence of the breaking of the ladder on which the patient was standing. I do not think a direct cause intervened in the production of the fracture. The upper fragment of the tibia, which has not the form of a V, projected at the time of the accident through a slightly oblique wound which was an inch and a half long, the reduction was easily made; the fracture does not seem to be comminutive, but there is a wound of considerable size which evidently communicates with the seat of this fracture.

The prognosis is much graver, and the treatment will be more difficult than in the preceding case.

I shall try occlusion again; but although the edges are not much contused, I do not hope for immediate union of the whole wound, and suppuration of the bone seems inevitable. I shall leave the collodion dressing in place until I am warned by spontaneous pains and those excited by pressure that pus is collecting under it and should be let out. As soon as the presence of pus becomes incontestable I shall continue to keep the limb as immovable as possible in the trough, which will be lined with oiled silk so as to avoid a contamination which would compel us to raise the limb too often in order to maintain the indispensable cleanliness; the dressings will be renewed morning and evening. How will these dressing be made? We have to choose between several methods. Those which are most used today are alcohol and carbolic acid (1 per mille solution). To use it we begin by carefully removing with sponges all the pus which has collected upon the sides of and behind the limb; sponges are not used for the wound itself, we content ourselves with carefully wiping it

with lint soaked in one of these liquids, and we exert pressure about
it so as to favour the escape of the pus which might collect in some
neighbouring pouch. If we find any of these pouches, which are not
too far from the skin, we open them, and, if possible, pass drainage
tubes. In these ossifluent suppurations which threaten pyæmia it is
important that the pus should not remain, for then it stagnates, decomposes, and may furnish for absorption the putrid materials which engender purulent infection.

When the wound has been cleaned, balls of charpie soaked in common alcohol unmixed with water, or in the carbolic acid solution, are
introduced into it, and into its cavities if they are accessible. Over
them are placed one or more compresses soaked in the same liquid, the
whole is covered with oiled silk, and then the apparatus destined to
keep the limb immovable is completed.

Are there any reasons for giving the preference to one or the other
of these agents? I prefer alcohol during the first fifteen or twenty
days, because its effect is to diminish suppuration, and the less abundant the suppuration the less does the patient weaken, and the fewer
the materials susceptible of putrid decomposition. It is also possible,
but it has not yet been demonstrated, that alcohol, by coagulating
certain albuminuous principles of the pus, modifies them in such
a way that their putrid alteration is rendered more difficult. Perhaps
also the alcohol, by its astringent action, obliterates some of the lymphatics and bloodvessels which might furnish passage to the putrid
poisons. All these opinions have been uttered with a certain enthu-
siasm by the partisans of alcoholic dressings; but only one of them
has been proved by clinical observation, that one is the diminution of
suppuration. For this reason alone alcohol should be used during the
first days. You will rarely see me continue its use after the twenty-
fifth or thirtieth day, for if it diminishes suppuration, it also retards
cicatrization. By long contact with it the granulations become small,
the wound grows pale, and becomes painful sometimes, and does not
dry over, if not in all cases, at least in a certain number.

I shall then begin with the alcoholic dressing; then if, at the time
when purulent infection is less to be feared, I find that cicatrization
advances too slowly, I shall substitute carbolic acid, which, without
increasing the suppuration, generally maintains on the surface of the
wound that rosy colour which indicates the regular work of repair.
Of course, during the dressings, I shall examine from time to time
with a probe to see if there is not some loose splinter to be removed.
All the abscesses which form will be opened freely, and a general
treatment with tonics prescribed. After the twelfth or fifteenth day I
shall give the patient a drachm of phosphate of lime morning and
night in his soup; he will also have five drachms of brandy daily, and
all the nourishing food which he can and will accept, and which we
have at our disposal in the hospital; finally, we shall try to obtain the
best possible aëration of the ward. In this respect we are not as well
provided for as I could wish. This patient is one of those for whom
an isolated, well-ventilated, well-warmed room is necessary, or for
whom, during the hot season, permanent or intermittent quarters in a

tent or cabin like those which have just been built at St. Louis, Cochin, and Lariboisière, would be of the greatest use. Remember this, that of all the means preservative against purulent infection, immersion of the patient in a very pure atmosphere is by far the most important.

I have not raised, gentlemen, an important question which is discussed by all our authors in the chapter of compound fractures, that of amputation. Why have I not mentioned amputation to this patient? Because, in my opinion, he may get well and preserve the leg, and indeed his chances of dying are a little less than if I should now make an amputation, which would belong to the category of *primitive amputations*, that is, those which are made before the appearance of traumatic fever.

Notice first that the dangers from which I should wish to protect him are exactly those to which he would be exposed after an amputation at the place of election. His wound exposes him to a traumatic fever, which may be severe and even fatal, that is true, but amputation exposes him to the same. His wound exposes him especially to purulent infection, but that also is what we fear the most after an amputation. His wound exposes him in a certain degree to traumatic erysipelas and to a consecutive hemorrhage. But would amputation preserve him from them? Would it not rather expose him even more to secondary hemorrhage? His wound may perhaps leave him with an infirmity and a limp, but would not the necessity of wearing an artificial leg also be an infirmity?

Amputation would be justified only if I was certain that he was more likely to die by the injury than by the mutilation, through one of these complications. Now, upon this point I am in the most complete ignorance. I see in the regularity, which is still considerable, of the wound, in the presence of a fracture but slightly comminuted, in the very moderate disorder of the soft parts, conditions which make me hope for a cure; I recognize that my hopes do not go very far, I will even admit that the chances of death are greater than those of recovery.

I should like to show you by figures the proportion which exists between these two chances, but I have not recorded all the facts which have passed under my observation with sufficient exactitude to offer you the figures. I know that in my hospital practice I have seen more patients with compound fracture of the leg with large wound die than recover. In my private practice, on the contrary, of six patients of this kind four got well and two died, one of them of tetanus, and I am convinced that when the conditions of aëration in the hospital become the same as in private practice, we shall have the same results. Furthermore, I do not think I am mistaken in assuring you that, even with these good hygienic conditions, the mortality after primitive traumatic amputation is a little greater than after attempts to preserve the limb.

Notice that this mutilation adds one cause of purulent infection to those which exist in consequence of the wound itself, I refer to the serious moral perturbation. The man who, in full health and unexpectedly, is obliged to suffer the loss of a limb, without having been

led to it progressively by long sufferings and a wretched existence in
a hospital bed, as is the case with those whom we amputate for suppurating white swellings, without having been led to consider this
mutilation a relief, is very much affected thereby. Now you may be
sure that this great moral shock is a powerful cause of the accidents
which follow amputation. Our patient, seeing that we have a strong
hope and desire to preserve his limb which he knows is dangerously
injured, is in this respect in better conditions, and for that reason I
think he is less likely to die than if I should amputate.

I recognize none the less that in the present state of surgery this
problem will not receive a rigorous solution until we learn from the
statistics of a great number of observations in what proportion
patients affected with such wounds as we have before us recover, and
in what proportion they die, so as to compare these proportions with
those given by primitive traumatic amputations. These statistics are
very difficult to establish, because no single surgeon has enough personal facts to be demonstrative, and because in statistics comprising
facts furnished by different surgeons, we can never be sure that the
observations are identical, that, for example, they do not include fractures with much and with little shattering and those with small
as well as large wounds. Moreover, success depends very much
upon the care which is given to the patient and upon hygienic conditions. Now if they place in the same statistics patients who have
not been properly dressed, or who have breathed a vitiated air, and
those who have been subjected to the opposite conditions, the general
result is not what it ought to be. In the lack of these rigorous
proofs I act according to the reasons which I gave, and I advise you,
whenever you meet with a compound fracture with a moderately large
wound like the one I now speak of, but without much crushing of the
soft parts and the bones, to do conservative surgery. I advise this
particularly if you practise in the country, in small towns, in small
hospitals, that is to say, in an atmosphere which is not vitiated by
crowding.

I do not mean to proscribe absolutely primitive amputation in all
cases of compound fracture of the leg.

If, contrary to my expectation, I saw gangrene appear in a few days,
especially gangrene with emphysema, I should not hesitate to propose
amputation. I do not think it will happen in this case, for the fracture
is by indirect cause, and in such cases gangrene is much less common
than when the fracture is by direct cause.

So, too, when the injury is accompanied by a considerable crushing
of the marrow, by extension of the fracture to the tibio-tarsal articulation, and imminence of suppuration in this joint, it is hardly to be
doubted that the patient will be carried off by intense traumatic fever
or by purulent infection, and that the chances of recovery are a little
greater after amputation. This then should be proposed to the patient. Gunshot wounds caused by large projectiles and with considerable shattering, direct fractures by a heavy body, such as the wheel
of a wagon, and certain V fractures, sometimes cause lesions which
authorize us to expect no good from conservative surgery.

Some of you saw me last year perform amputation the day after the accident upon a patient the lower part of whose leg had been caught under the wheel of a heavily laden cart and presented a comminuted fracture with laceration of the muscles and tendons and opening of the tibio-tarsal articulation.

I made another one at the same time in the environs of Montargis for a similar fracture with enormous shattering caused by the point-blank discharge of a fowling piece.

Both patients succumbed.

Let us suppose now that our patient in No. 5 has had only a moderate traumatic fever, that suppuration has set in regularly, and that from twenty to thirty days have passed without purulent infection, does that mean that he would be safe and that consecutive amputation might not become necessary?

You know, gentlemen, that suppurating osteitis takes in these cases the form of necrosis. Now, if this necrosis should invade a great part of the bone, if, in consequence, exfoliation should be very slow, if suppuration, having become very abundant, should undermine the patient's strength, if it was accompanied by continuous fever, with exacerbation at night, loss of appetite and of flesh, sweats, diarrhœa, if finally the patient seemed in danger of dying of hecticity, amputation would be indicated. It would be indicated all the more because, if, by chance and against all expectation, the organism should resist this drain, the patient would recover with fistulæ, a more or less painful hyperostosis, fresh necroses, more or less frequent attacks of inflammation, rebellious ulcers, in short, the whole series of permanent and re-curring complications which we see about large necrosed bones. He would not be able to walk, and would lead a miserable existence, from which amputation would certainly save him.

Notice, too, that we should no longer have to fear, as at the beginning, the moral effects of which I have spoken. The patient would see that the limb would not get well, the surgeon would show him little by little the impossibility of preserving a useless limb, and would lead him to accept imputation as a benefit. But it is probable that it would be necessary to amputate the thigh instead of the leg; for the supurative osteitis would undoubtedly have invaded the whole of the tibia, and it would be better to apply the saw to the healthy femur than to the diseased tibia.

No one would think to-day of discussing the question of amputation conformably to the prize subject proposed by the Académie de Chirurgie in 1755, under the title: "*Amputation being absolutely necessary in wounds complicated with crushing (fracas) of the bones, determine the cases in which the operation should be performed immediately, and those in which it is proper to defer it.*" Faure, who obtained the prize,[1] did not answer the question as it was asked, and applied himself only to proving, in a general way, that secondary amputations were more successful than primitive ones.

Modern statistics have not confirmed Faure's opinion; but it is not

___

[1] Faure, Prix de l'Académie de Chirurgie, tome iii. in 4to. p. 489.

the less true that, in practice, the problem cannot and ought not to be stated as the Académie de Chirurgie stated it.

I rejected primitive amputation because it was not indicated, and because I could hope that it would not become necessary; I rejected it, and did not postpone it. If later I propose amputation, it will be because complications which I knew to be possible, but the appearance of which could not certainly be foretold, have arisen and have caused an indication which might possibly have remained absent.

In a word, in these great traumatic lesions we propose amputation when it becomes necessary; but we are never free to say in advance that we shall perform it at any one period of the disease rather than at another.

(The patient who was made the subject of this lesson suppurated for more than six months, lost three large fragments, and recovered finally with a solid callus, consecutive to the bony transformation of the granulations, and with a hyperostosed tibia. He left us, walking with crutches, he came to see us twice during the following three months, still unable to do without crutches; since then we have not seen him.)

LECTURE XIV.

FRACTURES OF THE LEG.

I. Compound fracture of the lower third of the leg with small wound and emphysema. Distinction between primitive or aërial emphysema, and consecutive or gangrenous emphysema. II. Fracture with large vertical wound and commencing gangrene. Imminence of dangerous septicæmia—Amputation.

GENTLEMEN: I. *Fracture with small wound and emphysema.*—We saw this morning a man who was admitted yesterday with a compound fracture, the wound being a small one, below the middle of the leg very near the place of election, of which I have so often spoken. It is one of those cases in which we have a right to expect recovery without suppuration, by means of occlusion with collodion. I call your attention to-day to a peculiarity which is not often seen. Placing your fingers over the fracture and pressing lightly you feel the fine crepitation which characterizes emphysema. Light percussion by snapping with one finger, gives sonority. We have then here an infiltration of gas about the wound. This complication, or rather this coincidence, was pointed out for the first time by Velpeau in 1839,[1] was well studied by one of his students, Dr. Boureau, in 1852,[2] by Morel-Lavallée,[3] and lastly by M. Demarquay.[4]

----

[1] Velpeau, Traité de Médecine opératoire, 2d édition, tome ii. p. 321.
[2] Boureau, Thèse de Paris, 1856.
[3] Morel-Lavallée, Gazette Médicale, 1863, p. 520.
[4] Demarquay, Traité de Pneumatologie médicale, p. 289.

Whence comes this gas, and what is its signification in the prognosis?

Opinions varied upon the first question because it is difficult to give a rigorous demonstration of the way in which this emphysema is produced. I admit, with M. Demarquay, that it might arise in two ways, either by the infiltration of the external air into the subcutaneous cellular tissue, or by the spontaneous production of gas consecutive to a perversion of nutrition causing either a decomposition of the tissues, or an exhalation similar to that which takes place in the stomach and intestines of nervous people. I think that here we have to deal with the first variety, infiltration of external air, and that this air was introduced through the wound by muscular contractions which during and since the accident have caused a sort of aspiration about the little wound, according to the mechanism so well described by Morel-Levallée. It is then a primitive and not a consecutive emphysema, as it would be if it resulted from the spontaneous formation of gas in the tissues.

I base this opinion upon two reasons: 1st. The emphysema appeared early, for twenty-four hours have not yet passed since the accident. Emphysema by decomposition and exhalation rarely appears before forty-eight hours. 2d. Its appearance was accompanied by no serious general symptom; neither chill, nor quickening of the pulse, nor augmentation of the temperature, nor delirium, etc. Emphysema by decomposition, preceding traumatic gangrene, is accompanied by grave general symptoms which announce a speedy death.

For the second question, that of the clinical signification, I hesitate no more than for the first. This emphysema indicates nothing serious. Velpeau and Boureau, in saying that it indicated approaching death from which the patient could be saved only by prompt amputation, committed an error which it is easy to understand. Writing at a time when no one had yet spoken of this phenomenon, they remained under the impression of the facts which they had witnessed, in which the injury ended promptly in death. They were led into error by one of these circumstances: either the death was caused by the wound itself, without the emphysema having added anything to the gravity of the situation; or instead of a primitive emphysema by the entrance of the outer air, they had perhaps to deal with a consecutive or gangrenous emphysema, which they were not able to distinguish from the first.

To-day we are perfectly informed upon this point by the observations of the clinicists, and by the experiments of M. Demarquay upon animals. Infiltration of air giving rise to this primitive emphysema without fever is in itself not dangerous, adds in no way to the gravity of the wound, and by no means indicates amputation.

Watch this patient carefully, and I can assure you that if, as I hope, the small wound cicatrizes without suppurating, the infiltrated air will be slowly absorbed, the emphysema will disappear in four or five days, and the fracture will behave like a simple one.

(These predictions were verified, and the patient left the hospital three months after his admission.)

8

II. *Fracture of the leg with long vertical wound and commencing gangrene; amputation.*—We have had, gentlemen, for two days in No. 45, a teamster 45 years old, quite vigorous, but addicted for the last ten years to the use of alcohol, over whose right leg one of the wheels of his heavily-laden wagon passed. We found yesterday morning, the first day of the accident:—

1st. A fracture of both bones, of the toothed variety, a little above the junction of the middle and lower thirds, with very few splinters.

2d. A wound upon the anterior part of the limb five inches long, and parallel to the axis of the limb; or, if you prefer, to the adjoining crest of the tibia.

3d. A quite extensive loosening of the skin on the outer and inner sides of the wound.

4th. A denudation of the two fragments of the tibia, that is, a disappearance of the periosteum from the outer and inner faces of these fragments for a distance of at least an inch from the fracture.

This compound fracture is one of the most dangerous that you can meet. It does not owe this gravity to the multiplicity of the fragments, and to the crushing of the bone and the medullary substance. If this crushing existed with the other conditions of which we are witnesses, we should be in presence of the variety which is unquestionably the most dangerous of all fractures of the leg. That which gives the prognosis in this case an unfortunate character is first the alcoholic habit, a habit which, without our being able to explain it, renders the subjects much less likely to recover from great traumatic lesions; and second, the action of the body which produced the injury. This evidently is a fracture by direct cause; now in all these fractures the effects of the contusion of the soft parts are necessarily added to those of the solution of continuity of the bone, and as the wagon was very heavy, we may fear that the contusion has been severe enough to ultimately produce gangrene, if not of the whole limb, at least of a notable part of the skin. Now, at the time of the first examination it was precisely gangrene of the loosened skin which I declared possible and even probable. Upon what did I base this fear? First, upon the commemoratives which indicated the passage over the leg of a very heavy body.

Notice well, gentlemen, that the wound is a vertical one. Now how can the wheel of a wagon, passing transversely or obliquely across the leg, produce a vertical wound? It does so by forcibly pressing the skin against the crest of the tibia which becomes, in consequence of this pressure, the real vulnerant body, and cuts, from within outwards, the skin forcibly stretched over it. Certainly, it is not because the crest of the tibia has been the vulnerant body for the skin that the wound is dangerous; but this mechanism of the wound necessarily supposes very violent pressure, and consequently the most serious results of the contusion.

Notice, also, that the skin is loosened for a certain distance about the wound. You know what this loosening is, for I have often spoken about it; it is the result of great oblique pressure, that is to say, it is produced by very heavy vulnerant bodies which, instead of concentrating their action upon a point parallel to the axis of the leg, pass transversely or obliquely across this axis. The wheel of a wagon, a rolling cask, act in this way. Now, in passing obliquely, the vulnerant body slides the skin over the subjacent layers and causes more or less extensive rupture of the subcutaneous connective tissue. It is precisely this rupture which explains the loosening seen in our patient. You understand that by this loosening a large number of the blood-vessels which go from the subcutaneous layers to the skin are torn, and consequently this membrane loses a part of its means of nutrition. You know, also, that the pressure crushes and destroys part of the capillaries and nerve-filaments, another cause of the death of the skin. Consequently a patient over whose leg the wheel of a wagon has passed, causing a vertical wound, a loosening, and a violent contusion of the skin, is much exposed to gangrene of the latter. He may also, if the pressure has extended far enough to cause rupture of the deep vessels and nerves, have gangrene of the whole limb. You saw me yesterday seek the pulsations of the dorsalis pedis and posterior tibial arteries. Having found them easily, I concluded that the tibial arteries had remained intact, and that doubtless the patient was not exposed to general gangrene of the limb, gangrene which I should have considered imminent if I had not found these pulsations upon the wounded side and had found them on the other. But I still feared mortification of the skin, and for that reason I spoke to the unfortunate man of amputation of his leg. He refused and asked for twenty-four hours for reflection.

This morning you saw that the skin about the vertical wound was cold and insensible to the prick of a pin, and that it presented a yellow-brown or livid colour, which it did not have yesterday. We also found on each side and behind an emphysematous crepitation which I attribute to commencing putrid decomposition of the connective tissue. The patient has as yet no traumatic fever. But this fever will undoubtedly soon appear, and that is why I urged the patient to submit to amputation

Why did I urge this? First, amputation is indicated because, as the patient is destined to lose a part of the skin of the leg, the repair of the integument, supposing death not to occur, would be very slow, and all the more difficult because the bones would be very much enlarged by condensing osteitis; and if the cicatrix finally formed, it would be very thin and probably adherent to the bone, so that it would constantly tear and be covered with relapsing and rebellious ulcers which would constitute a deplorable infirmity.

Further, amputation is indicated now, and it is urgent. For to the other dangers which threaten the patient, we must add those of which the gangrene may be the occasion. For sometimes, although only the skin and subcutaneous cellular tissue have been destroyed, we see, after the third or fourth day, grave general symptoms arise, burning fever, delirium, jaundice, and prostration, followed by a rapid death.

I admit that these accidents may be attributed to traumatic fever, which is thought to-day to be a variety of septicæmia. But they would be much more intense than usual, and it is allowable to think that this greater intensity would be due to the worse character of the septicæmia, for the putrid gases which form under the skin, and there produce the consecutive emphysema, might be reabsorbed and become the cause of a more serious poisoning than that of the ordinary traumatic fever.   However that may be, in such a case, when gangrene has commenced with emphysema, death is imminent unless the putrefying part is removed in time.   That is why I urged the patient more strongly than I did yesterday to submit to amputation.

Fortunately the gangrene and emphysema have not extended to the upper part of the leg, and we can amputate at what is called the place of election, and still be beyond the limits of the trouble.

(Amputation was performed.   The patient did not succumb to the traumatic fever, but he was carried off by purulent infection fifteen days after the operation.)

LECTURE XV.

BI-MALLEOLAR AND SUPRA-MALLEOLAR FRACTURES OF THE LEG.

I. Bi-malleolar fracture—Obscurity of the mechanism—Two cases, one without displacement, the other with the displacement described by Dupuytren—Different indications for the two patients—Simple retention for the first—Retention with adduction of the foot for the second. II. Supra-malleolar fracture—Displacement difficult to correct—Possible eschar in cases of this kind—Explanation by more crushing behind than in front—Principal indication is to avoid an eschar.

GENTLEMEN: I. *Bi-malleolar fracture.*—We have at this moment in the wards two patients affected with simultaneous fracture of the lower extremity of the fibula and the internal malleolus.

I give this variety of fracture the name of *bi-malleolar*, although I recognize that sometimes in the fibula the solution of continuity occurs a little above the part which, strictly speaking, constitutes the external malleolus.

In both cases the fracture was caused by a misstep in which the foot was subjected to a certain degree of torsion.   I wish I could tell you if the foot, at the moment of the accident, turned about its vertical axis from within outwards, so that the outer facet of the astragalus pushed the external malleolus backwards and outwards, while strong traction was exerted upon the internal malleolus by means of the lateral ligament, and that we might, following M. Maisonneuve,[1]

[1] Maisonneuve, Fractures du Péroné (Archives Gén. de Médecine, 3d série, tome vii. p. 165).

explain the fracture of the fibula by divulsion, and that of the internal malleolus by traction. Nor can I tell you if at the time of the accident the foot turned about its antero-posterior rather than its vertical axis, nor if it took, to use Malgaigne's expressions,[1] the position of adduction, or that of abduction. For the patient could give me no precise information as to the way in which his foot turned.

Reading the works of the two authors just mentioned, and Dupuytren's[2] much earlier one on this subject, one would believe from the manner in which they speak of the mechanism of fractures of this kind, that they were able constantly and very easily to confirm by their patients the theories which they developed upon it. But it is not so. The patients can almost never say how the foot turned, and can give the surgeon no information upon this point which can clear up his diagnosis and prognosis.

I admit willingly that we can study upon the cadaver certain points of the mechanism of fractures of the fibula, and especially that which relates to the effects of torsion of the foot. But we can never know if, in an accident, everything has taken place as in our experiments, for two reasons: first, because the patients, as I told you, do not know what has taken place; and, second, because in the living body we have, added to the torsion of the foot, energetic muscular contractions, and the weight of the body upon the lower part of the leg and the foot while they are in a vicious direction. These difficulties render the results of experiments upon the cadaver inapplicable to the clinic, and cast, it must be frankly admitted, great obscurity upon the mechanism of fractures. But on this point, as on many others, I like better to tell you that we do not know, than to give you false and incomplete explanations.

In one of our two patients the double fracture is accompanied by no deviation of the foot, and no other deformity than that which results from the swelling. The diagnosis, nevertheless, is incontestable. Not only have we found that sharp pain on pressure above the external malleolus and at the base of the internal one, which is one of the probable signs, but we were able to feel crepitation by the three principal manœuvres recommended for that purpose :—

1st. For the external malleolus, pressing with one finger upon the point of this malleolus while the other hand holds the lower part of the leg firmly; for the internal malleolus, seizing it between two fingers, and moving it backwards and forwards.

2d. Raising the leg, holding it firmly with one hand, seizing the foot with the other, the palm of which embraces the sole, while the thumb and middle finger are placed by the ankles, and moving it alternately outwards and inwards, sometimes without rotation, that is, carrying it bodily sideways, sometimes with rotation about its antero-posterior axis.

3d. Fixing the leg upon the bed, without raising it, with one hand, the fingers of which are placed over the ankle, and moving the point

[1] Malgaigne, Traité des Fractures et des Luxations, tome i. p. 808.
[2] Dupuytren, Leçons Orales de Clinique Chirurgicale, tome i.

of the foot outwards with the other, thus giving it a movement of rotation about the vertical axis of the astragalus.

In the other patient, on the contrary, you saw most notable deformity. When the two limbs are compared without raising them we see that the right foot (the injured side) is distinctly carried out wards, that its external border is slightly raised, and its internal border lowered, in consequence of the rotation about the antero-posterior axis which coincided with the abduction. Two finger-breadths above the external malleolus is a depression which Dupuytren compared to an axe-cut. The internal malleolus projects below the skin; which is very tense and seems threatened with rupture. But this projection is a little above the point of the malleolus, and is formed by the irregular surface of the upper fragment of a fracture which passes near the central part of this eminence.

You saw that I reduced the deformity by fixing the leg with one hand, and carrying the foot inwards with a double movement of bodily transportation and rotation about its antero-posterior axis. I showed you that during this manœuvre the point of the internal malleolus, forming the lower fragment, returned to its place, and that after the reduction, the skin was much less tense and no longer threatened with gangrene or perforation.

The prognosis in these two patients is very different.

In the former we have to fear neither trouble on the part of the skin, nor consecutive suppuration. We are sure that the patient will recover without deformity. The only ultimate troubles will be those of tibio-tarsal arthritis and synovitis of the neighbouring tendons. These troubles, of which I often speak (see p. 70), are inherent to all fractures near articulations, and of course to these which communicate with the joints, as these two must inevitably do. These arthrites and synovites differ in being accompanied by lesions, sometimes temporary, sometimes of very long duration, or even incurable, which limit the movements, render them painful, and make it difficult to walk. These lesions are a thickening of the synovial membranes, and consequently a rigidity; or, if you prefer, a loss or a notable diminution of their extensibility, artificial union by means of false membranes, between the articular surfaces and the parietal synovial between the tendons and their sheaths. In order that the articular movements and the gliding of the tendons may resume their physiological conditions, it is necessary that these lesions should disappear. That never occurs in less than from four to six months, and often much later. The length of time that is necessary depends especially upon the age. Especially during youth, and until about the age of forty years, the synovial membranes lose quite promptly these consecutive inflammatory lesions. After forty, and especially after fifty years of age they disappear much less rapidly, particularly if the subjects are rheumatic or gouty. It is then that you see the patients, especially the women, walk for years slowly and painfully with the help of a cane. In this respect the condition of our first patient is favourable. He is thirty years old, and is not rheumatic; we may then hope that he will feel the consequences of his articular fracture

for only five or six months. I do not mean that he will be confined
to his bed during all this time; on the contrary, fractures of this
kind, like those of all the small bones, like those of all the extremities
of long bones, consolidate rapidly, and it is not necessary to keep the
limb immovable for more than thirty days. After that immobility is
no longer of any use to the fracture, and it may have disadvantages
for the articulation already inflamed by proximity, and especially for
the small articulations of the foot. In this respect, I make a distinction, as I have already shown you, and as I shall again show you
hereafter, between the joint or joints which are near the fracture, and
those which are more or less removed from it. The first present the
·lesions and symptoms of arthritis; but as these lesions are the result
either of the propagation of the inflammatory process from the fracture to the synovial membrane, or of the traumatism in which the
articulation has participated, we cannot tell to what extent the immobility has contributed, and in this respect M. Teissier (de Lyon)[1] invoked a number of facts which are not demonstrative, when he cited
examples of arthritis of the knee with neighbouring fracture of the
femur. The second, on the contrary, those which are more or less
distant from the seat of the fracture, and which we may suppose not
to have participated in the effects of the traumatism, may alter in
consequence of prolonged immobility, and they alter the more as the
articulations are smaller and tighter, such as those of the hand and
foot. There would then be reason to fear that by keeping the foot
immovable too long, we might produce in the small articulations of
the tarsus and metatarsus the lesion pointed out by Teissier and
Bonnet de Lyon,[2] which are followed by more or less painful prolonged rigidity.

To return to our first patient. I say then that he will have an inevitable tibio-tarsal arthritis; but that as he is young and not rheumatic
this arthritis will remain subacute, and will not pass to the state of
curable but prolonged chronic arthritis, nor to that of incurable dry
arthritis, and as I shall not leave him very long in the immovable
apparatus, he will also escape those arthrites caused by immobility
and the consecutive stiffness which we see especially in the small
articulations.

As for our second patient, if we should do nothing or if we should
not treat him properly, the prognosis would become very serious.
First, if we should not make the reduction an eschar might easily form
over the upper fragment of the internal malleolus and cause its suppuration and that of the articulation itself. If suppuration did not
occur consolidation would take place with the foot in its present position. That would be a deformity, and at the same time an infirmity,
for the patient would walk upon the inner border of the foot and not
upon the sole. The internal lateral ligament and the inner portion
of the synovial membrane would be constantly strained, causing re-

[1] Teissier, Mémoire sur les Effets de l'Immobilité des Articulations (Gaz. Médicale, 1841).
[2] Bonnet, Traité des Maladies des Articulations, tome i. p. 67.

peated sprains and incessant tibio-tarsal arthritis, which would compel the patient to walk very little and to rest himself frequently.

Treatment.—That of the first patient will be very simple. In a few days we shall wrap his foot and the lower part of the leg in a silicated apparatus which will be removed about the 25th or 30th day, counting from the accident. After having taken it off we shall permit the patient to walk with crutches; we shall advise him to move his foot while lying in bed, and we shall ourselves communicate some movements to it every morning, in order to restore suppleness to the articulations and tendons. We shall apply prolonged frictions, either with the naked hand and grease, or with a flannel, and finally we shall give him some sulphur baths.

For the second one we have to make and maintain reduction. You saw that reduction was quite easy, but that the foot, abandoned to itself, returned promptly to its vicious position. It is then necessary to apply an apparatus which will hold the foot firmly in place. Dupuytren understood this indication perfectly, and met it with an apparatus which was as perfect as was possible at a time when they did not use immovable bandages. This apparatus, which I have applied temporarily upon this patient because there was too much swelling to allow of the immediate application of an immovable one, and which I am glad to show you, because you may be obliged to use it yourselves sometimes, is composed :—

1st. Of a very long bag filled with chaff and folded at the middle, which is placed, thus folded, upon the inner side of the leg, taking care that it does not descend as low as the internal malleolus and that it leaves it free; for you understand that from the moment we fear an eschar at this point we must abstain from compression.

2d. Of a wooden splint long enough to cover the bag and extend beyond the sole of the foot, so as to leave a gap between itself and the foot.

3d. Of two bands, one of which is rolled about the upper and middle portion of the leg and fastens the bag and splint there, and the other, as soon as the foot has been brought inward by the manœuvre of reduction which I indicated a little while ago, forms a figure of 8 about the lower part of the leg and the foot, holding the latter close to the splint.

This dressing meets the indication very well if it is sufficiently tight over the foot and is renewed almost every day, for it gets loose very easily. You saw that after the apparatus had been applied I placed the limb upon a large and rather high cushion of chaff, resting the limb upon its outer side, as Dupuytren advised in cases of this kind, and as, before him, Pott advised for all fractures of the leg. This position has no advantage when the limb is in the Scultet bandage, but it is much more convenient when it is set with an inner splint. A hoop to keep off the weight of the bedclothes completes the dressing. Of course if the bands are too tight and the patient suffers, or if the inner border of the foot is pressed so tightly against the splint as to give pain, it would be necessary to loosen the bandage or to renew it before the end of the twenty-four hours. There is, however, no reason to fear gangrene by constriction, for the fractured region is not entirely comprised in the apparatus, since on the inner side the band passes over the splint and not over the foot itself.

If after forty-eight or seventy-two hours, I find that the inflammatory swelling does not increase, I shall apply an immovable apparatus. I should wait longer if there were any small wounds, phlyctenæ, or scratches which I wished to see cured before thus inclosing the limb. This delay would be no disadvantage if the Dupuytren apparatus were renewed every day, and if it certainly maintained the reduction.

It has happened to me sometimes, and some day you may meet with cases in which you will be obliged to do the same thing, to apply an immovable bandage on the first or second day. Once it was because the patient had violent alcoholic delirium, and disarranged his apparatus and reproduced the displacement of the foot by his movements. On two other occasions it was because, notwithstanding the care with which I placed the splint and bag, the displacement of the foot reappeared in a few hours, and the skin over the internal malleolus was so pressed upon as to render perforation or eschar imminent.

The application of an immovable apparatus having been decided upon, to which should we give the preference? Unhesitatingly to the plaster apparatus without the addition of gelatine. Why? Because it dries most rapidly, and if the foot is well drawn inwards and the reduction maintained during its application, I am sure that when the operation is terminated the bandage will be dry and will keep the parts as I placed them.

If by chance, in a case of this kind, you do not have proper plaster at your disposal, apply a bandage of starch, dextrine, or silicate of potash; but take care to keep the foot turned in during its application, and add to the inner side of the leg two thick linen cushions, one below the knee, the other above the internal malleolus, place over them a long inner splint like that of Dupuytren's apparatus, and fasten the leg and foot in the same way until all is dry.

The immovable apparatus should not remain more than 30 days in place. After that time the consecutive treatment is the same as that described in the preceding case.

II. *Supra-malleolar fracture.*—The patient in No. 26 is a man 61 years old, a little weakened by age, who, while descending a staircase in the dark, thought he had reached the bottom when he was still three steps from it. He fell, having, he says, his left foot and leg caught under his buttocks. You saw that the deformity resembles that of the preceding patient in this, that the foot is turned outward, that its outer border is raised, that there is the "axe-cut" depression above the external malleolus, and abnormal projection of the internal malleolus with a depression below. The foot is drawn backwards as well as outwards so that the skin is pressed upon and endangered by a very large bony prominence formed by the upper fragment of the tibia. For it is easy to see, by taking the leg in one hand and the foot in the other, and trying to restore their normal shape, that the principal line of the fracture is above the line of the malleoli, and passes through the inferior extremity of the tibia a few lines above the articulation, and through the adjoining part of the fibula. It is then one of those fractures which, on account of their position, Malgaigne[1] named *supra*-malleolar. You noticed that, after having made an almost complete reduction, I saw the displacement immediately reappear, and that after having placed the limb in a wire trough I saw, notwithstanding the anterior splint, the foot again turn outwards and backwards. I then placed two graduated compresses along the anterior and inner portion of the tibia, after having first applied a layer of cotton; then, adding the bag and anterior splint, and tightening the straps over them, I managed to maintain, if not the whole, at least a very great part of the reduction. We are here then in the presence of a supra malleolar fracture with complex displacement, difficult to correct.

It is not always so in supra-malleolar fractures; I have seen some, and Malgaigne also gives examples, in which there was little or no displacement, and in which reduction was easily maintained. On the other hand, the present case is not uncommon. Malgaigne quotes two similar ones from Dupuytren's work in which the splints, the only apparatus used at that time, did not prevent the displacement from obstinately reappearing, and the upper fragment of the tibia from causing a large eschar followed by suppuration and serious accidents. The patients recovered with a deformity and an infirmity. I myself had at the Hôpital de la Pitié in 1866 a man 66 years old, in whom a similar fracture was followed, in spite of all my care, by an eschar, suppuration of the articulation and bone, and finally by purulent infection and death.

To what is the difficulty of retention and consequently this gravity due? The authors have not explained it, but this is the explanation which I reached by autopsical examination of my last patient and a study of one or two specimens in the Musée Dupuytren. The fracture is undoubtedly produced, or, if you prefer, completed by the mechanism of crushing, that which takes place in most of the fractures of the extremities of long bones, and which has been well studied, especially for fractures of the lower end of the radius and upper end of the femur. At the moment of the accident the upper and lower fragments are pressed against each other by the weight of the body and by contraction of the muscles. This reciprocal pressure has caused the crushing of the cancellous tissue, a crushing favoured by its greater fragility which is the consequence of age, and which appears much sooner in some subjects than in others.

Remember that this patient is sixty-one years old, and that the one at La Pitié was sixty-six. The crushing is not regular, it is greatest at those points where there was most pressure, and those points are the ones where the muscular action was most energetic. The action of the peronei, the gastrocnemius, and soleus predominated, and was undoubtedly favoured by the abduction and extension of the foot at the moment of the accident. In consequence of this predominating action the sinking and crushing of the cancellous tissue were greater

---

[1] Malgaigne, *loc. cit.*, p. 818.

on the outer side and behind than in the other directions. When we replace the foot in its natural position, it can maintain it only if the fractured surfaces are interlocked at some points, but if this condition is lacking, and an empty space exists there where the crushing has been greatest, it is plain that the effect of the tonicity of the muscles is to draw the foot in the direction indicated by the irregular form of the fragments.

If, in other patients, the deformity is less, or if retention is easier, it is because the crushing has not been so great, the cancellous tissue not having yet acquired great fragility, or because it has taken place more evenly, the foot not having turned outwards at the time of the accident.

However that may be, we must not expect in this patient recovery without deformity. Whatever we may do, there will remain a deviation of the foot outwards and a projection forwards of the upper fragment of the tibia. The interfragmentary callus which will be produced, as in all fractures of the cancellous tissue, will partly fill the gaps, but will not efface them entirely. It will be the less able to do so because these crushings of the spongy tissue are followed by a process of absorption which removes part of the bone. Great as may be the power of repair, it is not sufficiently so, especially in a subject advanced in age, to reproduce all that has been lost, and so much the less so because the surfaces left by the loss of substance are constantly drawn towards one another by the tonicity of the muscles.

That which we desire most of all, and that towards which we shall direct all our efforts, is to prevent the formation of an eschar which would transform our fracture into a suppurating osteo-arthritis. The indication to be met is that of preventing the upper fragment from pressing upon the skin, since we cannot meet that of entirely correcting the deformity. How is this end to be reached? By repeated reductions, and by compression all along the upper fragment, the limb being kept in a metallic trough. I would not apply the plaster apparatus very early in this case, for I fear the displacement might be reproduced below it, and that the dreaded eschar might be caused. I prefer the trough, which lets me see what is going on.

If after a few days I saw the skin endangered by the incessant reproduction of the displacement forward of the upper fragment, I might perhaps use Malgaigne's point. At the end of his article upon supra-malleolar fractures, this surgeon expresses great confidence in his process. "As for apparatuses," he says, "the inefficacy of splints and of bands is shown by the preceding observations, and I do not know any which, under such circumstances, can take the place of my screw apparatus." I should have preferred to this affirmation the exhibition of one or two cases in which the screw had succeeded. This kind of fracture presents special anatomical conditions which might well make it fail. Still, I repeat, if we cannot keep the fragments well enough in place to prevent an eschar we shall make use of it. Would it not be better to give the preference to the section of the tendo Achillis, and to hope that, as after this section the foot and lower fragment would no longer be drawn upwards and backwards, the upper fragment would no longer project so much forwards? I ask the question, but I do not yet possess any fact upon which I could support the use of this little operation.

(The patient recovered without eschar and without suppuration, by the aid of the trough and compression distributed all along the upper fragment. There remained an abduction and a deviation backwards of the foot, with marked false anchylosis of the tibio-tarsal articulation.)

LECTURE XVI.

CONSECUTIVE AND LATE PHENOMENA OF SIMPLE FRACTURES OF THE LEG.

L. Fracture of the leg eight years before—Complete restoration of shape and function—Slight persistent muscular atrophy—Considerations upon this atrophy. II. Another fracture dating from eighteen months—Deformity due to the persistence of the projection of the upper fragment. III. Old fracture with hyperostosis of the tibia. IV. Consolidation since a year ago—Persistence of neuralgic pains (osteo-neuralgia). V. Fracture with persistence of tibio-tarsal arthritis. VI. Recovery with outward rotation of the upper fragment.

GENTLEMEN: Chance has permitted us during the week to see here five patients who had been treated for simple fractures of the leg, either by myself or by other surgeons. This is an opportunity to call your attention once more to the remote consequences of these fractures, consequences of which I have often spoken to you without having any examples to show you.

I. The first is a young man of 25 years, admitted for a wound of the left arm, who had his right leg broken in the lower third at the age of seventeen years (eight years ago). You saw that the conformation of the bones was excellent, that there was no pain along them, that all the articulations of the foot had their normal suppleness and motions, and that his walk was free, and without limping. Here is, then, an excellent recovery with restoration of shape and of functions. It is due to the fact that the fracture was without displacement, or that, if the displacement existed, it was easy to reduce and keep reduced, and it has appeared early because the subject was young, for at this period of life, when the constitution is not scrofulous, the tendinous and articular synovial membranes quickly recover the suppleness and extensibility which are destroyed in cases of fracture by the neighbouring synovites and the lesions caused by the immobility. I showed you only that the muscles in front and behind were smaller than those of the opposite side. We recognized it: 1st, with our eyes, when the patient was lying down and when he was standing;

2d, with the hands, by comparing the two calves. There is, then, in this patient, a little atrophy of all the muscles of the leg.

Do not wonder at it; this atrophy is very common after fractures of the leg.

It was twenty years ago that I discovered it for the first time, and showed it to the students at the Hôpital Cochin. I also told you that Dr. Lejeune,[1] by my advice, chose this atrophy for the subject of his inaugural thesis. Since then, I have noticed it very often, and have produced it artificially in animals, especially in guinea-pigs whose thighs or legs I had broken. It would be difficult for me to say what parts of the muscles this atrophy specially affects. Is it the muscular fibre itself, or is it the interfibrillary connective tissue? In the studies which I made upon guinea-pigs, not having had occasion to make them upon men, it seemed to me that both parts were diminished. Having weighed, immediately after death, the principal muscles of the thigh, and found a difference between their weight and that of the corresponding muscles of the opposite side, I macerated both in ether, taking care to renew the liquid often; at the end of seven months the muscles were freed of almost all their fat, those of the fractured side had lost as much of their weight as had those of the other, and there remained the same difference between the almost exclusively muscular parts which remained. Thence I concluded that the diminution of weight was made in both the constituent parts of the muscles, but more especially in their contractile part. I should, however, say that it was impossible for me to thoroughly appreciate the new anatomical condition of this contractile part; with the naked eye I saw that it was less red and less vascular than on the unaffected side, and M. Lejeune remarked the same fact. On microscopical examination, I found the usual longitudinal and transverse striæ. Upon some of the fibres of the guinea-pig, it seemed to me that the transverse striæ were a little less apparent or masked by fatty granulations, but it was not so evident that I could affirm the chief lesion of the muscular fibre to be a granulo-fatty transformation. It is probable, but thus far I have not been able to determine it rigorously with the aid of the microscope, that this capital lesion is a diminution of the volume of the fibrillæ, and that the general atrophy of the muscle is the result of the atrophy of each one of its fibrillæ, which, however, have lost neither their normal structure nor their function of contractility.

Notice, gentlemen, that although the diminution of volume is appreciable by the eye through the skin, the contractile power seems to be as well developed as that of the opposite side. Examination with the dynamometer would perhaps be necessary to form a precise opinion upon this subject. I have never made it, because I did not think it would lead to any important practical results. What you ought to know is, that after fractures in general, and those of the leg in particular, the muscles diminish in size, without diminution of their functions, so far as the patients can tell. You should know this fact

[1] Lejeune, see page 71.

and forewarn the patient and his friends of it, for otherwise they would not fail to say that the diminution of the size of the limb was the result of bad therapeutics.

I shall have said everything that should be said upon this subject, after having reminded you that muscular atrophy, after fractures, is inevitable and irremediable. Inevitable, because, whatever you may do, it will always result; it seems to me to be the consequence, both of the immobility and of the irregular distribution of the nutritive materials which go in excess to the bone before and after repair, and in less quantity to the other parts; now, you are not able to prevent this irregularity of distribution, which, moreover, is necessary for the formation of the callus. Irremediable, for I have often prescribed gymnastic exercises and electrization, and I have not brought the muscles to their original volume. Still it is evident that if anything can be obtained and if they wish to try, it is to these two means that recourse must be had. But you must expect to succeed very imperfectly.

II. The second patient is a man, thirty-five years old, who was treated nearly eighteen months ago, in another hospital, for a simple fracture of the right leg. He walks very well, and seldom has any pain, feeling only a little when the weather changes. There is the same muscular atrophy as in the preceding case. But he has, in the lower third of his leg, an abnormal bony prominence, which ends in a point, and still has the form of a V. You know this prominence. It is that which is so often formed by the upper fragment. It could not be corrected, undoubtedly because the transverse displacement was irreducible. Consequently, this patient has a deformity without functional trouble. The patient, of course, thinks that his fracture was badly set. Do not believe it, and never criticize your confrères by attributing this imperfect result to them. Undoubtedly, it might be due to carelessness, but much more probably to that irreducibility to which I have already, on different occasions, called your attention.

III. The third patient is forty years old, and had his leg broken three years ago. He has recovered well; has no projection of the upper fragment, and since the sixth month, has been able to walk quite easily, and is free from any articular or tendinous stiffness. But the tibia has remained voluminous about, above, and below, the line of fracture. It is not the peripheral callus alone which causes this excess of volume, as it sometimes does, from the sixth to the twelfth week after the accident. No, if the callus (the one which Dupuytren called provisional) has at any time been very large, it is no longer so to-day, for, as is usual, it has been absorbed. But the tibia has been hypertrophied, and has remained so since the end of the treatment, that is to say, the osteitis, which was developed during, and for the purpose of the consolidation, has surpassed, though we cannot say why, the limits which were necessary for the formation of the callus; it has extended to nearly the whole of the shaft, and has there assumed the characters of hypertrophying osteitis, while about the fracture it has preserved those of reparatory osteitis. To-day it is no longer an osteitis, since there are no longer any continuous pains; it is what we call hyperostosis, and this lesion, which, however, causes no trouble, is absolutely irremediable.

IV. *Fracture consolidated since a year ago; persistence of neuralgic pains (osteo-neuralgia of the tibia).*—We have recently seen at our consultation (Pitié, 1866) a woman, 32 years old, whom I treated a year ago for a fracture of the left leg below its centre. The displacement was slight. I first used the Scultet apparatus, and then the plaster bandage. We noticed, during the treatment, more prolonged and continuous pains than in other patients. She complained every morning of having slept badly and of having had throbbings and shooting pains about the fracture. You know that these pains are very common during the first eight or ten days. You know that, ordinarily, they grow weaker and weaker, and cease about the twelfth day, or only reappear if the patients move too much or sit up in bed; in any case, they are temporary. Well, in this patient the pains continued until the end of the treatment. They appeared without any previous movement, were almost continuous, but became much worse at night. Furthermore, when I removed the plaster apparatus on the forty-fifth day, the consolidation was not finished; I had to keep the limb immovable upon the cushion-trough of which I have sometimes spoken, and I prescribed from 30 to 60 grains of the phosphate of lime daily; it was only at the end of three months that abnormal mobility could no longer be found. Ordinarily, this delay coincides with a painful consolidation I attribute it to this that the reparatory osteitis is troubled, and assumes this continuously painful form with which the slow organization of the callus coincides.

This woman left us a year ago; she walks without crutches, but with difficulty, and has come to consult us for the pain which she still feels in the leg. This pain is much more endurable than it was during the treatment; it is moderate while the patient is seated, but becomes notably intense after she has walked for from twenty to thirty minutes. She has then to sit down that it may diminish. It reappears sometimes during the night without appreciable cause. The slightest blow causes fresh intensity.

We examined this leg together. You saw a very regular callus, and with the exception of a very slight swelling about the fracture, to which I cannot give the name of hyperostosis, the conformation is excellent. But pressure at this point causes pain. What is this persistent pain? I cannot locate it elsewhere than in the tibia, and as we have agreed to explain by an osteitis all the anatomo-physiological phenomena which occur in the bone after fractures, and during their consolidation, I have to say that this woman has had an osteitis, like all those who have had a fracture; but that this osteitis, without having taken on the suppurative form and without showing any tendency towards it, has differed from those which we see in similar cases by the intensity and the continuance of the pain. For a long time I have made use of the expression, *osteitis of neuralgic form*, to indicate this variety, which we also see sometimes independently of fractures, and of which it is impossible for me to give you a satis-factory anatomical or physiological explanation.

As for the prognosis, I hope, basing the hope upon some similar cases, that this abnormal sensibility will disappear in time. But will it need one, two, or three years? I cannot say.

I advised friction with the chloroform liniment, and the use of a roller bandage or cotton wadding. I have sometimes seen this compression lessen the pain sensibly, and the apparatus has the other advantage of protecting the limb from those slight shocks which cause pain, the repetition of which undoubtedly aids to keep up the painful condition.

This fact reminds me of two analogous ones.

I saw the first in 1857 and 1858, at the Hôpital Cochin, upon a mechanic, 41 years old, named Pierre D. His fracture, which was of the left leg, kept him in the hospital from the 18th September, 1857, until the 20th March, 1858 (six months). At the end of this time it was not yet consolidated. The patient, wearied of the hospital, wished to leave with a new plaster apparatus which I removed three weeks afterwards, the 8th April. It was then that, finding mobility no longer, I considered the consolidation made. Seven months, less ten days, were needed to obtain this result. Well, during all this time the patient, who was neither pusillanimous nor a deceiver, did not cease to complain of daily and nocturnal pains, sometimes with cramps, sometimes without them, which resisted opium or were only slightly diminished by it, and of sleep broken by these sufferings.

We might have supposed a deep abscess of the tibia, but there was none. Nothing in his constitution or antecedents could explain these rebellious pains; he was not even nervous. Like the woman previously mentioned, he had never had syphilis. I questioned and examined him on this subject a number of times, and obtained a negative result. Nor was there anything in the wound to explain the problem. There had been little displacement, and reduction was very easy. We remarked only that the fracture had been produced by direct action. A large wooden gate which he was helping to raise had slipped, and its edge had struck his left leg obliquely. But how many fractures by direct action do we not see recover without this prolongation of the suffering!

I saw this patient for more than a year, for he continued to suffer, less and less, it is true, but always very notably, while walking. I prescribed the rolled cotton dressing, frictions with the chloroform liniment, and iodide of potassium and valerianate of ammonia internally. I cannot say that one of these measures was more efficacious than the others; I only know that little by little the pains diminished. Since then I have not seen the patient, and suppose that finally the sensibility disappeared.

The other patient was a lady, 39 years old, impressionable, and very nervous, who suffered cruelly for three months, during which, the fracture, a very simple one of the right leg, did not consolidate. It was only during the course of the fourth month that the mobility disappeared. Three years have passed since then, and the patient still walks with pain and with the help of a cane. Every movement, every touch, awakens suffering, and yet there has been no abscess, and syphilis cannot be for a moment supposed.

What other name than that of *osteitis of neuralgic form* for the first period of the disease, and osteo-neuralgia for the later period, in which it is difficult to believe in the persistence of an inflammatory process in the absence of suppuration and fresh swelling; what other name, I ask, can we find to indicate these unusual painful forms?

V. *Fracture consolidated since six months ago ; persistence of painful arthritis.*—This patient is a woman, 58 years old, whom I treated for simple fracture of both bones of the right leg, in the lower third, six months ago. Consolidation was neither very painful nor slow. At the end of two months and a half, the patient left the hospital, unable to walk without crutches, and evidently suffering in the tibio-tarsal articulation. I then expressed the fear that the arthritis would last for a long time, that perhaps it would never disappear, for the age of the patient and the rheumatic pains which she had often felt, made me think her arthritis might take on the chronic and incurable form of the dry arthritis of old people. To-day, six months after the accident, the lower part of the tibia and the internal malleolus are hypertrophied, there is also a notable swelling of the ankle; the spontaneous movements of the articulation are very limited ; communicated movements also are limited, cause pain, and are accompanied by some crackling. There is then, here, a persistent arthritis which seems to me to belong to the category of dry arthritis. The patient will be kept quiet, with soothing frictions and poultices for two or three weeks. I shall also give her some douches and sulphur baths. We shall thus obtain an amelioration ; but I do not dare to hope for an entire cure, which, however, I should consider possible if the patient were younger. I fear that this woman is condemned to walk always with crutches, and very slowly, and that admission to La Salpêtrière[1] is the only useful thing we can offer her.

VI. *Fracture of the leg cured with rotation outwards of the upper fragment (consecutive displacement).*—I have again called your attention to a patient whom I treated here for a V fracture of the left leg, a simple fracture, but one which I could not reduce completely, as indeed happens quite often in V fractures. I placed the leg in a wire trough, and established compression all along the upper fragment, except at its point, where an eschar might have been produced. This patient, who is only forty years old, still suffers in walking, and as there is a notable swelling of the ankle, I consider him still affected with the remains of arthritis " by proximity," which we see after fractures, and especially after those which have a fissure extending to the articulation, as often happens in the V fracture. I have admitted him to let him rest for a few days, and to show you a deformity left by the fracture, deformity which I have seen several times, but which is not very frequent. When the patient is lying down and is asked to place his feet side by side, he does it easily, but by turning his thigh and

---

[1] An Asylum for Incurable and Indigent Old Women.

knee outwards.   If asked to place his knees in the same position, we see the foot and lower part of the leg turn inwards, that is to say, consolidation has taken place in this patient, not only with the slight projection of the upper fragment which you see, but with a rotary displacement, the upper fragment having turned about its axis from within outwards, and the lower one, with the foot, from without inwards.

This is a deformity, but it causes no trouble in walking.   As soon as he gets rid of his arthritis he will walk, but with his foot turned inwards ; and after all, when dressed, the deformity will not amount to much.

It was more than ten years ago that I first noticed this variety of deformity, which, so far as I know, has not been pointed out by our authors, and since then I have seen it five or six times.

I should like to be able to tell you what causes it, how it happens, and how it can be prevented, but I don't know much about it.

The rotary displacement does not exist at the beginning, or if it does exist, it is so easily corrected that we do not pay much attention to it.   It appears especially in fractures with transverse displacement of the upper fragment difficult to reduce and to keep reduced.   Thus far, I have seen it only in V fractures.   It appears from the eighteenth to the twenty-fifth day, after the patients have been long under treatment, and all has been done that should have been done, and care has been taken to place the inner border of the foot and of the patella in the relations which I have indicated.   If the surgeon continues, while watching the patient, to occupy himself only with the position of the foot, all seems to be going on well, but if, at the period of which I speak, he compares the position of the foot with that of the patella, he sees that the latter is turned outward.   He then removes the apparatus to make sure of the fact, and finds that, the foot being kept in place, it is the upper fragment, and the femur with it, which have turned outwards.   It takes place little by little, without pain ; the patient does not notice it, and when the surgeon discovers it the effect is irremediable; for it is useless for you to try to correct this consecutive displacement.

For me, at least, whatever plan I have tried has failed ; and it is easy to understand.   The consolidation is already too far advanced to permit the deformity to be corrected.   We might make the callus yield by violent manœuvres, but we might also fail, and even if we did succeed, the consecutive displacement might be reproduced during the new consolidation.   Perhaps also the exaggerated osteitis thus produced might cause dangerous suppuration.   I have, therefore, considered it prudent to confine myself to moderate attempts at reduction, and they have not succeeded.

From the notions which I have given you, you should draw this conclusion, that, notwithstanding all possible attention, deformities, which could not be prevented, are possible after fracture of the leg, and instead of attributing them to the carelessness of the surgeon, as non-professional people are so prompt to do, we must consider them due to peculiar and inevitable conditions which our authors have not made sufficiently prominent. I shall add this other conclusion, that we cannot, in these cases of difficult fractures, give too much care and watchfulness during the first two or three weeks to the situation of the foot, with reference to that of the patella and knee. Perhaps, if you recognized this rotation from the beginning, you might remedy it, at least in part, and be more fortunate than I have been, for thus far I have only discovered it when it was too late to correct it.

LECTURE XVII.

FRACTURES OF THE LEG.

I. Fracture of the left leg more than a month old—Obliteration of the veins. II. Consolidation retarded. III. Pseudarthrosis with angular displacement ; suture of the tibia ; purulent infection.

GENTLEMEN : I. I called your attention during the visit to the patient, in No. 39, who has been treated for more than a month now in the wire trough for a fracture of the right leg. I could not apply an immovable apparatus on account of the numerous phlyctenæ and two small superficial eschars, the dressing of which required the leg to be left uncovered. The patient has had considerable œdematous swelling of the leg and foot for several days. This swelling, which occurred without pain, is not very rare in the course of fractures of the leg. You will find it rather upon adults and old men than in young people. What does it mean, and what will it become? It means that the venous circulation is obstructed in consequence of the coagulation of the blood. I do not think there is thrombosis of the femoral vein, for I did not feel a hard cord along its course, and pressure upon it did not cause the pain which is rarely absent in such a case. It is rather a thrombosis of the anterior and posterior tibial veins. We do not here find the pains which spontaneous phlebitis, with coagulation, often causes ; but this pain is generally absent when only veins of the second order are involved. We cannot feel the hard cord because the veins are too deeply placed to be reached by our fingers, and the existing œdema increases the difficulty. I can- not, therefore, prove the existence of the thrombosis by physical signs ; but I admit it because I know it has sometimes been demon- strated in autopsies after fracture, and also because I cannot otherwise explain the œdema. Notice that this is not an inflammatory swelling of the first period, for the tumefaction did not appear until towards the 27th day, long after the inflammatory phenomena had disappeared. On the other hand, we cannot attribute it to a disease of the liver, nor of the heart, nor to albuminuria, for the other foot is not œde- matous, and the patient presents no symptoms of these different diseases. This little complication is instructive from two points of view; first, because the thrombosis will undoubtedly last a long time, several months; the œdema will increase when the patient begins to walk, and this swelling will join the other causes, with which you are acquainted; rigidity of the articulations and tendons, weakness of the muscles, to oppose the re-establishment of the functions; second, because it explains the possibility of the fatal emboli, of which Professor Velpeau[1] and M. Azam, of Bordeaux,[2] have published cases. We ourselves had here, two months ago, a woman who, on the 27th day of her treatment for a fracture of the leg, was suddenly taken with oppression, precordial pain, and lipothymia, which we attributed to a pulmonary embolus too small to cause death, but which, if it had been a little larger, would have completely obstructed the pulmonary artery and killed the patient promptly.

I wish I could point out, as a complement of these facts, a way to prevent the detachment and passage toward the heart and pulmonary artery of clots which I suppose to exist in the tibial veins inflamed by their proximity to the osteitis of the callus. But I am not acquainted with any prophylactic measures against embolus. That is one of those unfortunate complications which the practitioner should know of, but which, in the present state of our science, he can neither prevent nor cure when it appears.

II. *Delay of the consolidation.*—Since I am speaking of the consecutive and tardy phenomena, I want to call your attention to two patients with broken legs, the consolidation of which is delayed.

One of them, No. 5, Ward St. Vierge, is a young man 23 years old, who was admitted with a compound fracture. Thanks to the occlusion which we made with collodion, there was no suppuration, and then I hoped everything would pass as in a simple fracture; the limb was placed in a trough; the patient suffered no pain, but, when at the end of forty-five days I removed the apparatus, I still found very marked mobility; the 20th January, two months after the accident, as the mobility persisted, I applied the immovable apparatus which is still upon the fractured limb.

The other is a woman in No. 17, Ward Sainte Catherine; her fracture is more recent than the preceding one, dating from only forty-five days ago; however, the mobility and the pains which, from the beginning, have been greater than usual, still persist and compel us to use restraining apparatus.

Here are two examples of consolidation that has made but little progress; but notice, gentlemen, that I do not say non-consolidation, pseudarthrosis. For we must not confound a delay with a non-existence of consolidation, and, like Norris, perform operations in cases which would doubtless have been caused by immobility. As for myself, I claim that at least a year must elapse before the word pseudarthrosis is to be pronounced in a fracture of the leg. But to what can we attribute the delay in our patients? I admit that I

---

[1] Velpeau, Comptes Rendus de l'Académie des Sciences, 14 April, 1862.
[2] Azam, Bull. de la Société de Chirurgie, 7 June, 1864.

find no cause. Syphilis, scurvy, pregnancy, nursing, have been invoked to explain pseudarthrosis; I cannot discover here the existence of any of these general causes; and if it is possible for syphilis to delay consolidation, our patients have not had it. If we examine the local causes we find, as a possible explanation of the delay, defective fixation of the fragments; but here immobility has been too well maintained for us to admit this cause. Finally it might be permitted to believe that there is, between the fragments, a piece of tendon, muscle, or aponeurosis, or a splinter which, by its interposition, prevents the callus from forming, but that is a thing which we cannot recognize, and which, indeed, we could not remedy.

We shall continue then to keep our patients' limbs completely immovable, and we shall give phosphate of lime internally, to hasten the formation of a long callus.

III. *Ancient non-consolidated fracture, or pseudarthrosis, with angular deformity of the leg; suture of the bones; purulent infection; death.*— Gentlemen, pseudarthroses due to non-consolidation of fractures of the leg are exceedingly rare. You sometimes hear me speak of delays, but you have never seen any of our patients remain without consolidation. During more than twenty years that I have practised in the hospitals of Paris, I have not seen a single one of the fractures of the leg which I have had to treat, remain in the condition of pseudarthrosis. I am surprised then to find in Malgaigne's work the statistics of an American surgeon, Norris, in which are found—

30 pseudarthroses of the humerus,
18   "   of the femur,
14   "   of the leg and tibia alone.

I wish to put you on your guard against the interpretation which has been given to certain observations in this table, and against the abuse which has been made of operations designed to cure pseudarthrosis.

The error is due to two causes: first, because, at a certain time, at the beginning of this century, when the operations of seton and resection had been proposed, some surgeons in America confounded delay in consolidation with non-consolidation, and considered fractures which still gave mobility during the second or third month, as having passed to the condition of pseudarthrosis. Now we know to-day that those fractures end by consolidating after four, five, or six months of treatment. The second cause is that they did not distinguish, among the pseudarthroses, those which they observed, or thought they observed, in patients who had been regularly treated, and those presented by patients who had remained without treatment, and whose limbs had never been set. Now you may be sure, gentlemen, that pseudarthroses, not only in the leg, but also in the humerus and femur, are exceedingly rare in patients who have been properly and perseveringly treated. If we remove from Norris's statistics the patients in whom they despaired of consolidation too soon, there would remain only those whose injury had not been treated at all. Now, those are extremely rare, for generally, fractures of the leg are so painful, that the patients have to keep quiet, and so easily recognized that the diagnosis must be made, and lead to treatment by immobility.

You may, however, meet with patients who suffer little, and in whom the diagnosis is rendered difficult by certain anatomo-patholo-gical conditions.

I once treated a child, six years old, who had had a fall three weeks before I was called to see him. At Geneva, where the little patient then was, the surgeon who was consulted had not detected the frac-ture, and had allowed the child to walk, which he did with a little difficulty at first, but afterwards quite easily. He was brought to Paris, where one day he made a misstep, and felt a new pain in his leg (it was the right one). I found, near its middle, a slight swelling, which I was told had existed since the first fall; also pain on pressure at this point, where there was, however, no ecchymosis; and, finally, after several unsuccessful attempts, I felt very distinctly a mobility and a crepitation which left me no doubt as to the existence of a frac-ture of the tibia, and probably of the tibia alone. I did not doubt that this fracture had existed since the first fall, and had been consoli-dated not at all, or so incompletely that the new accident had caused the imperfect callus to yield.

Several conditions in children and young people may render diag-nosis difficult, not only of a fracture of the tibia, but also of a simul-taneous fracture of the tibia and fibula. The first is the preservation, at the place of fracture, of the periosteum, which acts as a means of union. The second is the toothed disposition, with reciprocal inter-locking of all the points, and little excavations which correspond to them upon the other fragment. These two conditions, which, more-over, may very easily exist together, not only oppose displacement, but may prevent detection of mobility and crepitation.

In a young man whom I treated in 1865, at La Pitié, and over whose right leg the wheel of an empty cab had passed, I was unable at first to recognize a fracture, and after several examinations, I made the diagnosis, *contusion of the leg.* The patient kept the bed because he suffered while standing, but he moved as much as he liked in it. It was only on the eighteenth day that, a small abnormal prominence appearing, I was led to examine it again, and I then felt a fine crepi-tation and a mobility, indicating a fracture of the tibia which I had mistaken at first for the reasons I have given. Suppose that in my little patient and in this latter, at La Pitié, new examinations had not been made, and they had continued to walk. Undoubtedly, consolida-tion would have been possible, but it might also have failed and a pseudarthrosis been established.

This is what probably took place in the young man, 19 years old, who was admitted into Ward St. Louis, No. 50, the 27th November, 1866. He told us that in December, 1864 (he was then 17 years old), one of his comrades had given him a violent blow with a stick upon the lower part of his left leg. He suffered, but did not fall; was not obliged to keep his bed, and continued to walk, though limping, without consulting anybody. He only knows that a small lump appeared at the place where he had been struck. A month after this accident he fell while trying to jump over a ditch. The same leg gave him a great deal of pain ; he was carried home, where he kept the bed for several days, and then resumed his work in a factory. But he could no longer endure the fatigue; his leg caused him pain after a few hours of walking.

A little later he fell again, and was admitted to the Hôtel-Dieu, where he remained ten days without anyone speaking to him of fracture. After that he walked with more and more difficulty without being able to bear his foot upon the ground; then he saw that his foot turned outwards, and that his leg bent, forming an anterior and internal angle. This bad conformation was increased by the manipulations of a bone-setter.

To-day we are struck with the deformity of this limb. The foot and the lower part of the leg are turned outwards, and the leg presents, at its anterior and inner portion, an angle, the opening of which is directed outwards. Grasping the leg above and below this angle, we feel a mobility from before backwards and transversely which is not very marked, but which does not allow us to doubt the existence of an imperfectly consolidated fracture, of a pseudarthrosis with incomplete vicious callus. For the last six months the patient has been able to walk only by the help of a wooden leg, upon which he rests his knee. He declares that he will not remain in this state, and that at any price he wishes his leg to be straightened and solidified ; he has repeated this declaration so often during the week he has been here, that I have determined to make an oblique resection followed by suture of the two bones.

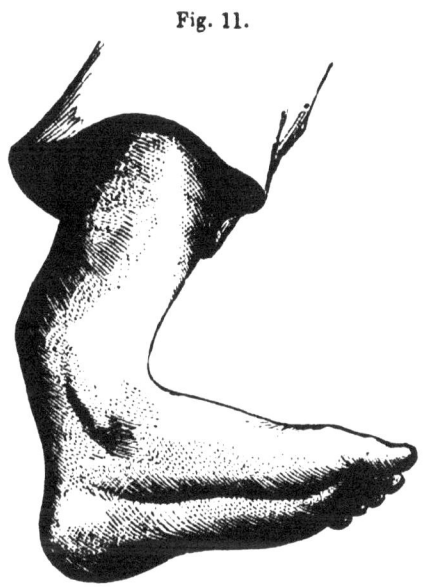

Fig. 11.

Angular pseudarthrosis of the left leg.

The operation was performed in the following way : An incision about three inches long, and parallel to the axis of the limb, was made along its anterior portion, and crossed by another about two inches long. The four flaps made by these incisions were dissected backwards, and the angle formed by the two fragments of the tibia exposed. I then divided the intermediate fibrous tissue which united the fragments, and, exposing the lower one, I made, with a small saw, an oblique section downwards and inwards on the inner and posterior faces of this fragment. I then made the upper fragment project, and made, on its outer face and anterior border, a similarly oblique section downwards and inwards, so that, the two sawn surfaces facing one another, I could bring them exactly together. I then replaced the limb in its proper position, and with much difficulty perforated the fragments with a drill, and then passed a double silver wire through the holes, with which I fastened the bones together. The limb was then placed in a wire trough with cotton and oiled silk, and the wound, which was not united, was covered with a simple cerat dressing.

In short, the operation which you saw me perform was a mixture of resection and suture. Resection, without suture, was made in 1760, by White, and afterwards by a certain number of English and American surgeons. Then resection, followed by suture, was made in 1825, by Kearney Rodgers, an American surgeon, and by Flaubert, of Rouen, whose two cases were reported by Dr. Laloy.[1] It is true, that in all these cases the pseudarthrosis was of the humerus, and in all, except Flaubert's second, the section was perpendicular to the long axis of the bone. My operation was peculiar in this, that it was performed for a pseudarthrosis of the tibia, and that, conformably to the precept given by Flaubert after his second case, which was, if I am not mistaken, a case of vicious callus, and not of pseudarthrosis, I made oblique sections in the two fragments in opposite directions, and united them with a suture.

My patient, unfortunately, was attacked with purulent infection ten days after the operation, and died the 27th December. I show you here his lungs and spleen, in which you see numerous metastatic abscesses. There was also a sero-purulent effusion in the two pleural cavities, suppurative arthritis of the knee above the fracture, and an abundant suppuration between the fragments, which, though still held in contact by the suture, are not united by the beginning of a callus.

<hr />

LECTURE XVIII.

FRACTURES OF THE PATELLA.

Non-consolidated fracture of the left patella, dating from 18 years before; separation of two and a half inches—Study of the movements and functions of the limb.

GENTLEMEN: I stopped for a long time this morning at No. 25, Ward Sainte Vierge, to study and to show you the results of an old fracture of the patella, the fragments of which are widely separated from one another, and do not seem to be united by an intermediate fibrous substance.

The man, who is 50 years old, tells us that 18 years ago (in 1850) he was brought to the same ward for a fracture of the left patella.

Velpeau applied an immovable bandage, with which the patient

[1] Laloy, Thèses de Paris, 1839.

was allowed, he says, to walk after the tenth day. He assures us that the apparatus remained in place for four months, and that when it was removed the distance between the fragments was considerable. They then applied another apparatus which he cannot very well describe, but which seems to have consisted of two vertical straps fastened, one about the thigh, the other about the leg, with a circular bandage, and tied together over the patella; they were intended to keep the fragments near one another. This apparatus was removed every five or six days for about two months, and then, that is, six months after the accident, the patient left the hospital, walking with crutches, and with a considerable separation of the fragments.

He spent six months in the country, during which his walking improved so much that when he returned to Paris he could walk easily and without a cane, take long walks without being fatigued, and did not hesitate to resume his former occupation of bar-tender.

He comes to us to-day for a small contused wound of the right leg, and would not have spoken of his former fracture, of which he no longer thinks, if we had not noticed it ourselves.

You noticed a notable deformity of the left knee. Two small bony prominences appear over it, separated by a long depression. We can feel that these two prominences are nothing else than the fragments of an old transverse fracture of the left patella, and by pressing back the skin over the intermediate depression we can feel the condyles of the femur. When the limb is extended, the separation is two and a half inches; when bent, it is five inches. When the leg is bent, we can see the outlines of the condyles of the femur under the skin between the fragments.

The patient complains of no pain, and has never had any inflammation. There is the usual amount of flexion and extension, and no abnormal lateral mobility.

We studied the movements, and found that the patient made all of them easily except those which require the almost exclusive intervention of the quadriceps femoris. For example, while he was lying down, I asked him to flex and extend the knee; he did it quite easily, but I showed you that the extension might be explained by the relaxation of the flexors, and the pressure of the heel upon the bed. To see if he used the quadriceps normally, I asked him to raise the heel from the bed without previously bending the knee. He was not able to do it. I then told him to bend the knee and then raise his foot from the bed and carry it into the air. He could not do that either. It is true, that all the muscles of the thigh, and especially the quadriceps, are less voluminous than those of the opposite side, as is the case, I have often told you, with almost all muscles after fractures. But although diminished, these muscles are not paralyzed. You saw that they hardened during the attempts he made to do what we asked of him, and that even the lower fragment was drawn up a little. If the movement of elevation of the foot, in the production of which the psoas and iliacus aid a little, but for which the action of the quadriceps is absolutely necessary, cannot be executed, it is because this action is not sufficiently transmitted to the tibia through the ligamentum patellæ.

I then made the patient rise and walk before us. He did it without the slightest hesitation or limping.

While he was standing with his feet together, I asked him to move the left one forwards; he did it, but by flexing the knee. I asked him several times to bring the foot forward without thus bending the knee, but he was unable to do so. Why? Because as soon as the foot is detached by the action of the psoas, iliacus, and adductors, the knee is held too feebly, and the foot falls either by its own weight or by the action of the flexors which are not counterbalanced. In fact, it is the quadriceps alone which can keep the knee extended whilst the foot is carried forward.

Although the physiological analysis of the functions of the limb shows us the loss, or at least a great diminution of the contractions of an important muscle, it is nevertheless true that the patient makes up for this loss by means of the psoas and adductors, and has no great difficulty in walking. He mounts staircases quite easily, descends them with a little more hesitation, placing both feet upon each step; can easily walk five miles without a cane, and continues uninterruptedly his fatiguing occupation.

The anatomical deformities, or, if you prefer, the morphological vices of a fracture of the patella with separation, are here carried to their greatest degree. I should tell you that you will find similar ones in many patients, but to a much less degree.

We often see a smaller separation, of not more than an inch, for example, cause at first functional troubles as great as those of our patient, and then gradually the patient becomes able to use his leg almost as well as the other. He feels his infirmity only when descending a staircase, and the surgeon detects the lesion only by telling the patient to raise his heel from the bed or to move his foot forward without bending the knee. These two equally difficult movements indicate an old fracture of the patella. That is the ordinary result. Do not forget it, whether the separation is greater or less, the limb is neither more nor less weak; it remains weakened, that is incontestable, but the patients, except, perhaps, those who have to do heavy work, do not perceive it, or habit has taught them to counterbalance the defect of contraction so well, that they pay no more attention to it.

Bear in mind, however, that this proposition, relative to the mode of cure of transverse fractures of the patella, is not absolute, and does not apply to all cases.

I establish, like our classic authors, a distinction between fractures without separation, or a separation of a few lines only, in which part of the surrounding fibrous tissue remains intact, and fractures with separation of half an inch or more, in which the fibrous tissue is completely torn across.

In the first case the fracture heals without separation, and with a bony callus, and the functions of the quadriceps are entirely re-established.

It is in the second case only that persistence of the separation is the rule, that its increase during the first weeks is not very rare, and that the cure is not by a bony callus. A cellular or cellulo-fibrous substance is formed between the fragments, and if it is dense it allows partial transmission of the effects of the contraction of the quadriceps to the ligamentum patellæ; but if it is not dense, and it almost never is, it does not permit this transmission.

Such is the rule; but I add at once that exceptions are possible, and that you may be fortunate enough to obtain, by a well-directed treatment, or by the existence of favourable organic conditions in your patient, the exception which we always seek, that is, the cure of a transverse fracture with separation either by a bony callus, or by a fibrous one strong enough to permit perfect extension of the limb.

Now two questions naturally arise here. Why these results? Why do our methods of treatment succeed only exceptionally in getting better ones?

1st. Why do we have recovery with separation and a too soft fibrous callus, or none at all? On account of local and general causes.

The predominant local cause in the case of an unopposed or unsuccessfully opposed separation, is the communication of the fractured surfaces with the articulation, and with an articulation which, participating in the consecutive phlegmasia, fills up with blood and synovia, and remains full of liquid for several weeks. The materials which would serve for the formation of a callus fall into this liquid and are lost in it. This explanation was first given long ago; you will find it in all your books, and it is always true.

A second local cause is the absence, before and behind the fracture, of tissues which might help to form the callus. For I have supposed that the fibrous tissue, which performs the part of periosteum and establishes the continuity between the end of the triceps and the beginning of the ligamentum patellæ, is broken. What remains in front of the patella? Connective tissue and the synovial bursa; but these tissues, not having been torn, do not undergo the consecutive inflammation which would enable them to exude the materials of the callus, or if by chance they furnish some, they fall into the articulation, and are not kept between or about the fragments. This absence of torn tissues, in front of and about the fracture, serves for an answer to the objections of those who say you attribute the difficulty of consolidation to the effusion of the reparatory liquids into the synovial cavity; how then does it happen that the vertical and transverse fractures without separation, or with very moderate separation, recover with a bony callus? The answer is very simple; it is that there remains about the fragments in the last two cases a fibrous portion which keeps them together, which has been sufficiently torn to furnish reparatory materials, and which serves as support and gangue to the callus, which having begun in it extends gradually between the fragments. Furthermore, when the latter remain almost in contact, we may suppose that the reparatory glutinous substance of the first days is retained upon their surfaces in sufficient quantity to furnish useful materials to the callus.

The general causes are inherent to the constitution. Remember, gentlemen, that this is a contest between two opposing forces; a tendency to repair, which exists for this bone as for all the others, and an effort constantly exerted by the tonicity of the quadriceps to keep up, and even augment the peculiar displacement which exists in this variety of fracture, displacement by separation through muscular action. Now, by increasing the separation, the quadriceps elongates the reparatory substance, disarranges it, and opposes its calcareous transformation.

Consequently, in fractures with considerable separation, you can have a bony or a very solid fibrous callus only if the surfaces of the fragments furnish materials capable of being rapidly transformed into solid substance, and if the muscles will remain inactive for a sufficient length of time during the treatment which you have instituted. We occasionally meet with patients in whom the reparatory tendency is sufficiently strong to furnish a solid intermediate substance during the time that we are acting upon the fracture. But we find more in whom the intermediate substance has not been able in this time to get the necessary solidity.

2d. Why do not our means of treatment always succeed in preventing this imperfect consolidation? You know why, if you have well understood the preceding details. We do not succeed for three reasons.

The first is that we find it difficult to bring the broken surfaces together, and to successfully oppose the action of the quadriceps. We sometimes succeed in bringing them into contact with the aid of certain apparatuses of which I shall speak. But this contact does not last very long. The quadriceps ends by slightly overcoming our opposition. If by chance it does not reproduce the entire separation, it reproduces it partially; or the fragments remain together in front, but separated behind. The second cause is that, in spite of the retention, the patient instinctively flexes the knee a little on account of the pain, and thus reproduces some of the separation. The third reason is that the contention is so exact that the patient suffers and loosens the apparatus, thus allowing the separation to again take place.

All three causes, or only two of them, often act at the same time, and in any case the same effect is produced, effusion into the articulation and immersion of the reparatory materials in the liquid which it already contains.

But that is not all; suppose that the mechanical problem has been solved, and that the fragments have been kept in place by the apparatus which you have chosen. If the consolidation is not complete when you remove this apparatus, from the 60th to the 80th day, for example, the quadriceps will recommence its unfavourable action. Its tonicity separates the fragments again, the intermediate substance yields, lengthens, and if the patient moves a little (and how are we to prevent him from moving after so long a time?), consolidation is arrested, and you have a separation with a soft intermediate substance, which amounts to about the same as if you had no intermediate substance. It is only in young and healthy patients that, during the eight or ten weeks of the application of the apparatus, the exudation has the time to organize into a strong fibrous or fibro-calcareous tissue so solid that the quadriceps can no longer act successfully against it and reproduce or increase the separation.

LECTURE XIX.

FRACTURES OF THE PATELLA.—Continued.

I. Recent fracture of the patella with a separation of nearly three-quarters of an inch—Difficulty of the cure—Indications to be met—Different treatments by two kinds of apparatus ; some closed, others open—Preference given to rubber rings. II. Sprain of the callus, and apparent relapse a year after a fracture of the patella.

Gentlemen: I. A man, 35 years old, a carpenter, whom we saw this morning during the visit (Ward Sainte Vierge, 28), caught his foot yesterday morning in his workshop among some pieces of wood which were lying on the floor. He fell forward, made a violent effort to save himself, and then fell backwards, feeling a painful sensation in his left knee. He was lifted up, and tried to walk, but could only take a few steps backwards, dragging his leg and leaning upon a comrade. He was at once brought to the hospital, and this is what we find :—

As physical signs :

1st. A notable swelling of the knee with a fluctuation that leaves no doubt of the existence of an effusion.

2d. A transverse depression in which the finger can easily lie, indicating a separation of nearly three-quarters of an inch, and increasing when the knee is bent.

3d. Above and below this depression a bony fragment, each of which can be easily moved sideways, and is evidently formed by one of the halves into which the patella has been divided.

As functional signs :

1st. Moderate pain when the patient does not move.

2d. Ability to flex the leg upon the thigh.

3d. Inability to then extend it without using his hands or pressing his heel forcibly upon the bed and making it slide downwards.

4th. Utter impossibility of detaching the heel from the bed, and notable increase of the pain in the knee when he makes the attempt.

By these signs you all recognize a transverse fracture ef the patella with a separation which indicates the complete rupture of the fibrous tissue in front of it.

This fracture has been produced by muscular action, for the patient fell, not forwards, but upon his back. I ask myself if these indirect fractures, by muscular action, should not be explained by a premature rarefaction and fragility of the cancellous tissue of the patella? However that may be, the lesion is not complicated by a sprain with lateral mobility, such as I have twice met with in fracture of the patella ; but it is accompanied by an effusion into the articulation which, considering the rapidity of its production, must be principally formed of the blood furnished by the patella and the lateral fibrous tissues which were torn at the same time to a certain extent. But such an effusion does not take place after a traumatic lesion of the knee without causing the synovial membrane to inflame and promptly secrete an excess of synovia which increases the quantity of the effusion. There is then, together with the fracture, a beginning of the traumatic arthritis which is inevitable under such circumstances.

What is the prognosis and what will be the consequences of this fracture?

The prognosis is not serious, in this way, that life is not at all endangered, and in all probability the patient will recover the use of the limb to such an extent that he will be able to stand up, walk, and gain a living by the trade which he has heretofore exercised.

But the prognosis is bad in this respect, that the injury will compel the man to remain in bed for about two months, then to walk with crutches for one or two more, and finally to walk slowly with a cane for at least as much more. It is impossible to fix exactly the number of days, but it will be very long.

You will hear of patients who, after fracture of the patella, have remained only four or five weeks in bed, and have been able to walk without a cane at the end of two months. But those were patients who had fracture without rupture of the anterior fibrous tissue and without separation. In naming the approximative limits of the duration, I recall what I have observed in patients who, like this one, had fracture with considerable separation.

It may even happen that this duration will be longer than I said. I showed you that we have here also a traumatic arthritis ; now, this arthritis may remain painful for a longer time, and compel the patient to take care of himself and not to work for six, eight, or ten months. I ought to tell you that I have but little fear of this prolongation, for he is still quite young, healthy, and not rheumatic.

The prognosis is also bad in this way, that the arthritis may possibly leave behind it an incomplete anchylosis, with very notable diminution of the movements of the knee, or even a complete anchylosis.

I had occasion to show here last year, a man, 56 years old, who after a well-managed treatment of a fracture of the patella, recovered without separation and with, very probably, a bony callus, but with almost complete anchylosis of the knee. I should have more fear of such consequences if our patient was older.

Suppose that the concomitant arthritis does not last long and is not followed by anatomical modifications injurious to the functions of the limb, the prognosis is still bad, in this sense, that this limb will not recover the integrity of its functions and the strength which it previously had. It would recover them if we should be so fortunate as to obtain either a bony callus or a fibrous one sufficiently short and solid to transmit the full effects of the contraction of the quadriceps to the ligamentum patellæ and the leg. Certainly such a result is not impossible.

I have preserved notes upon 20 patients whom I have treated during the last fifteen years for fractures of the patella with separation varying from one-third of an inch to an inch and a quarter, and in only two of them have I obtained a bony or fibrous callus, solid enough to allow the heel to be raised from the bed without bending the knee, and to cause the transmission to the lower portion of the patella of movements communicated to the upper portion, and reciprocally. And as one of them was twenty-two, and the other twenty-five years old, I ask myself if youth was not the principal condition which allowed this fortunate result to be obtained.

In the others recovery took place with considerable separation. The patients lost their ability to raise the heel from the bed or the sole from the ground without a previous involuntary bending of the knee. Their patellæ were composed of two pieces which could be moved independently of each other, and all had the same difficulty in descending the stairs when the knee was not supported by a kneecap. Without that help they could only go from one step to the next by placing both feet upon the first and then advancing the uninjured one.

I fear still more a persistence of the separation when, pressing the two pieces towards one another with my hands, I do not succeed in bringing them into contact. That is the criterion which I recommend to you. When with your two hands you can bring the fragments into contact, there is hope of recovery without separation. This hope has less foundation when this contact cannot be obtained.

Dr. Lecoin, a former interne at the Vincennes Asylum,[1] had the good idea to record[2] the results which he observed during more than two years upon patients who, after having been treated in the different wards of the Paris hospitals, had been admitted to the asylum at Vincennes for their convalescence. These patients were 26 in number, but as one of them had had an iterative fracture of the same patella, the author makes the number 27. Well, in 23 of these there was a separation which varied from one-third to one and two-thirds of an inch, with independent mobility of each fragment. They had been treated by various apparatuses, some by the trough and elevation only, most of them by an immovable apparatus, two by M. Trélat's apparatus, one by this apparatus with Verneuil's modification, one by Laugier's rubber rings, two by Valette's (of Lyons) apparatus.

---

[1] Situated outside of Paris, and designed for the reception of convalescents coming from the hospitals.

[2] Lecoin, Thèses de Paris, 1869, No. 249.

Notwithstanding the incontestable advantages of these methods, which I shall explain more fully in a moment, notwithstanding the talent and care of the surgeons, the separation persisted with an imperfect consolidation which left the patients in conditions nearly the same as those of non-consolidation.

As for the other four, they are given as recoveries with a bony callus. But the author could not learn in each case whether the fracture had been originally with or without separation. In one of them alone was it known that M. Cusco had made the diagnosis of fracture without separation, a fact which easily accounts for that callus being favourable.

On this point we know nothing in the other three. I will admit that all of them owed their bony callus to successful treatment of a fracture with notable separation; we should thus have three **good** results out of twenty-six, a proportion similar to mine (two **good** results out of twenty).

Can we obtain a better proportion? I believe so; but the proof is yet to be given.

Malgaigne[1] perhaps darkened a little the list of the inconveniences left by fracture of the patella which was healed with separation. Undoubtedly the limb remains weakened, in this sense, that the contractions of the quadriceps are no longer utilized except by means of the transmission of their effect through the fibrous tissues on each side of the patella, and by an elongated patella, the movable upper fragment of which consumes most of the effort which is communicated to it, and transmits but a very small part to the lower fragment.

We must also take into account the muscular diminution which I have often mentioned when speaking of fractures of the thigh and leg, and of which I showed you an example in a patient affected with an ancient fracture of the patella. But, nevertheless, most of the patients, all those who have retained neither arthritis nor anchylosis, and who suffer only the consequences relating to the quadriceps, become able to walk very easily without a cane, to take long walks without fatigue, and, in short, to no longer notice their fracture or the weakness of the limb, except when they go up, and especially when they come down staircases. Perhaps Malgaigne, in the estimate which he made of the results, did not sufficiently distinguish between that which was the consequence of the arthritis, and that which was the consequence of the weakening of the triceps, which was undoubtedly because he examined the patients too soon after the accident.

To exactly appreciate the consequences of a fracture of the patella they should be studied several years after the accident, and after being satisfied that the arthritis has left no bad result.

I must now mention another unfortunate element of the prognosis. The patient may perhaps break the other patella, and break it in the same way, by muscular action, and with separation of the fragments. I have seen an example of this, as have also Malgaigne,[2] Demarquay,[3]

[1] Malgaigne, Journal de Chirurgie, t. 1er, p. 201 ; and Traité des Fractures, p. 751.
[2] Demarquay, Gazette des Hôpitaux, 1866, p. 523.
[3] Malgaigne, Gazette des Hôpitaux, 1853, p. 312.

and M. Trélat.[1] Now, if the second fracture should give the same results as the first, the patient would be really infirm. With one bad patella and a good one upon the opposite side, the functions are well enough re-established, as I told you; but with two bad patellæ the weakness is very much greater. The walk is uncertain, needs artificial support, and cannot be long continued.

The patient whom I treated in 1869, and who is now forty years old, had had his right patella fractured nine years before. There remained, after treatment by the dextrine bandage, a separation of from one to one and a half inches, and very little or no intermediate fibrous substance. The left patella was broken in June, 1869, in consequence of a mis-step and a fall backwards. The separation was more than three-quarters of an inch before the treatment. At the end of a fortnight we treated him, Dr. Philippeaux and I, by means of an apparatus invented by the former which resembled in some points Fontan's and Vallette's. The fragments were kept almost in contact, but the pressure occasioned sometimes so much pain, especially at night, that the patient turned the screw and allowed the separation to be reproduced, tightening it up again the next day. This apparatus remained in place for seventy-eight days, at the end of which time we removed it, hoping that the intermediate substance had become solid. The patient remained in bed fifteen days longer with the leg raised upon an inclined plane; commenced to sit up on the ninety-third day, and to walk with crutches, still without bending the knee, on the one-hundredth day. Little by little the fragments separated by the lengthening of the intermediate substance which was too soft to resist the action of the quadriceps. This separation finally amounted to one and a quarter inches, the patient could walk only with a cane and slowly, go up and down stairs with difficulty, and could not take long walks.

These consecutive fractures of the patella are not so frequent that we are authorized to believe them due to a peculiar predisposition of the subject, or to the insecurity of the walk, and the exposure to falls after the first fracture, rather than to chance. But in any case there is no harm in remembering the possibility of the fact in making the prognosis and in choosing the method of treatment.

Treatment.—How shall we treat this patient?

We have to distinguish two periods: a first, of from fifteen to twenty days, during which we have to occupy ourselves only with the arthritis and articular effusion; and a second, during which, the inflammation having gone down and the effusion having diminished or disappeared, we may think of some apparatus for bringing the fragments into contact.

1st. For the first period, the patient will be kept in bed with his foot raised as high as possible, so as to relax the quadriceps femoris; for that purpose we might use simply large cushions of chaff. But on these cushions it is probable that the knee would soon flex a little. A resisting surface, to prevent, or at least to greatly diminish this

---

[1] Trélat, Gazette des Hôpitaux, 1862, p. 523.

flexion, is necessary. We might follow the example of Gerdy, and place a chair in the bed, so that its back, covered with a cushion, could support the leg. I have sometimes used this, and would do so again if I did not have other means at my disposal. I gave it up because the chair takes up too much room and troubles the patient, and also because it happens quite often that the heel sinks into the interval between two of the rungs so as to produce the flexion of the knee which we are seeking to avoid. Still the limb might be placed in a trough and then rested on the back of the chair.

Desault recommended a long posterior splint and an appropriate cushion. This splint extended from the middle of the thigh to beyond the foot; a long cushion of chaff was interposed between it and the skin, and it was kept in place by a roller bandage. But this bandage has the double disadvantage of getting loose too soon, which permits a lateral displacement of the splint and consequently a flexion of the knee, and of masking the injured region. This might be avoided by fixing the splint with three long bands of diachylon rolled about the thigh and the upper and lower parts of the leg. But diachylon easily irritates the skin and causes erythema with itching, and for that reason I do not like to use it.

I prefer an inclined plane, made like a trough, which I have made by any carpenter, to suit the size of the patient and the dimensions of the limb. Our patient will be placed upon a plane of this kind, by which the knee will be kept extended and the quadriceps relaxed. Poultices sprinkled with lead-water will be placed every morning and evening upon the knee. As the articulation is greatly distended by the effusion, we may be tempted to make a puncture, as Professor Jarjavay recommended and did several times for traumatic effusions in the knee without fracture. I have not thus far been a partisan of his operation, for here the inflammation is more intense than in simple contusions, and there would be reason to fear that puncture might cause it to become suppurative. Now, suppuration of this large articulation is too dangerous for us to expose the patient to it.

2d. For the second, I shall have to choose between two methods of treatment: simple elevation, or a uniting apparatus.

I understand perfectly that surgeons, who, like myself, have been struck with the rarity of recoveries without separation, have proposed to treat fracture of the patella by simple elevation of the limb. This is the advice which Valentin[1] and Sabatier[2] gave.

I would willingly adopt this method, which has the advantage of avoiding the constrictions and painful pressures of most bandages, if I could be sure of curing my patient without separation. But from what I have already told you, we have at least one chance in eight or ten of obtaining, by means of a uniting apparatus, a better result, that is to say, a very short and solid intermediate substance, and consequently a more prompt recovery and a complete restoration of the functions of the limb. It is all the wiser to take this chance

[1] Valentin, Histoire Critique de la Chirurgie Moderne, 1772.
[2] Sabatier, Mémoires de l'Académie des Sciences, 1783.

because we can reduce the pain to almost nothing by multiplying the precautions and care.

It now remans to choose a uniting apparatus.

A great many have been invented. I counted fifty from an interesting memoir by Dr. Bérenger Féraud.[1] Do not wonder at this abundance, gentlemen; it is explained by the difficulty which has always existed to obtain a good result, and by the eagerness to explain this difficulty by the insufficiency of the treatment; whereas a large, the largest, part should be attributed to the anatomical and physiological conditions of which I have spoken, and which no apparatus can completely suppress. The uniting means meet satisfactorily one important indication, that of bringing the fragments together and overcoming the action of the triceps; but while doing it they produce pain which causes the knee to bend instinctively, and thus re-establishes a certain degree of separation, which is one of the causes of non-consolidation. And then, whatever may be the patience of the patient, the apparatus cannot be kept long enough in place for the intermediate substance, at the time of its removal, to be solid enough to resist the traction exerted by the quadriceps. We succeed, as I told you, only when the subject is one of the few in which this solidity is promptly acquired.

Which one shall we choose?

I leave out first all completely closed bands which hide the injured region from view, and I advise you not to use them unless you find yourselves absolutely unable to procure the rather more complicated means of which I am about to speak. For whether it is a roller bandage with a double headed compress above the patella, and another one below perforated to receive the ends of the upper one, the bandage which you know under the name of *the uniting bandage of transverse wounds*, or whether it is a roller bandage with crossed compresses placed above the upper fragment and below the lower one, you will always have this disadvantage, that if you do not tighten sufficiently over the knee the fragments will not be brought near enough together, and if you do tighten sufficiently you will have a painful compression. On the other hand, the apparatus soon loosens and the displacement is reproduced. It is in vain that you renew it every day or every second day; if you have taken care, by making it only moderately tight, not to cause pain, you allow the separation to be reproduced to a certain extent. Of course, if the roller bandages are used they must be accompanied by Desault's posterior splint and elevation of the limb. These two adjuncts correct the insufficiency of the method by at least relaxing the quadriceps and extending the knee.

Immovable closed apparatuses, made with dextrine, plaster, or silicate of potash, and applied about the fifteenth or twentieth day, when the articular swelling has gone down, have been much employed recently. These bandages are inferior to the preceding ones for the following reasons: during the first few days they keep the fragments

---

[1] Bérenger-Féraud, Revue de Thérapeutique Medico-chirurgicale, 1868, p. 481.

well together, then they grow loose because the compression diminishes the volume of the muscles, and as soon as this diminution commences the upper fragment is drawn upwards by the quadriceps. If
you employ an immovable bandage do not forget to place a posterior
splint between its layers and keep the foot elevated.

I give the preference to open uniting apparatuses, that is to say, to
those which leaving the patella uncovered enable us to see if the
separation is corrected or not, if the skin is excoriated, and to modify
the situation of the pieces according to the results of this examination.
These apparatuses are of recent invention, and will meet the indication of bringing the fragments together. But I establish a distinction
between those which have to be made by a workman, and those which
the surgeon can easily make himself.

In the large cities this distinction is of little use, since we can easily
obtain the things we need; but it is not so in the country. Of course
if fractures of the patella were frequent we might always have at our
disposal one or the other of the uniting instruments which I am about
to mention. But these fractures are rare; a busy practitioner will
hardly see two a year, many will not see more than one or two in
three years. Now it would always happen, if you kept the instrument on hand, that it would be rusty and would not work when you
had need of it. Undoubtedly the remedy would be easy, for you
would always have the time to have it repaired, or even to have a
new one made during the fifteen or twenty days of the inflammatory
period; but what is the use of having this trouble if these manufac-
tured apparatuses do not give any better results than those which you
make yourself? And that is just what happens.

I. Among the uniting instruments I will mention Malgaigne's
hooks, the modification in their use proposed by M. U. Trélat, Vallette's instrument, and Fontan's.

1st. Malgaigne's hooks (Fig. 12) which I now show you, and
which it is sufficient to see to understand, are composed of two pieces

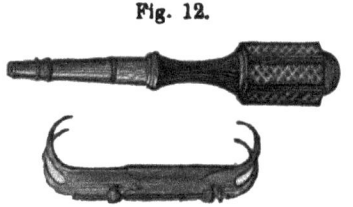

Fig. 12.

which can be moved along one another
by means of a screw. Each piece
ends in two hooks which are implanted
above and below the fragments, traversing the tendon of the quadriceps
and the ligamentum patellæ. After
having been properly implanted, the
two pieces are brought nearer by
means of the screw and thus the frag-
ments are held together. If the patient suffers too much it is loosened;
if, after a few days, separation is reproduced, it is again tightened.

If I intended to advise you to use this instrument I should enter
into longer details upon the manner of applying it, upon the difficulty
of properly implanting the upper hooks, upon the considerable effort
which is needed to do so, upon the pain of the first hours, upon the
tolerance which is afterwards established, upon the possibility of
phlegmonous and consecutive lymphangitis, of which I have had an

example, and even upon that of an arthritis, like the one which I find reported in the *Union Médicale*.[1]

But I do not dwell upon it for two reasons.

First, the hooks, as applied by Malgaigne, because they traverse the skin offered many disadvantages, and were very disagreeable to the patients; they could not remain in place long enough for the consolidation to take place. They were applied on the fifteenth or twentieth day, and had to be removed by the fiftieth, and often sooner, because they held no longer; now at this period, as I have told you, the intermediate substance is not solid except in very exceptional cases. Consequently this gives the patient pain and annoyance without any profit.

Secondly, if you wish to use the hooks, you can now do so without traversing the skin, thus suppressing most of the disadvantages of Malgaigne's original method. For this we use Prof. Trélat's modifications.

2d. *M. U. Trélat's Method.*[2]—Dip in boiling water two pieces of gutta-percha five inches long, two and a half inches wide at one end and one and a quarter at the other. Apply one of them above, the other below the patella, modelling them exactly upon the anterior and lateral faces of the limb and upon the patella while the leg is completely extended. Then apply compresses dipped in cold water to

Fig. 13.

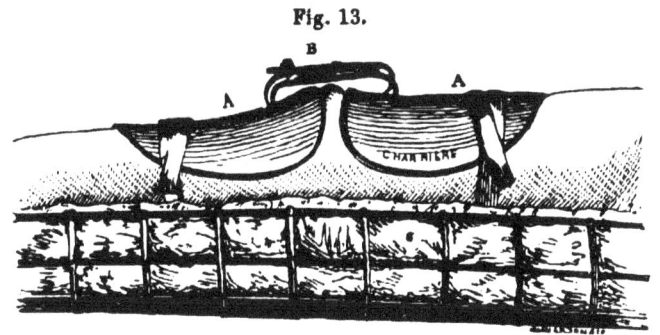

Trélat's apparatus for fracture of the patella.

harden the gutta-percha, and when it has lost its softness plunge it into a basin of cold water. Then while an assistant holds the fragments together, the surgeon places one of these pieces above the upper fragment, and fastens it there with a strip of diachylon long enough to go thrice around the limb. The same is done for the lower fragment. It only remains to implant the hooks in each of these plates without going through to the skin, and to screw together the two pieces of the instrument, thus bringing together the two pieces of the patella near to one another.

It cannot be denied that this modification is ingenious, but is it

[1] Union Médicale, 18 December, 1871.
[2] Trélat, Note sur le Traitement des Fractures de la Rotule par un Nouvel Appareil (Bulletin Thérapeutique, 1862, tome lxiii. p. 447).

not also a little illusory?   Does not the upper plate slide over the
fragment without pushing it along?   Is there no reason to fear that
the hard gutta-percha may cause excoriations and eschars?   I feared
so, and for that reason I have not used it.   It is true that I was also
turned from it by the preference which I gave to apparatuses made
with vulcanized India-rubber, which had been proposed at about the
same time, and which seemed to me to offer more security.

3d. *Fontan's Apparatus* (Fig. 14), *and Vallette's (of Lyons)* (Fig. 15).—
I shall show you these without describing them.   They are more
complicated than the preceding ones, but both of them meet very
well the main indication.   Vallette's has the disadvantage of breaking
the skin.   Fontan's does not do that, but by the pressure it exerts it
may cause eschars, consequently it needs to be carefully watched,
especially when the skin is fine and thin, as in women.

Fig. 14.

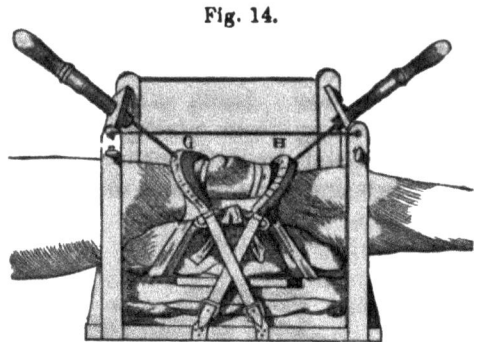

Fontan's apparatus for fracture of the patella.

In my opinion these are not superior to Malgaigne's and Trélat's,
and they are inferior to those of Morel-Lavallée and Laugier; and
therefore I have not used them and advise you also not to.

Fig. 15.

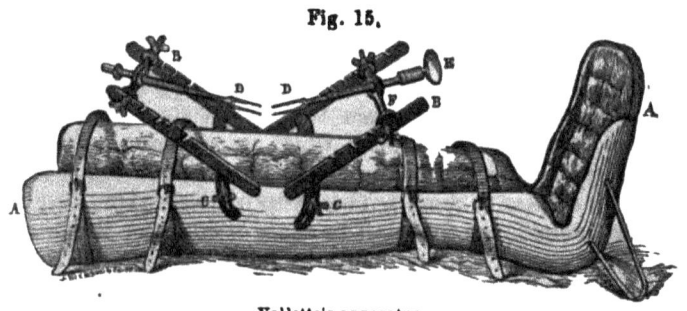

Vallette's apparatus.

II. Among the uniting apparatuses which leave the patella uncovered and which the surgeon can make for himself, I first mention
Mayor's;[1] which consisted of a wire trough upon the sides of which
were attached four non-elastic well-padded bands, two above and two

---

[1] Mayor, Gazette Médicale, p. 184.

below the knee. The limb being placed in the trough, the two upper bands are brought over and crossed above the upper edge of the patella and tied together on the side, and the two lower ones are crossed below the lower edge. The bands, thus tightened, ought to keep the fragments together. But to make it still surer three ribbons are sewed to each of the transverse bands and tied together, each upper one with a lower one, so as to draw the transverse bands nearer together, and with them the fragments. Morel-Lavallée's apparatus, well described by M. Bosia,[1] differs from Mayor's in this, that the transverse bands above and below the patella are made of India-rubber webbing, like that of suspenders, and that these bands, instead of crossing above and below the patella, cross on the edge and, at the same time, the anterior face of the fragments, so as to prevent them from tipping. Their action is also completed by the same vertical bands.

4th. *Laugier's Method: Oblique pressure by means of two rubber rings.*—In the two preceding apparatuses the fragments were kept in place by pressure perpendicular to the axis of the limb, applied above and below the patella, and by parallel pressure. Professor Laugier[2] had the idea of using two vulcanized rubber rings which, placed obliquely, would press, by their elasticity alone, each fragment towards the other. The apparatus (Fig. 16) is arranged in the following way:—

Fig. 16.

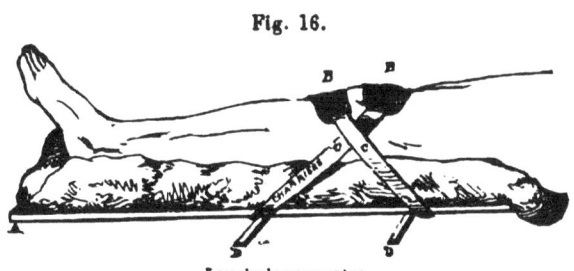

Laugier's apparatus.

The limb is placed upon a board covered with a thick cushion. The board and the cushion reach an inch or two beyond the leg on each side. Two cross-pieces are fastened to the board, one of them three inches above, the other three inches below the patella. The board itself lies upon a cushion as long as the leg, the lower end of which is much higher than the other. The limb is placed upon the cushion, and two pieces of gutta-percha, after having been dipped into boiling water, are moulded upon the upper and lower ends of the patella. Then one of the rubber rings, in the form of a flat ribbon, is passed over the leg and the board and stretched from the lower cross-piece to the piece of gutta-percha which is over the upper fragment of the patella. The other ring is stretched from the upper

[1] Bosia, Gazette des Hôpitaux, 1860, p. 413.
[2] This apparatus has been described by M. Gaujot (Arsenal de la Chirurgie Contemporaine, tome ler, p. 246), and by M. Dubreuil (Gazette des Hôpitaux), 1869, p. 433).

cross-piece to the lower fragment. As the rings have to be stretched to take this position, their elasticity tends to draw the pieces of gutta-percha and, through them, the fragments together.

I have used this apparatus twice; but fearing lest the hard gutta-percha might cause pain, excoriate the skin, and produce eschars, I substituted for it two cotton pads. In one case the result was excellent. In the other the separation reappeared when the apparatus, which had remained in place for forty-five days, was removed. In both patients I found that the pressure was sometimes very painful, and I had to allow them to remove the rings for a few moments and then replace them. I also found that the pressure was not sufficient, and I had to put more cotton under the rings to bring the fragments together.

To remedy these disadvantages, and to give the limb a greater and more certain elevation, I modified Laugier's method, for a private patient, in the following manner:—

I had the strong inclined plane, of which I have already spoken, made by a neighbouring carpenter, and had six hooks placed on each side, three turned towards the thigh, three towards the foot. I then made two rolls of cotton enveloped in coarse cloth, and sewed loosely on them two tubes of very elastic vulcanized rubber, to each end of which was tied a stout string. The limb being laid upon the inclined plane, I placed one of these rolls over the upper fragment, and while an assistant pressed the latter as near to the other fragment as possible, I stretched the tube by drawing on the strings and then fastened them to one of the lower hooks. I then placed the other roll below the lower fragment and fastened its strings to the upper hooks.

By this means I could modify the pressure at will, increase it when I found separation, and diminish it, without removing it entirely, when the pain was too great. After a few days I found that, notwithstanding the great pressure, the separation reappeared and the fragments tended to tip upwards. I then completed the apparatus by passing two elastic tubes longitudinally in front of the patella and hooking them to the oblique ones. In this way the fragments were kept exactly together. But I often had to yield to the entreaties of the patient, who suffered very much, and allow the vertical tubes to be removed for several hours at a time and replaced as soon as the pain was over.

Pain and eschars are always to be feared with these apparatuses, as with all those that exert a strong and steady pressure upon the same surface. It thus becomes necessary to watch carefully and to loosen the cords whenever the pain becomes great and the skin reddens. This last patient, who was a young man of 23 years, is one of those in whom I think I obtained bony consolidation. At the end of sixty days he walked without a cane, descended the staircases easily, and, when lying down or standing, could raise his foot without bending the knee. The separation, which at the beginning of the treatment was three-quarters of an inch, was only about one-eighth of an inch, and the substance which filled it was so solid that transverse movements communicated to the upper part of the patella were easily transmitted to the lower part.

In short, the two best results which I have obtained in treatment of fractures of the patella with separation, I have owed to apparatuses in which vulcanized rubber played the principal part, and that is why I give it the preference. Before that I had often used bands dipped in collodion.

I do not refuse to admit that other methods might give equally good results, but it seems to me that with vulcanized rubber, which can be so easily procured, the apparatuses have a simplicity of construction which should cause their adoption by every one.

In any case, do not forget, gentlemen, that, whatever may be the mode of treatment, recovery with separation will always be the exception, because the quadriceps will most often end by overcoming the still insufficient resistance of the intermediate substance, as soon as the six or eight weeks, beyond which it is very difficult to have the treatment borne, have passed, and the fragments have to be left to themselves.

To recapitulate, the treatment of our patient will be directed as follows:—

For about a fortnight I shall keep the foot elevated and apply poultices; during the following thirty days I shall use the bandage of vulcanized rubber; after which, still keeping the patient in bed and the foot raised, I shall see if the fragments separate. If they do not separate, I shall try to keep him in bed until the sixtieth day. If they do separate, I shall propose to the patient to apply the rubber bands for another month, which would give us in all eighty or ninety days of confinement to the bed, and in case he should not willingly accept the proposition, I should not urge it very strongly, for I am not at all certain that consolidation of this bone, if not obtained in forty-five days, can be obtained in sixty-five. Still, the attempt may be made.

After this period of confinement to the bed, the duration of which I cannot previously determine, I shall allow the patient to get up, and give him crutches.

I shall then occupy myself with the stiffness of the knee; if it is very great, I shall order moderate movements of flexion and extension to be made every morning and evening, and shall advise the patient himself to make some; in addition I shall prescribe massage and sulphur douches. If it is not very great, I shall tell the patient to execute movements of flexion himself, but with moderation.

There is one danger here which you foresee and which must be avoided. The intermediate substance, whatever its length and resistance, must be very carefully treated at this time. Already drawn upon by the tonicity alone or by the voluntary contractions of the triceps, it would be still more so by a flexion carried a little too far. Care must then be taken not to go beyond a moderate limit.

Then, when, fifteen or twenty days later, walking becomes a little easier, is possible, for example, with a cane, I shall advise the patient to support the knee while walking with a small roller bandage cover-

ing the lower third of the thigh and the upper third of the leg, and
containing a posterior wooden splint. This dressing is intended to
prevent a too great involuntary flexion, which might cause rupture
of the intermediate substance or renew the arthritis; it is also intended
to make walking easier and to allow a little beneficial exercise, and
is to be worn only while the patient is walking.

This precaution will be taken for only five or six weeks if we find
that the intermediate substance is solid, and if the separation has not
increased. After that I shall prescribe the use of a rubber knee-cap
during the day.

On the other hand, in case the separation should increase, and the
knee, notwithstanding the disappearance of the arthritis, should
remain very weak, the patient might use one of the more complicated
knee-caps which by an arrangement of elastics or springs assist the
action of the quadriceps, or may even supply its place entirely.

Whichever may be the apparatus used, you may be sure that after
a few months it will be no longer necessary, and the knee will have
recovered enough strength and solidity to no longer need any help.

III. *Sprain of the callus and appearance of relapse in a patient who
had a fracture of the right patella a year ago.*—Here, gentlemen, is a
woman whom I treated a year ago for fracture of the right patella,
with bands dipped in collodion.

There remained, in spite of all my care, a separation of three-fifths
of an inch, independent mobility of the fragments, and inability to
raise the foot from the ground while keeping the knee extended.
Flexion of the knee had not recovered its full extent, not going beyond a right-angle; nevertheless walking was easy, and I had advised
the patient to wear a knee-cap, but she had soon neglected its use.
Yesterday she made a mis-step, fell, and felt a slight crack and
pain in the knee; she was, however, able to take a few steps, and
then, thinking she had again broken the patella, she had herself taken
to the hospital.

You may have noticed an ecchymosis on the anterior and inner
portion of the right knee, and a very moderate swelling without
appreciable effusion in the articulation. Movements are painful;
flexion and extension are possible however, but the foot cannot be
raised from the bed.

Let us not here commit the error which I have sometimes seen
committed, that of believing in a complete rupture of the intermediate
fibrous substance, and the reproduction of a fracture, and thence
conclude that the patient ought to be subjected to a treatment of two
or three months in order to re-establish the broken callus.

Instead of an iterative fracture this is simply a sprain with very
limited rupture of the new tissue which unites the fragments, and it
is because the bloodvessels of this tissue are numerous and fragile
that a considerable ecchymosis has been produced by a very limited
fibrous rupture. I say that this rupture is not complete, and even
that it is very small, because the separation is not greater than when I
last examined the patient, and because I still feel between the fragments a certain thickness of tissue which prevents my touching the
condyles of the femur.

I also base the opinion upon two analogous cases, both in women, which the physicians first consulted supposed to be iterative fractures. As I had treated the cases fifteen months before, and as I found the parts in the same anatomical condition in which I had left them, I declared that it was only a sprain, and that the patients would be able to walk in a day or two, just as before the accident. The events justified the prediction.

In the present patient the lesion is the same, sprain of the fibrous callus, probably rather vascular, of the patella. The patient will remain three or four days in bed with poultices sprinkled with spirits of camphor, then she will replace her knee-cap and be able to walk.

The ecchymosis will gradually disappear, and furnishes no special indication.

LECTURE XX.

SIMPLE FRACTURES OF THE SHAFT OF THE FEMUR.

Simple fracture of the shaft of the femur—Commemoratives—Attitude of the patients —Deformity—Apparent shortening, real shortening—Abnormal mobility—Double manœuvre to seek it—Crepitation—Exact point of the fracture—Consecutive arthritis of the knee, of the hip-joint—Overlapping irreducible by the bands and simple bandages—Employment of chloroform—Scultet apparatus—Continuous extension—Reasons why it is not generally used in practice, its utility in certain cases—Preference given to Hennequin's apparatus.

GENTLEMEN : We have at this moment in the wards several patients affected with fracture of the shaft of the femur. I take the oppor-tunity to show you the peculiarities presented by this lesion, which is quite common in practice.

I take as types the patients lying in Nos. 5, 11, and 46. All three represent their injury as caused by external violence. The first was run over by an omnibus, the others fell from a high place. Only one of them heard a crack at the time of the accident; the other two do not remember the circumstances of their fall. Neither was able to rise after the accident, and all were brought to the hospital by their comrades on stretchers.

You saw them lying in their beds, each one on his back and a little on one side, and they have kept that position since they were admitted; it is the one in which they suffer least. Raising the bed-clothing, we see a slight bending of the body, towards the right side in No. 5, towards the left side in the others. I told them to lie straighter, squarely upon the back ; they were not able to do so, and the attempts which they made caused much pain. I asked them to raise the heel of the injured limb from the bed. This attempt also remained unsuccessful and caused renewed pain, while the uninjured limb executed the little manœuvre perfectly.

You noticed how the shape of the injured thigh differed from that of the other one, how it is gathered up and twisted about its axis. You also saw that the foot, as well as the leg, lay on its outer side. Here then are two signs of fracture: deformity, and outward rotation of the limb.

On a superficial examination our eyes detect only a slight shortening; but if we stretch a string from the spine of one ilium to that of the other, we see that its direction is oblique with reference to the axis of the body, and that the iliac spine on the injured side is sensibly lowered, whence we conclude that, although the shortening seems slight, it is really greater than it seems.

Then stretching the string from the anterior-superior spine of the ilium to the external tuberosity of the femur, and then to the external malleolus, and then making the same measurements upon the other side, we find that the injured limb of No. 5 is shortened at least an inch and a quarter; then measuring both limbs from the spine of the ilium to the internal malleolus, we find the same difference; there is then a very considerable real shortening, and as the patient assures us that he did not limp before his accident, this sign has a great value.

I then sought for abnormal mobility by two manœuvres. You saw that one consisted in raising the heel and the leg with one hand whilst the other was placed transversely over the middle and anterior portion of the thigh. Then giving a lateral movement to the limb with the first hand, I saw that the lower part of the thigh moved with the leg, while the upper part remained immovable, and I felt with my second hand that no movement which might have escaped detection by my eyes was transmitted to the upper part, and that the hinge or centre of movement of the movable part was a little below the middle of the femur. The same manœuvre executed upon No. 11 showed us that his fracture was situated at the centre of the bone, and in No. 46 the femur was broken high up, just below the great trochanter (Malgaigne's sub-trochanteric fracture).

To seek mobility by the second manœuvre, I passed my hand, by depressing the bed, under the injured thigh, and then raised it a little. By this movement the thigh was bent at the point of fracture, forming a projecting angle in front, while the same experiment repeated upon the uninjured leg did not give this result.

During these two manœuvres I had also felt crepitation. I am therefore perfectly sure of the lesion; our patients have fractures of the thigh, and it is not necessary to prolong the examination to make the diagnosis.

Our three patients have presented the same symptoms; but the prominence formed by the overriding of the two fragments of the femur seemed to us much higher in No. 11 than in No. 5, and much higher still in No. 46. In all the pain is greatest over the point of this prominence.

I have called your attention especially to the deformity of the thigh; but the knee also is increased in size. It is appreciable by the eye and by direct measurement. Passing a string around the condyles of the femur and the middle of the patella, I find that in one patient the circumference of the knee upon the injured side is two-fifths of an inch greater than on the other, and in the other two patients the difference is three-fifths. Suspecting the presence of liquid in the articulation I grasped both its sides with my left hand, a little above, and with my right hand, a little below the patella, and then without changing the position of the hands I brought my right index finger upon the centre of the patella which yielded under the pressure and was forced backwards against the condyles of the femur. During this manœuvre I distinctly felt the other fingers raised up, which could be due only to the presence of liquid. Our three patients then have a considerable effusion within the knee-joint, and it is greatest in the one, No. 5, whose fracture is the lowest. Perhaps you think that this lesion is due to a concomitant contusion of the knee produced by the violence which caused the fracture.

It is not so; first, you find upon their knees no sign of a contusion, and then, our internes, who saw them when they were admitted yesterday, an hour or two after the accident, will tell you that the effusion did not then exist, and it is very probable that you will find that No. 11's effusion, which is very small to-day, will increase considerably to morrow and the following days, with more pain on pressure.

It is too evident that the articular lesion which has so soon followed these fractures of the femur has not been caused by the prolonged immobility which Tessier, of Lyons, has indicated too absolutely as the cause of consecutive arthritis. It is the consequence of an early arthritis which might have been due to a concomitant contusion of the knee, but which, in these cases, seems to me to have been caused by the extension to the synovial membrane of some of the lesions belonging to the injury of the bone. In an autopsy of a recent fracture which I made in December, 1868, I found an infiltration of blood which, starting from the interfragmentary space, extended almost into the sub-synovial tissue of the knee, although the fracture was in the middle third. During our late war we had occasion to notice this same sub-synovial infiltration of blood, which M. Berger, Demonstrator of Anatomy, has further studied and confirmed by experiments upon animals, in a work not yet published.

I cannot say whether this dropsical arthritis, occurring upon these three patients soon after the accident, and which I have found during the last twelve years upon nearly all the patients whom I have treated for fracture of the thigh, is always the consequence of an infiltration of blood into the sub-synovial connective tissue, or whether it is not due in certain cases exclusively or principally to the propagation towards the articulation of the violent phlegmasia starting from the seat of the fracture. I only call your attention to this early arthritis, because, without being dangerous, without interfering with consolidation, it explains the principal origin of the articular rigidities which are one of the principal causes of the trouble in the movements after fractures of the thigh.

I looked to see if pressure was painful and if there was an appreciable swelling over the articulation of the hip. I found nothing there, and cannot say that there is a coxo-femoral as well as a femoro-tibial arthritis.

Moreover, it is to be noticed that the articulation placed above the fracture, in this bone as in others, is more rarely affected with consecutive inflammation than is the articulation below. I do not say that it is never affected, for I have found in several patients after fracture of the thigh a prolonged stiffness of the hip which indicated the consequences of an arthritis. I only say that this complication is not common, while arthritis of the knee is almost constant.

We noticed at first sight that the thigh was gathered up on itself like a leech, and that it seemed to swell out forwards. Let us try to interpret this disposition and to determine what ought to be the reciprocal position of the fragments. It is clearly understood that the fragments have undergone a rotary displacement, for the leg and the knee lie upon their outer side, and an angular displacement for the centre of the thigh is very prominent. Moreover, since the limb is shortened, there is a third kind of displacement, that is, an overlapping or longitudinal displacement together with a transverse displacement. Shortening exists always in the adult, and can be explained, as our predecessors understood, by the obliquity of the fracture; but it is also found in cases where the fracture, instead of being purely oblique, is toothed, with or without fissure, described by Gerdy as spiral fracture. It is produced when the fragments, whatever may be the direction of the fracture, no longer meet one another directly, and it is due to the action of all the muscles of the thigh which draw the lower fragment upwards and inwards, and sometimes backwards, causing it to overlap the upper one more or less, and in any case, to an extent which will increase during the following days, as it will be easy for you to see in these patients. At the same time the upper fragment is drawn upwards and outwards by the psoas. We found the shortening in Nos. 5 and 11 to be an inch and a quarter, and in No. 46 it was about two inches and a quarter. This difference is due to the latter fracture being trochanteric, that is to say, situated much higher than in the two other cases, and to the upper fragment being drawn much more forcibly forwards and outwards by the psoas, while the lower one is drawn upwards, inwards, and backwards. In this case then there is not only overlapping, but also great angular displacement which increases the shortening.

The *prognosis* in these cases is not bad, in the sense that they will recover, but *they will probably not recover without shortening.* You still see in our wards a fourth patient who has been there for seventy-five days. He is beginning to walk, but his right thigh is two inches shorter than the left. Well, there is reason to fear that, notwithstanding all our care, those of whom I am speaking to-day will retain a shortening, and it is even probable that this shortening will be a little greater at the end of the treatment than it was after the limb had been set. That unfortunately is the rule in fractures of the thigh in the adult.

It is true that it will be corrected in part by the instinctive lowering of the pelvis, and in part by wearing a heel a little higher upon the injured side, and that ultimately the deformity will scarcely be perceived.

Does that mean, in a word, that these patients will be lame?

Here, gentlemen, we must distinguish between the primitive or temporary, and the definitive results.

As for the first, there is no doubt; after the seventy-five or eighty days of confinement to the bed which are generally necessary for the consolidation of fractures of the shaft of the femur in adults, we shall allow the patients to walk. But they will only be able to do so with the aid of crutches, which they will continue to use for two, three, or four months. Three principal causes will prevent their doing otherwise; these are:—

1st. The difference in the length of the limbs, of which we have just spoken.

2d. The feebleness of the muscles resulting from the prolonged inaction, and from the slight atrophy which broken limbs always undergo, as I often have occasion to tell you (see page 71).

3d. The persistence, in the chronic condition, of the dropsical synovitis of which I spoke a moment ago. For if this synovitis resembles the others of this kind which I have seen, it will not be of short duration, as it is in children. It will continue during the whole time of treatment, and for a so much longer time thereafter as the patients are older. Thus I expect it to last much longer in No. 11, who is 56 years old, than in the two others, one of whom is 35, the other 41 years old.

After having walked upon crutches for a time, which will vary, according to the subjects, from two to six months, our patients will begin to use a cane, and will certainly limp very distinctly for several months. I estimate at about a year the time that is necessary for the walk to become what it can be and will be during the rest of the life. It is at the end of that time that we shall be able to determine what I called a moment ago the definitive results. I expect them to vary in these three cases.

No. 5, who is 35 years old, and whose fracture is in the middle of the femur, will undoubtedly limp very little, perhaps not at all, notwithstanding the shortening of from one to one and a half inches, which I presume he will retain, and this absence of limping will be due to this, that his muscles, although remaining slightly atrophied, will have recovered enough energy of contraction to correct the disadvantage resulting from the shortness of the lever. It will also be due to the fact that this shortness will not be excessive, and that the knee will have recovered all its movements, the synovial membrane not having retained any consecutive rigidity.

In No. 11 I expect the lameness to be more distinct, not on account of the shortening, which I presume will be about the same as in No. 5, but because he is older. For I fear that the muscles, after their prolonged inactivity and in spite of the integrity of their innervation, will not recover their former contractile energy; and I am also less certain about the consequences of the arthritis; for experience has taught me that subacute, spontaneous arthritis, passing to the chronic

condition, as arthritis following fractures almost always does, is
followed by a synovial rigidity of which we see frequent examples
in fractures of the lower extremity of the radius. Now these rigidities,
as I have often told you and shall tell you often again, are more
marked and permanent as the subjects are older.

Finally, in No. 46, the one who has the sub-trochanteric fracture,
I expect, as a definitive result, a very marked lameness, partly on
account of muscular weakness, partly on account of a certain degree
of synovial rigidity which may remain, but chiefly on account of the
shortening which is now two and a half inches, and may ultimately
be three or three and a half, since, during the whole inflammatory
period, that is to say, so long as the fragments are not united by a
substance possessed of a certain solidity, the muscular tonicity will
continue to act and will constantly increase the shortness.

My fear will not be justified in this patient if I can obtain by
continuous extension a notable diminution of the shortening.

But I argue on the supposition, which may become a reality, that
the apparatus for making extension will not be supported, or, if supported, will be insufficient.

Treatment.—In these three patients we have to meet the same indications as in all other fractures: make and maintain reduction.

To make the reduction, you saw to what manœuvre I had recourse:
an assistant, placed on the injured side, pressed firmly with both hands
upon the patient's iliac spines so as to fix the pelvis firmly. Another
one, placed at the foot of the bed, grasped the foot as in fractures of
the leg. He first straightened the foot which was rotated outwards,
then by drawing it towards himself he made what is called extension,
while the first assistant made counter-extension. Meanwhile I, standing beside the limb, tried with both hands to correct the deformity,
pressing the upper fragment inwards and the lower fragment outwards.
These two manœuvres caused great pain, and you saw what results
I obtained.

The rotary displacement (rotation of the foot outwards) was perfectly corrected in all three patients. The angular displacement was
also corrected in Nos. 5 and 11, but only imperfectly so in No. 46,
who has the sub-trochanteric fracture, and in whom, as you know,
the angular displacement is much greater on account of the powerful
action of the psoas, which is inserted into the upper fragment and
draws it forwards and outwards, and whose contraction it was impossible for us to overcome entirely.

But in no one of the patients were we able to correct the longitudinal and transverse displacements, displacements closely allied with
one another, or of which the second, at least, is essentially dependent
upon the first. For you understand perfectly that the contact of the
lateral faces of the two fragments can only end when the femur has
recovered its length.

I mention the impossibility of correcting the shortening by the
manœuvre of simple reduction, because many of your classical authors
do not lay sufficient stress upon this impossibility. Some of them
speak of reduction as a thing which always succeeds if properly

made; others intimate that in a certain number of cases the only indication is to correct the angular and rotary displacements, and that nothing is to be done about overriding because it does not exist. This is perhaps true for some children, but it is not exact for adults. In them fracture of the shaft of the femur is always accompanied by overriding or, what amounts to the same thing, shortening or longitudinal displacement, and if in some cases it has not been recognized, it is because the surgeon has not measured the limb and has been deceived by the inclination of the pelvis which makes both legs seem of the same length. Not only is there shortening in fractures of the shaft of the femur in adults, but it cannot be corrected by ordinary simple reduction, such as is made with the hands, according to the indications of the authors, and during the first days which follow the accident.

Can it be afterwards corrected by other means? We shall examine that question in a moment.

But I wished first to formulate, from what has occurred in our three patients and from what I have seen in many others, these propositions: 1st, that the immediate correction of the shortening by the hands alone, and without the aid of anæsthesia, is impossible in most cases, and it is through prudence that I do not say in all cases, of fracture of the thigh in adults; 2d, that if this correction can be obtained early, it is by anæsthesia. It may be obtained tardily and slowly by the prolonged use of continuous extension combined with that of retention, but unfortunately this method encounters difficulties of execution which make us fear we shall not reach the desired end.

I now resume the history of our three patients, and I say that in all three I made the ordinary reduction without obtaining a satisfactory result so far as the shortening was concerned. But there is one of them, No. 5, the youngest of the three, and the one who seemed to me to be the least affected with alcoholism, upon whom you saw me use chloroform the next day and renew the attempt at reduction. A Scultet apparatus, arranged like the one for the leg, but extending from the groin to the foot, had been previously placed below the broken limb, and while an assistant held the foot firmly and was ready to make extension, and another pressed upon the pelvis for counter-extension, the patient was brought under the influence of chloroform with the ordinary precautions, and especially the ordinary intermittences. We had some difficulty to obtain resolution, and it was preceded by a period of great agitation, during which the patient moved the broken limb as freely as the other one, caused the upper fragment to project under the skin, and increased by the violent contraction of his muscles all the displacements with which you are acquainted. Standing on the outer side I had to hold the fracture very firmly with both hands to oppose this powerful muscular action, and you saw, nevertheless, that at certain moments my opposition was overcome, and I was obliged to ask another assistant to help me hold the fragments. Finally quiet was obtained, the muscles became soft, and I made the reduction. I measured the limb rather rapidly,

11

and it seemed to me that there remained barely an eighth of an inch of shortening; I then applied the Scultet apparatus.

In the other two cases I did not have recourse to anæsthesia to make the reduction, and for these reason : one of them, No. 11, is a teamster more than 56 years old, and greatly given to drink; now you know that in such patients muscular resolution is difficult and slow to obtain. It is necessary to give a great deal of chloroform and consequently expose the subjects to the dangers of this agent, dangers which exist especially during the days which follow great traumatic lesions. It is also necessary to pass through a much longer and more intense period of excitation, during which perforation of the skin by the fragments is not impossible. This accident happened to one of my patients in the Hôpital Cochin in 1858. Two of us held the fragments as firmly as possible, but the patient struggled so violently several times that the limb slipped through our hands and a point of the upper fragment pierced the skin. This perforation healed by first intention, thanks to the occlusive dressing immediately applied. But it is none the less true that this possible complication and even the danger of increasing the tearing of the muscles and periosteum during these struggles, necessitates a certain reserve in the use of anæsthesia in cases of this kind, and are even a contra-indication in patients who are rather old and alcoholic.

The other patient, the one with the sub-trochanteric fracture (No. 46), has so much shortening that I could not hope to obtain a permanent diminution of it by means of anæsthesia. The little that I might have obtained would certainly not have lasted, and therefore it was useless to expose the patient to the risks of chloroform.

Let us now examine the second question, that of reduction. How shall these fractures be confined and immobilized, and what precautions shall we have to take during this retention?

For two of the patients, Nos. 5 and 11, the problem is already in great part solved. I have applied the Scultet apparatus, to one of them after having made reduction during anæsthetic sleep, to the other without this preliminary precaution. I took care—after having wrapped the leg in the compresses and bands which form the inside of this apparatus, and after having applied a very long external cushion of chaff which reached from above the crest of the ilium to below the edge of the foot, after having also applied internal and anterior cushions, then the three splints corresponding to these cushions, and after having closed the femoral and tibial portions of the apparatus with the buckled straps—I took care, I say to complete the dressing with a body bandage applied about the pelvis and sewed fast to the outer envelope of the Scultet apparatus, and then placed the patients on the mechanical bed.[1] I shall not use the water-bed unless sores appear on the sacrum and make me fear an eschar.

I have also told the patients not to sit up in bed, to eat while lying down, and to move as little as possible. I shall prescribe in a few days one or two drachms of the phosphate of lime daily.

I shall renew the apparatus every third or fourth day during the

---

[1] See page 83.

first fortnight, and each time that I do so I shall make fresh attempts to overcome the shortening. I do not hope to diminish it very much by these repeated reductions, but I shall at least be able to oppose the increase which tends to take place during the first two or three weeks.

After the twentieth day I shall renew the apparatus only every eighth or tenth day; I shall only have to tighten the outer straps when I find them relaxed.

On the sixtieth day I shall see if any mobility remains, by making with precaution the manœuvres which you saw me employ the first day to detect this sign. If I no longer find mobility I shall leave the limb uncovered and tell the patient to make a few movements of his toes, foot, and knee. I shall myself communicate some from time to time to combat rigidity of the articulations, especially of the knee. If I still find mobility, I shall reapply the apparatus and leave it, renewing it from time to time, until consolidation is obtained.

At what period will I allow the patients to get out of bed and walk with crutches? I shall wait at least until the eightieth day, and probably until the ninetieth. For one of the things which I fear, and which should be most feared after fracture of the thigh, is the breaking of the callus by a fall, even a very simple one, while walking or standing. I have seen these iterative fractures on the seventieth and seventy-fifth days, in patients who had left their bed too soon, in opposition to my advice, and then it required three months more to get consolidation.

In general, I let the patients get up only after I have demonstrated by several trials the absence of abnormal mobility and the patient's ability to raise the heel five or six inches from the bed without bending the knee.

You will perhaps ask why I have given the preference to the Scultet bandage, with the limb extended; why I did not choose, as has been recommended, and as you have seen me do, the same apparatus with the limb bent upon a double inclined plane; why I do not speak of an immovable bandage, and why I do not use continuous extension for all three of our patients, as I am going to do for the last one of them.

These are my answers:—

1st. As for the Scultet apparatus with the limb in semi-flexion, I recognize in it one advantage, which is that this position of the knee seems to cause a less rebellious arthritis and less consecutive rigidity.

Nevertheless the fact is not yet established by sufficiently numerous observations, to serve as a basis of treatment; and, on the other side, I have often seen this position of semi-flexion cause intolerable pain in the calf of the leg, so that the inclined plane had to be removed and the limb placed in extension. Indeed, in two of my patients, this compression of the calf of the leg was followed by obliteration of the popliteal vein and painful œdema of the leg.

I know that this obnoxious compression can be avoided by using, instead of the wooden inclined plane, one made with bags of chaff, as Dupuytren and Sanson did. But I saw that these bags yielded readily, and that to replace them and re-establish the semi-flexion the limb had to be moved three or four times every day, which is a disadvantage. And as finally consecutive rigidity is not completely prevented by semi-flexion, and as that which follows extension disappears, I do not see any real utility in adopting semi-flexion as an absolute rule.

2d. I do not intend to employ an immovable apparatus, because it would no more prevent shortening than will the one which we have chosen, and because it would perhaps permit the reproduction of angular displacement. For sixty to eighty days of immobility are necessary. If the limb was enveloped in a plaster, silicated, or dextrinated bandage, the application would be made by the fifteenth or twentieth day; for, if applied later, it would be of no use. It would have to remain in place for from forty to fifty days. Now during this time the limb would diminish in size, a gap would result, and the fragments, being less well supported, might undergo longitudinal displacement. I much prefer the movable bandage, which I tighten when relaxed, and which I renew entirely from time to time. I thus support the fracture much better, and avoid more surely very vicious consolidations.

3d. Why not an apparatus to make continuous extension? Theoretically, this mode of treatment is reduction, for if we cannot, with our hands and in a single attempt, overcome the resistance of the muscles which produce the shortening, it is logical to hope that this resistance can be conquered by a long-continued mechanical traction. That is the thought which guided Brunninghausen, Desault, Boyer, Baumers, F. Martin, and all the surgeons who, before and since their time, have invented apparatuses for continuous extension for the treatment of fractures of the femur.

Notice this well, gentlemen:—

The idea of continuous extension is very rational; many apparatuses inspired by this idea have been invented. None of them thus far have been able to take definitive rank in practice. From time to time a new one is invented because the inconveniences and insufficiency of the others are recognized.

Whence comes this difficulty of making the practice accord with the theory? It comes from this, that to overcome the very energetic muscular resistance against which they have to contend, these apparatuses for continuous extension have, on the one hand, to permanently exert strong tractions which are in themselves painful, and, on the other hand, to apply the extension and counter-extension at certain parts of the limb where the pressure causes pain, and sometimes eschars. That which has prevented, then, the use of these apparatuses from becoming general is found first in these two results: pain and eschars.

There is also a third reason; in many cases, after having subjected the patients to these inconveniences, the shortening has persisted. Those who have not given close attention, and who have not measured, may have been deceived by a lowering of the pelvis which hid the real shortness; but those who measured have almost always found a shortening of from one to one and a half inches, and have been obliged to recognize that by these sufferings, supported for several weeks, they have barely gained from one-quarter to three-quarters of an inch.

There is also a fourth reason. When the patients are young, the shortening, if not more than one and a half inches, does not make them limp permanently. Why then expose them to the pains of continuous extension? When they are old the shortening will certainly make them limp, but they will also be much less able to bear extension; they will have eschars more easily, and, in consequence, incur greater danger. Is it not better, then, to be satisfied with simple retention, which will leave a little more shortening, but will give more tranquillity to the patient and surgeon?

Such are the reasons, gentlemen, which have prevented, and will long prevent, the use of apparatuses for continuous extension from becoming general in practice.

Fig. 17.

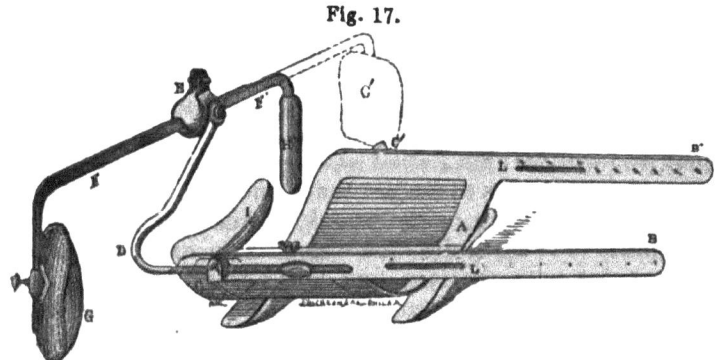

Hennequin's Apparatus. D, bent rod which can be placed on either side of the trough A; E, clasp, through which slide two rods, one of which bears the iliac pad G, the other, the pubic pad H; I, ischiatic pad in the form of a crescent.

But these reasons are not sufficient to cause us to reject them absolutely. I understand why they should try continuous extension in cases where the shortening is very great; but it should be done only on the condition of watching the apparatus attentively, so as to avoid eschars and to diminish as much as possible the pain caused by the tractions. These are the ideas which have guided me in the treatment of our last patient. I might have used Baumer's method, in which counter-extension is made upon the pelvis at the genito-crural fold, or that which is known as the American splint, in which the axilla on the side corresponding to the fracture is used for this purpose; but I preferred the apparatus now more generally used in the Paris hospitals (Fig. 17), which was invented by Dr. Hennequin.[1]

Fig. 18.

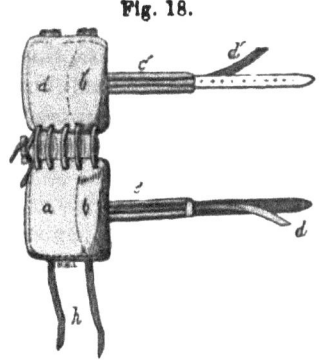

Hennequin's Apparatus a a', band to surround the leg, thickly padded at b b', which corresponds to the condyles of the femur; c c', elastic bands ending in straps perforated with holes; d d', ribbons graduated to show in pounds the amount of traction.

[1] Hennequin, Quelques Considerations sur l'Extension continue et les Douleurs dans la Coxalgie (Archives Générales de Médecine, Dec. 1868, à Pevrier, 1869).

I shall not give you a minute description; it is sufficient to show it to you, and to recall in a few words its principal points and advantages. It consists of a trough in which the thigh rests, allowing the knee to be flexed, the leg being outside the bed and the foot upon a chair.

Counter-extension is made by means of pressure exerted—1st, upon the ischium by a curved pad (I, Fig. 17), attached to the upper part of the trough; 2d, upon the outer iliac fossa by another pad, G; 3d, upon the horizontal ramus of the pubis by another pad, H. The two latter are attached to the rest of the apparatus by two rods sliding through a hinged clasp, E. Counter-extension is made by means of the bracelet represented in Figure 18, which surrounds the thigh, and from which extend two elastic bands, $c\,d$, $c'\,d'$, a sort of artificial muscle, which are attached to buttons on the two long lateral parts of the main apparatus.

I shall apply this apparatus about the twelfth or fifteenth day, after the inflammatory period is ended. If things go on as in three other patients upon whom I have had occasion to employ this mode of treatment, you will see that I shall have to change the situation of the pads several times, so as to render them endurable; that the patient will be tormented by the pains caused by extension; that it will be necessary, from to time, to diminish the traction exerted by the elastic bands; and finally, that the foot and lower part of the leg will become œdematous, notwithstanding the roller bandage which will previously have been placed about them. If the patient is not too sensitive, and if he bears the pain bravely, we shall perhaps succeed in curing him without shortening, or with a shortening of about an inch. But if the pain is intolerable, and if, to diminish it, we are obliged too often to loosen the elastic bands, the result will be less fortunate, and there will remain a shortening of two inches or more. Everything here depends upon the degree of sensibility and energy of the patient; and it is precisely because we find only few who are able to bear the pain caused by this and by every other apparatus for continuous extension, that it cannot be adopted in all cases. Above all, do not try it upon children, women, or old people; for to the pain you might easily add eschars, which would increase the suffering and might be dangerous.

LECTURE XXI.

FRACTURES OF THE NECK OF THE FEMUR.

Two fractures of the neck of the femur in old women—Difficulty of determining upon
what point the fall occurred—Functional and physical symptoms—Impossibility and uselessness of the diagnosis between intra- and extra-capsular fractures—Astley Cooper's error as to the influence of age—Obscurity of the authors
upon the differential signs—Be satisfied with presumptions upon the seat of the
fracture as upon the penetration—Simple treatment in all cases—Indication to
avoid pain—Rejection of apparatuses for continuous extension.

GENTLEMEN: We have at this moment in ward Ste. Catherine two
old women, one of whom was brought to us the day before yesterday,
the other a week ago. Both of them fell while walking, without great
violence.

The first (No. 6), 69 years old, slipped in her room, and, after
several efforts to keep her balance, fell upon the right side.

The second (No. 20), 71 years old, made a misstep in the street and
fell upon her left side.

I asked them particularly what part of their body received the force
of the fall; they answered that it was the side, and indicated with the
hand, the one more especially the hip, the other the hip and buttocks.
But both showed a certain hesitation in it, and said they did not know
very well, but that they thought they fell in such or such a way.

However that may be, neither was able to get up and walk, and
they were brought here upon stretchers.

On examining them we find in both the following symptoms:—

1st. *Functional Symptoms.*—Both suffer when they try to move in
bed. If the hips are raised for the purpose of passing a bed-pan, they
cry out; when not moved they suffer little. The one who has been
here for a week suffered during the first two nights, but scarcely at
all now. The one who was admitted the day before yesterday suffers
a great deal, and had a bad night on account of the pain.

I told them to raise the foot from the bed; neither one was able to
do so. No. 6 took her thigh in both hands and raised it, but at the
same time she bent her knee, and her foot slid along the bed without
being raised above it. No. 20, who suffers more, was able to make
no movement.

Both of them have an imperfectly circumscribed swelling of the
upper part of the thigh; the one who was admitted most recently has
an extensive ecchymosis in the trochanteric region.

2d. *Physical Symptoms.*—I called your attention first to the attitude
of the patients. They were lying upon the back, and a little on the
painful side, and begged earnestly not to have the position changed.
The injured limb was rotated outwards, so that the outer edge of the

foot rested upon the bed, and the heel corresponded to the space between the internal malleolus and the heel of the other foot.

The better to appreciate this attitude, I persuaded the two patients to allow themselves to be placed flat upon their backs, and then I showed you that the rotation of the limb outwards persisted, and that there was also a notable lowering of the pelvis. For, stretching a string from one spine of the ilium to the other, I showed you that its direction was oblique with reference to the median line of the body, the end on the injured side being half an inch lower than a line cross-ing at right angles from the other spine.

Finally, there is in both a shortening which can be seen and meas-ured; it can be seen, because the heel of the injured side is clearly higher than the other; and by measuring the distance between the spine of the ilium and the malleoli on each side, I find a difference of about three-quarters of an inch in No. 6, and one inch in No. 20. I say about; for whatever care you may take, it is difficult to place the measure so accurately upon the different points as to be sure that you do not make a mistake of a line or two. But the important fact is to determine the existence of shortening; now, it certainly exists here, and the measurement shows it to be a little greater than it seems. You understand why; the pelvis is inclined, as it is in almost all painful diseases of the hip and of the upper part of the thigh, and this incli-nation hides part of the shortening.

I did not look for either mobility or crepitation; for, gentlemen, with the signs which I have just pointed out, doubt is not possible. These two women have fracture of the neck of the femur.

A simple contusion might indeed cause the trouble in the move-ments and the pain which we find here, but it would not cause rotation outwards and shortening. We could be mistaken only if the contu-sion happened to a patient who, for a long time previously, had had dry arthritis or *morbus coxæ senilis*, which had caused rotation outwards and shortening. It was to guard against this error that you heard me ask if they had limped or suffered in the hip for several years, and it was because they answered negatively that I do not have to believe this is a fresh contusion superadded to an old dry arthritis.

Nor have you reason to think of a traumatic dislocation. For, in addition to the fact that dislocation is rare in old people, and that it is produced by a fall from a high place rather than by causes so slight as those which have intervened here, we do not find the symptoms of the most frequent, the iliac, dislocation, since in it the rotation is inwards, not outwards. Supra-pubic dislocation is the only one which is accompanied by rotation outwards and shortening, and it is easily recognized by the prominence formed by the head of the femur as it lies upon the pubes.

We have decided now the most important point of the diagnosis. These patients have fracture of the neck of the femur.

But there is another point which, if I turn to the descriptions of our best authors, ought also to have a certain clinical importance. Is the fracture *extra capsular*, *intra-capsular*, or *mixed*, that is, both intra- and extra-capsular?

If you read the works of Astley Cooper and Malgaigne you will find different chapters for extra- and intra-capsular; if you read those of Vidal de Cassis and Nélaton you will not find, it is true, a separate description of the two varieties, but they insist so strongly upon the differences and the diagnosis that one ought to conclude in the utility and possibility of a differential diagnosis.

I see, with pleasure, that M. S. Duplay[1] has not followed the same road, and passes over in silence the diagnosis of intra- and extra-capsular fractures. I like to think that this is due to my clinical lessons at La Pitié, in which he heard me develop the idea that a rigorous diagnosis between extra- and intra-capsular fractures is both impossible and useless. Impossible, because the differential signs given by the authors are inexact or cannot be detected upon the living subject. Would you like the proof? Examine any one of the differential points given by A. Cooper and Malgaigne.

Astley Cooper insisted upon one means of diagnosis, which, if it was true, would be very convenient. He said : Almost all fractures of the neck of the femur, after 50 years, are intra-capsular, and before 50 years, extra-capsular; and he adds in proof of this assertion, that of 225 persons over 50 years of age, in whom he found fracture of the neck of the femur, in only two was it extra-capsular ; in the 223 others the fracture was intra-capsular. Our two patients, being more than 60 years old, should therefore have intra-capsular fracture.

Astley Cooper here fell into a great mistake, from which he drew, fortunately, an excellent therapeutical conclusion. I explain this error by these two circumstances, that he scarcely found in his autopsies anything except intra-capsular fractures, and that he found them in old people. For, in his time, they did not very well understand fractures with penetration, they did not know that in order to detect them upon the cadaver it is necessary to split the neck of the femur vertically ; those who examined the pieces without taking this precaution, failed to recognize extra-capsular fractures. Astley Cooper then reasoned thus : When I make autopsies of fracture in old people, I find only intra-capsular fractures ; that is undoubtedly because they are peculiar to old people ; and without occupying himself with other differential signs upon the living subject, he thought that age was sufficient to establish the diagnosis.

But facts soon appeared to show that Astley Cooper was mistaken. Bonnet (de Lyon), Rodet, and others after them, found in well-conducted autopsies with vertical section of the neck, extra-capsular fractures with or without penetration, so that to-day it would be difficult to say whether, after 50 years, the intra- or the extra-capsular fractures are most frequent.

A word, now, upon some of the differential signs given by Malgaigne in the table placed at the end of his paragraph upon fractures of the neck of the femur.

---

[1] Follin & Duplay, Traité de Pathologie externe, tome ii.

1st. The intra-capsular, he says, is caused by a fall upon the foot, or the knee, or the buttocks; the extra-capsular, by a direct blow upon the great trochanter. But you will not find out from my poor old women, and you will never find out from other old people who have broken the neck of the femur, whether they have fallen upon the great trochanter, or upon the buttocks. These two regions are too near each other for the patient to be able to say whether it was upon the one or the other that he fell; and suppose that he fell upon his feet or knees—as, after such a fall, there is almost always another backwards and sideways—how are you to know whether the fracture was made before or after the fall upon the side?

I should also like to know how often the diagnosis has been verified upon the cadaver. I doubt if it has ever been done. Malgaigne, in writing these lines, was evidently inspired by a work of M. Rodet,[1] who had published this opinion after experiments made upon plaster femurs. A piece of plaster in the shape of a femur does not at all resemble a cancellous bone whose compact tissue has been thinned, and whose cells have been enlarged by senile rarefaction; for it is due to variations of resistance in different points of its length resulting from these anterior lesions, that the femur, after a blow, yields in one point rather than in another.

2d. In the intra-capsular, adds Malgaigne, there is little swelling, no ecchymosis; in the extra-capsular, much ecchymosis. I complain here that the author did not contrast the swelling in the one with the swelling in the other. Undoubtedly he was embarrassed by the difficulty of being precise. As to the ecchymosis, the word *much* is very elastic. Has our second patient much or little? I could not say, and in any case, it is not impossible that intra-capsular fracture should be accompanied either by great contusion of the soft parts, or by a tearing of the bone which might cause considerable ecchymosis.

You see then that the ecchymosis cannot supply a serious element of the diagnosis.

3d. In the intra-capsular, continues Malgaigne, there is pain near the insertion of the psoas; in the extra-capsular, the pain on pressure is over the great trochanter.

Gentlemen, it is not possible to make pain on pressure a means of diagnosis, for two reasons: first, because if the pressure is slight or moderate it causes no pain, even where there is a fracture not far from it, and because if it is great, it may cause pain itself, and not by transmission of a shock to a neighbouring fracture; secondly, because, supposing the pain on pressure to be due to a fracture, it may be caused by fracture at the base as well as in the middle of the neck.

4th. In the intra-capsular, still according to Malgaigne, the shortening is limited to one and a quarter inches at the most; in the extracapsular, the shortening is from one-quarter of an inch to two and a quarter inches. Well, we have here four-fifths of an inch, and an inch; consequently we are within limits which allow us to believe in one as well as in the other.

[1] Rodet, Des Moyens propres à distinguer les différentes Espèces de Fracture du Col du Fémur (Thèses de Paris, 1844).

I do not wish to carry this critical examination any further. Mal-gaigne gives us four more differential signs, all of them as difficult to determine as the preceding ones, and from no one of which can the clinicist draw a rigorous conclusion, and do not think that by group-ing them all you can reach a conclusion. For, in this group you have a certain number which are as much in favour of one as of the other variety.

Furthermore, that which obliges me to retain and allow you to retain no illusion upon this point, is that pathological anatomy has often shown fractures which were at the same time extra-capsular and intra-capsular; by what signs are they to be distinguished? No one has given them, and yet it is not logical to give the means for recog-nizing the intra- and extra-capsular, and not give the means for recog-nizing a mixture of the two.

The truth is that upon this part of the diagnosis we may reach presumptions, but never a certainty. Thus, in our first patient, I may presume the fracture is intra-capsular because there has been no ecchy-mosis and the pain has been moderate. In the other, I may presume that the fracture is extra-capsular, because there is an ecchymosis, the swelling is considerable, and the pain more severe. But, the reasons which I give in favour of these presumptions might be completely contradicted by an autopsy, or the fracture might prove to be a mixed one.

I said also that this rigorous diagnosis between an extra- and an intra-capsular fracture was useless for the prognosis and treatment, and consequently useless from a practical point of view.

I say that it is useless for the prognosis. Here I find myself in the presence of two contestable opinions which were advanced by Astley Cooper, and upon which he established his distinction between extra- and intra-capsular fractures. The first was that intra-capsular fractures did not consolidate, or consolidated only by a very thin fibrous callus; the second was the conclusion, or rather the intimation (for Astley Cooper did not express himself categorically upon this point), that the patients were condemned to an inevitable infirmity by the fact of this entire or partial failure to consolidate. You see the utility which this question of diagnosis would then have for the prognosis.

This one of our patients, who seems to me to have an intra-capsular fracture, would not get consolidation, would henceforth walk only with the aid of crutches, or at least with a cane and with great diffi-culty, would be, in a word, condemned to an infirmity, while the other one, who seems rather to have an extra-capsular fracture, would, unless I am mistaken in the diagnosis, have bony consolidation and walk very well. And as for the treatment, you see at once the consequence; if intra-capsular fracture does not consolidate, it is useless to treat the patient by confinement to the bed intended to assure the immobility which is a necessary condition to the formation of a regular bony callus.

Gentlemen, it is very true—and the facts invoked by Astley Cooper and before him, it must be admitted, by other authors, especially by J. L. Petit and Boyer, are demonstrative upon this point—it is very true, I repeat, that intra-capsular fractures sometimes remain without consolidation, or heal only by means of an intermediate fibrous substance, for the following reasons: 1st. Because the upper fragment is short and no longer receives a sufficient quantity of nutritive material, since it is supplied exclusively by small vessels accompanying the round ligament; 2d. Because the materials of the callus are poured out into and lost in the articular cavity, as is the case in fractures of the patella. It is equally true that extra-capsular fractures, especially when accompanied by penetration, consolidate by means of a bony callus.

But besides these facts, which are common, there are many exceptions which do not allow us to establish absolute rules for the prognosis. Thus, certain intra-capsular fractures form a bony callus; Astley Cooper himself distinctly says so. These are the ones in which a considerable part of the periosteum has remained intact about the fragments, and, on the one hand, supports the vessels which feed the upper fragments, and, on the other hand, opposes the escape of the reparative materials into the synovial cavity. These are also the ones in which, notwithstanding the rupture of the periosteum, bony stalactites form at the edge of the fragments and unite them at some points, although inter-fragmentary consolidation is lacking. Furthermore, the interfragmentary fibrous callus, when it forms, is sometimes strong enough to give the neck of the femur as much solidity as if it had been bony. You see then that if, after an intra-capsular fracture, the bony or fibrous callus can be as solid as that of an extra-capsular fracture, there is no reason, so far as the prognosis is concerned, to maintain that the diagnosis would be of any great value. It would be if, to the knowledge of the precise seat of the fracture, we could add that of the other anatomical and physiological conditions, that is, the amount of periosteum that has been preserved, the aptitude for the formation of stalactiform prominences. Now, as to these points, no author has ever claimed to be able to make a rigorous diagnosis.

Moreover, it must not be believed that all extra-capsular fractures consolidate with a bony callus; in some of them also it remains fibrous.

I have seen two positive examples of this, and regret that I did not preserve the specimens. In both cases it was fracture with penetration, and the injury had been received six months before in one case, and eight months in the other. Taking the head of the femur in one hand and the shaft in the other, an abnormal mobility could be found, and one might have supposed that a bony callus united the fragments. But, to examine the mode of reunion, I made with a saw a vertical section through the bone, a section without which it would be impossible to exactly appreciate the condition of the parts. This section having been made, I first noticed the penetration of the upper fragment into the lower one, the complete disappearance of the bony substance that had been crushed, the diminution of the length of the neck in consequence of this loss of substance, and finally an irregular fibrous line of demarcation between the upper and lower fragments. This line was about one-fifth of an inch thick. Its tissue was quite dense and adhered firmly to the two fragments, so that the femur thus repaired was perfectly able to sustain the weight of the body. It is none the less true that the callus was fibrous as in many intra-capsular fractures. I proved this by macerating the piece for several weeks, at the end of which the fragments separated.

You see then there is nothing absolute, as to the method of consolidation, in one or the other variety, and we are authorized to-day to say that the rigorous diagnosis between them is not useful for the prognosis.

It might be, however, if the method of consolidation was the only means of explaining the ease or the difficulty of walking after fractures of the neck of the femur. For I could understand that one should say: the old man affected with intra-capsular fracture will probably never walk, because his consolidation will be insufficient, and vice versâ for the extra-capsular. But our anatomo-pathological studies have shown us that the difficulty in walking after this fracture, as after all those which are near articulations, depends greatly upon the consecutive arthritis and the diminished power of the muscles. All patients who have fracture of the neck of the femur have traumatic arthritis almost inevitably when the lesion is wholly or in part intra-articular; it is also very common, if not constant, in extra-articular fractures. How is it possible to prevent the articulation which is so near the solution of continuity from taking part in the consecutive phlegmasia? The intensity and the effects of this arthritis vary according to the subjects, and the varieties depend much more upon their idiosyncrasies than upon the seat of the fracture. At the beginning, then, it may be presumed with certainty that the patient will have an arthritis; it may also be presumed, on account of the age (fracture of the neck of the femur being, as you know, an affection of old people), that this arthritis will become an incurable dry arthritis, or if it does not pass to that state, it will leave for many months a painful rigidity of the synovial membrane. I will admit, if you wish, that these results are more probable after intra-capsular than extra-capsular fractures; I wish to establish, only, that they are possible after both, and that from this point of view also, a perfect diagnosis would not have the value which is claimed for it.

Under the supposition that our second patient has an extra-capsular fracture, I ask myself if this fracture is with or without persistent penetration. For the works of Hervez de Chegoin[1] and Alph. Robert[2] demonstrated plainly that in fractures of the neck of the femur, and especially in those at the base, or the extra-capsular ones, the upper fragment might penetrate the great trochanter and split it, in which case fracture of the neck is complicated by fracture of the great trochanter. They also showed that, without splitting the great trochanter, the upper fragment might lodge within it, crush its cancellous tissue, and remain implanted there (Fig. 19); an important fact, for it leads

[1] Hervez de Chegoin, Journal Général de Médecine, 1820, tome lxxii. p. 3.
[2] Alph. Robert, Mémoire sur les Fractures du Col du Fémur accompagnées de pénétration dans le Tissu spongieux du Trochanter (Mémoires de l'Académie de Médecine, 1847, tome xiii. p. 486).

to this conclusion, that there are fractures of the neck of the femur in which attempts at reduction cannot succeed, or if they succeed are followed by a prompt return of the displacement. It is the same here as in fractures with crushing of the lower extremity of the tibia and of the lower extremity of the radius.

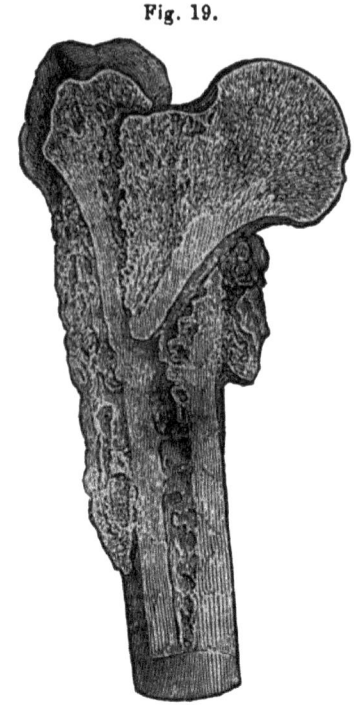

Fig. 19.

Extra-capsular fracture of the neck of the left femur with complete penetration of the cancellous tissue of the trochanter.

From the moment when the pressure exerted by one of the fragments has hollowed out the other by crushing it, the resultant gap is necessarily filled by the muscular action which draws the fragments into contact. If they should succeed in re-establishing the natural length and direction of the limb, it would be by removing the fragments from one another and substituting for their contact an empty space which cannot persist, and towards which the pelvi-femoral muscles would very soon draw the lower fragment. Moreover, under such circumstances the interlocking of the fragments is such that our efforts cannot disengage them, and for consolidation their connection is rather advantageous than not.

From this point of view there would be some use in recognizing beforehand the existence of penetration; for the therapeutical corollary would be to make no exaggerated attempt to remedy the shortening and the outward rotation   But here again we reach only presumptions. When the pain and the ecchymosis make us think that the fracture is extra-capsular, we may at the same time suppose that it is with penetration, because it is especially in such cases that penetration is met with.

The presumption becomes greater, if by making an assistant stand at the end of the bed, grasp the limb, and try to lengthen it and rotate it inwards, we see that the two principal displacements (rotation outwards and shortening) do not yield, and that the attempt causes pain. For in fracture without penetration it would seem as if the assistant's hand ought not to encounter the same resistance as in fracture with penetration. I have again to regret that I cannot give you this mode of exploration as one leading to a positive conclusion. For, if the limb lengthens, and the outward rotation is overcome easily, that will be a proof that penetration, or at least irremediable penetration, does not exist. But inability to correct either of these displacements may be due to two causes; either to penetration, or to muscular resistance. Now, to which of these two causes should we attribute it? This is precisely the question which we have to ask in the case of our second patient.

We have not been able by a gentle effort to correct either of the two displacements. I presume, but I am not certain, that this is due to penetration. The question will be cleared up in a few days. If it is only a muscular spasm it will disappear with the pain, and then if there is no penetration we shall be able to correct at least the rotation outwards, and probably also part of the shortening; if, on the contrary, there is penetration we shall remain unable to correct the displacements.

To recapitulate: you see, gentlemen, that if the etiological, anatomical, and physiological studies relative to fracture of the neck of the femur, which have been made since the beginning of this century, have enlightened us upon the mode of production, the varieties of location, the symptoms, the difficulties, and the method of consolidation, the clinic has not found the means of recognizing, especially at first, all the anatomical dispositions revealed by these studies. The diagnosis upon the living subject is precise only as to the existence of the fracture, and is reduced, on the other points, to presumptions. I prefer to admit this before you rather than to transmit to you errors or useless opinions.

Prognosis.—Those who taught clinically twenty years ago, would undoubtedly have told you that the prognosis was bad for both women, and that death was imminent in a certain measure.

At the beginning of my studies, during my internat under Professors Roux and Blandin, I remember to have seen patients affected with fractures of this kind die after a few weeks, and to have had the opportunity to make the autopsy. But this has no longer been so during the last fifteen or twenty years; the patients survive, and we rarely have occasion to make the autopsical examination of recent fractures of the neck of the femur.

Since I have been practising as hospital surgeon, that is, since 1847, I remember only one case of death during the fortnight following the accident. It was at the Hôpital Cochin, a woman, 82 years old, whose fracture was extra-capsular with penetration.

The three or four other autopsies which I have had occasion to make, were upon subjects who had had their fractures for several months, who no longer suffered at all from them, and who died from some other affection.

To what is this change due? I attribute it to one single cause, that at the beginning of this century the surgeons, guided by false ideas upon the indications of treatment, subjected their old people to the pains of continuous extension. Hence insomnia, fever, loss of appetite, and an alteration of the respiratory passages which carried them off. They said the patients died of hypostatic pneumonia due to horizontal decubitus, and they did not see that this pneumonia was the ultimate lesion of a febrile affection consecutive to a painful condition which old people cannot support. These pneumonias have almost disappeared since we have ceased to make our patients suffer.

Does that mean, however, that our patients are exposed to no alteration of their health dependent upon the fracture? Although I have little fear of a fatal termination, still I ought to tell you here that of all fractures, that of the neck of the femur is the one which has seemed to me to cause the most fever during the first days. You know that after fracture we have a first period, called inflammatory, during which the predominant symptom is pain. I showed you, however, that, during this period, patients affected with fracture of the leg, or of the shaft of the femur, or of the arm or forearm, did not have any marked quickening of the pulse or elevation of temperature, or that, if this elevation took place, it was temporary. In old people who have fractures of the neck of the femur, on the other hand, we often see during three or four days the pulse rise to ninety, the axillary temperature increase two degrees, and in those who are more than 80 years old eschars form rapidly on the sacrum. I asked myself at the time when we saw these fractures terminate quite frequently by death, if this fever was not the consequence of a septicæmia starting from the crushed spongy tissue, and if it did not deserve the name of septicæmic bone fever, and if the death should not be attributed to a peculiar congestion of the bronchi and of the brain in the course of, and by the fact of, this septicæmia. Since the mortality has sensibly diminished I have given up these explanations, or at least I have recognized that, if it is permitted to invoke a septicæmia, we must admit that it is often slight, and that if we do not torment the old people with the pains of apparatuses, it limits itself to a few days of malaise.

Of our two patients, the one who was injured a week ago is entirely without fever; the one whose fracture was received forty-eight hours ago has a pulse of ninety-two, a little headache, loss of appetite, and thirst. But as there is no oppression, no dryness of the tongue, no delirium, no commencing eschar upon the sacrum, I have the right to hope that the fever will be temporary and mild.

If I have no fear for the life of our patients, I am not so certain about the restoration of the shape and functions of the limb.

As for the shape, I hope that the one in No. 6, the one in whom I suspect intra-capsular fracture, will recover without retaining rotation outwards, because in the few movements which I communicated, it seemed to me that this rotation outwards might be corrected.

The other, on the contrary, the one in whom I suspect an extra-capsular fracture with penetration, will undoubtedly retain the deformity resulting from the persistence of the rotation outwards, that is to say, that when standing or walking, she will have the foot turned outwards. This deformity will cause no great inconvenience, it is true, but it is none the less to be mentioned in the prognosis. We shall, moreover, have to direct some of our treatment towards it, for it is possible that we may ultimately correct it, since I do not consider it absolutely irreducible, although I am by no means sure of being able to make it disappear.

On the other hand, these two patients will preserve a shortening of the limb, for two reasons: first, because I shall not try to oppose it; secondly, because if I should try, I should not succeed, the muscles on the one hand, and the interlocking of the fragments on the other, (especially in the second patient), being obstacles against which we can contend advantageously only by means of excessive tractions, which the patients cannot support, and to which it would be cruel to subject them.

As for the functions, I am obliged to leave you in uncertainty, because their re-establishment depends upon individual conditions which I cannot produce, although all my efforts should be directed towards this end.

After a few weeks of confinement to the bed these women will begin to get up and walk with crutches. How long will that last? If affairs go on fortunately, if bony or strong fibrous consolidation is obtained, if the consecutive arthritis is resolved, if no false anchylosis remains after three or four months, and if the muscles are not too much weakened, the crutches will be replaced by a cane, and the patients will be able to walk quite easily, limping but little.

I know three old people, one of them 69, the other two more than 80 years old, who broke the neck of the femur at 68 and 70 years of age, and who for many years have walked without limping—can even walk several miles easily. It is true that they are men, and vigorous ones.

The old women whom I have known or still know in private practice, with fracture of the neck of the femur, have continued to limp, to suffer, to walk with a crutch or a cane, and for only short distances.

Nevertheless, I saw at the Hôpital de la Pitié, in 1866, a woman 66 years old, whom I had treated for a fracture of the neck of the left femur, by simple rest in bed for three weeks, and who, at the end of this time, had walked with crutches. She left the hospital seven weeks after her admission, using only a cane, not suffering, and able to walk without fatigue for about fifteen minutes. After her departure she continued to walk better and better, still with the aid of a stick, but taking walks of about half an hour without too much fatigue. The patient came to see us several times, and I presented her as an example of good consolidation after a fracture whose extra- or intra-capsular position I had not been able to determine strictly, for the reasons which you know. Seven or eight months later she was received into the service of my colleague and friend, M. Empis, for a disease of which she died. We made the autopsy, and, to my great surprise, I found an intra-capsular fracture which was consolidated neither by bony tissue nor by fibrous tissue. The fragments, held together only by a few pieces of periosteum, slipped upon one another, forming a pseudarthrosis like an arthrodia.

I fear then, because this is a quite frequent termination in both sexes, and still more frequent in women than in men, that our two patients will never walk without crutches, will have pain caused by movements, and, in a word, will remain infirm. But there is no certainty upon this point. For these bad results may depend either upon a non-consolidation, or upon an incurable dry arthritis, or upon muscular weakness, or upon all three causes united. Now, I cannot say definitively whether these causes will intervene; for the patients may not have dry arthritis. They may have a sufficient consolidation;

12

I have just told you that even with a pseudarthrosis it was not impossible to walk. Let us hope for a good result, let us try to obtain it, but without counting absolutely upon it. Such, in short, ought to be our prognosis.

Treatment.—What shall we do for these two patients?

Certainly it would seem rational to employ apparatuses which correct external rotation and shortening. P. J. Desault[1] formulated this indication perfectly, and invented a splint for continuous extension which still bears his name. Guided by the idea of Desault, Boyer invented another splint supplied with screw which answered the purpose still better, and which had a certain vogue.

It is a remarkable fact, but these apparatuses for continuous extension caused pain, fever, sometimes eschars, always sleeplessness and loss of appetite, and certainly the death of a good number of old people. Those who survived preserved none the less rotation outwards, shortening, and more or less infirmity; nevertheless they were so penetrated with the idea that the surgeon's duty was to oppose the deformity, and that the death was the result of unfortunate conditions in the patient, that they were finally led to abandon apparatuses for continuous extension by false theories rather than by the results of observation.

It is to two great surgeons, Astley Cooper and Dupuytren, that we are indebted for these theories, which, to the great profit of the patients, led to the abandonment of these apparatuses.

You already know Astley Cooper's: fractures are intra-capsular in old people, and intra-capsular fractures do not consolidate. Consequently, whenever the patients are more than 50 years old it is not necessary to subject them to the pains of continuous extension. We now know that in old people fractures are sometimes extra-capsular, and that intra-capsular fractures can consolidate, but we have retained the deduction, because observation has shown us, since Astley Cooper's fortunate modification of the treatment, that fractures of the neck of the femur treated without continuous extension heal just as well as, and even better than, with it.

On his side, Dupuytren, in proposing and employing treatment by means of semi-flexion, had the idea that in the semi-flexed position, counter-extension was made by the weight of the pelvis, and extension by the weight of the limb, and he asserted that as this position gave, without apparatus, continuous extension, it enabled us to obtain a cure without shortening. In this there was an error of interpretation and an error of observation. But the impulse given to the practice by Dupuytren was none the less very salutary, in protecting the unfortunate old people from the pain of continuous extension.

To-day, gentlemen, you may be very sure of two things :—

The first is that in old people apparatuses to make continuous extension cannot stretch sufficiently, and especially for a long enough time to oppose successfully the two causes of shortening of which I spoke a moment ago : muscular action and crushing.

[1] Desault, Cours théorique et pratique de Clinique externe ; Paris, an. xii.

The second is that, even while not exceeding certain limits, it produces, by the continuous pain, an alteration of the health which, at this age, is not always compatible with life.

We must then resign ourselves to seeing the shortening persist. We may try to oppose external rotation; but if this opposition is painful we must give it up, and await recovery with the persistence of this symptom also.

Pain is, above all, the thing which should be avoided in old people affected with fracture of the neck of the femur. With this object we leave the patient in No. 6 for the present without any restraining apparatus, and we apply linseed poultices sprinkled with laudanum. We prescribed a soothing potion for the day, and half a grain of the gummy extract of opium to be given if she suffers enough to make a bad night probable.

Furthermore, to avoid or diminish the pains which would be caused by movements, we have placed her upon a mechanical bed by means of which she can be raised for all necessary purposes without movement. If in a few days the patient complains of pain on the sacrum, and if, as her leanness may make us fear, we see an eschar is imminent, we shall place her upon a water mattress. The mechanical bed and water mattress, gentlemen, are the two great means of alleviation and, for a certain number of patients, of the preservation of life after fracture of the neck of the femur.

After the inflammatory period has ended, say in about a week, if the tenderness is greatly diminished, I shall place the limb in semi-flexion. I shall not simply use Dupuytren's two large cushions, one under the thigh, the other under the leg, for these cushions yield promptly and do not keep the limb flexed unless they are raised up two or three times daily, an act which causes pain.

I shall use a double inclined plane of wood, made of two planks united at an angle, upon each of which will be placed a bag of chaff. As soon as the limb has been placed upon it, a sheet rolled about the lower part of the leg, and pinned to the mattress or the side of the bed, will keep the foot in place after correcting its external rotation. I place the limb in semi-flexion because I have noticed, without being able to explain it, that in this position, rotation outwards was sometimes corrected easily, and much better than when the limb was extended. But I shall keep the patient in this position only if she does not suffer.

You will meet with old people in whom the semi-flexion causes prolonged pain either in the calf of the leg or in the groin. If our patient presents this complication, I shall remove the double inclined plane, leave the limb extended, and content myself with placing a cushion under the outer border of the foot to raise it a little. Above all, I seek to avoid pain, and to its dangers I prefer the slight inconvenience of the persistence of the rotation. I have all the more reason to prefer it, because the use of the double inclined plane gives me only the hope but not the certainty of recovery without rotation.

As to the other patient, I found her with a Scultet bandage well applied, and completed by a body band which partly immobilizes the pelvis. I left her in this apparatus after having examined the limb and applied the mechanical bed. As the rotation of the foot outwards is not very great, and the fracture seems probably to be with penetration, I shall not use the double inclined plane, and I shall continue the Scultet bandage, but remove it if I hear the patient complain that it causes pain.

It goes without saying that the nourishment of the patients will be as strengthening as circumstances will permit, and that the sacral region will be watched so as to prevent, by means of lotions of aromatic wine, starch powder, and cotton pads, the eschars whose approach would be indicated by erythema and excoriations.

I shall not leave the patients in bed very long. The horizontal decubitus weakens old people, and predisposes them to pulmonary engorgements. In about three weeks, if the pain has diminished sufficiently, I shall have them sit up in a chair. They will be lifted out and put back by means of the mechanical bed with great precautions. Experience has shown that these few movements do not prevent repair from going on to the extent to which it is possible.

I shall give them crutches at the end of five or six weeks, and a little later they will make use only of a cane.

LECTURE XXII.

FRACTURES OF THE LOWER EXTREMITY OF THE FEMUR.

I. Simple supra-condyloid fracture—Functional and physical symptoms—Projection forward of the upper fragment—Imperfect reduction—Probable penetration—Concomitant arthritis. · Treatment. II. Supra-condyloid and inter-condyloid fracture, its production by a wedge-like mechanism—Influence of age upon this mechanism and upon this diagnosis—Reduction impossible. III. Supra-condyloid and inter-condyloid fracture complicated with a wound and projection of the end of the upper fragment—Amputation—Examination of the piece.

GENTLEMEN : I. *Simple supra condyloid fracture of the right femur.* —The patient in No. 15, 32 years old, told us that yesterday evening he was knocked down by a wagon, and fell upon his right knee. He thinks he is sure that the wheel did not pass over his limb, and that he simply fell in a false position, although he cannot say in what this false position consisted. This, however, is certain, that after having fallen he was unable to rise, that he felt severe pain in the knee, and was brought on a stretcher to the hospital.

This morning, after having removed the Scultet bandage which was applied yesterday, we found :—

As functional symptoms : 1st. The absolute impossibility for the patient to raise his heel from the bed and to make any movement with his right leg; 2d. Quite sharp pain on pressure above the knee. *As physical symptoms:* 1st. A moderate swelling, but with fluctuation indicating an incontestable effusion in the femoro-tibial articulation: 2d. An abnormal prominence, a little irregular, but not pointed, at the anterior part of the thigh three finger-breadths above the patella; 3d. An unusual mobility in the transverse direction when I moved the foot alternately outwards and inwards with one hand whilst holding the centre of the thigh firmly fixed with the other.

I did not feel any crepitation, and, carrying my fingers behind into the hollow of the knee, I did not feel any abnormal prominence formed by a fragment of bone.

From these symptoms I do not hesitate to assert that we are in presence of a fracture of the lower extremity of the femur (*Malgaigne's supra condyloid*).

Undoubtedly, the functional troubles which I mentioned, and the considerable enlargement of the synovial cavity might have made us suppose it to be a violent contusion of the articulation,-a sprain, or a fracture of the patella. I do not admit the latter, because I found neither interfragmentary separation nor abnormal mobility of the upper and lower halves of the patella. I do not absolutely reject the idea of a contusion and a sprain; but if these lesions exist they are only a coincidence.

The main lesion is the fracture. The dominant symptom which proves it is the abnormal mobility in the transverse direction. This does not exist in the simple contusion; it is true it may be found in sprains of the severest kind, with rupture of the lateral ligaments. But the mobility which we find here is not that of a sprain, for two reasons: first, because it is much greater and more easily obtained than is that of a sprain; second, because the centre of these unusual movements is plainly above the articulation. Add to that the abnormal projection forwards of the upper fragment, which makes the diagnosis still more positive.

I shall not try to give you any notions upon the etiology, for I know but little about it. The patient, as is always the case, cannot tell us how he fell. His story permits us to infer that the fracture was not produced by a direct blow. But how did the indirect cause act, to produce a fracture at a point where the bone is so large and so strong? This is what remains problematical. I am disposed to believe that the lesion has been prepared by some alteration in the bone, similar to that which takes place in old people in the cells of the cancellous tissue, and which gives this tissue a fragility greater than at other ages. There may have been in him what I call *premature senile alteration.* But this opinion, which I offer here, as for certain almost spontaneous fractures of the shaft, is not thus far susceptible of demonstration.

One word upon the displacement. Since we feel a projection of the upper fragment forward, we infer the existence of a transverse displacement with projection, which we can attribute either to the direction of the fracture, or to the action of those parts of the triceps which are inserted into the femur. I do not think that there is at the same time longitudinal displacement or overriding; for I found a difference of only a line or two in the length of the two limbs, and this difference might be due as well to the difficulty of exact measurement as to a real shortening. I presume that the fragments have not slipped entirely past one another, and that consequently shortening could not be produced.

I looked carefully to see if there was tipping backwards and downwards of the lower fragment, a kind of displacement which was indicated by Boyer as being habitual in this fracture, and which he attributed to traction excited by the gastrocnemius. It seemed to me that nothing like that existed here, that the lower fragment simply extended beyond the upper one behind, and the upper fragment extended beyond the lower one in front.

Supra-condyloid fractures are not common enough for my own experience to enable me to know in what proportion this tipping backwards of which I have spoken appears. I have never met with it. M. U. Trélat[1] tells us that in nine cases, which he found described by the different authors, this tipping backwards occurred only once. I am, therefore, inclined to believe that it is rare. But as it may occur, I advise you always to see if it exists and if it does not exert, as it may possibly do, an undesirable compression upon the popliteal vessels.

The *prognosis* is simple, in this sense, that our patient's life is not compromised; but it is uncertain, and may be bad upon another point, that of persistent deformity on account of irreducibility.

I told you that there was a projection forward of the upper fragment. I add that I have made every effort to reduce it. While an assistant, placed at the foot of the bed, made extension upon the foot, and another held the middle of the thigh firmly to make the counter-extension, I tried to push back the upper fragment with my hands and to make this prominence disappear, but I did not succeed. I repeated the attempt several times, and it always failed. It is probable that I shall not succeed any better hereafter, and that, consequently, consolidation will take place with persistence of the transverse displacement. Fortunately, the prominence is not great enough to endanger the skin; fortunately, also, there is no considerable overriding, so that this deformity, in reality slight, will have no unfortunate consequences for the functions.

But to what is this irreducibility due? To an anatomical disposition which I have told you is often found in fractures of the extremities of long bones. To the penetration of the lower fragment by the posterior part of the upper one. M. U. Trélat has shown clearly that there is often crushing of the spongy bone found here, as there is in the lower extremity of the radius and in the neck of the femur near the great trochanter, and that one of the points on the circumference of the long fragment penetrates into the body of the lower one, and lodges there in such a way that it cannot be

[1] U. Trélat, Thèses de Paris, 1854.

disengaged. I do not mean to say that penetration always takes place in the supra-condyloid fracture, nor that, when it does so, it is always irreducible; I only say that it happens often, and that it has happened in this case.

The prognosis may be bad in another way, that of consecutive arthritis. I do not believe that the fracture sends a fissural prolongation towards the articulation of the knee. Still, it is not impossible. But the fracture is so near the articulation that, by proximity, the latter is already affected and full of liquid.

If we find arthritis of the knee after almost all fractures of the shaft of the femur, so much the greater reason is there for it to appear when the lesion, without being articular, is so near the joint. It is not that I fear that which would be more dangerous, suppuration. Such a termination, strictly speaking, would be possible; but we find it so exceptional after simple fractures that there is no reason to fear it in the present case. Still, non-suppurative arthritis is the more severe and the more likely to leave behind it a prolonged stiffness, or even incomplete anchylosis, as the articulation is nearer the inflamed seat of the fracture. This part of the prognosis in this case is diminished, it is true, by the circumstances that the patient is young and apparently neither rheumatic nor gouty. But, nevertheless, I cannot guarantee that he will not have a false anchylosis, and that the means with which we can oppose this result will be successful. Upon this point we should always warn the patients or their friends, so that they shall not accuse us, as so many people are disposed to do, of having allowed, through insufficient care, this false anchylosis to be established.

Treatment.—At present we have but one thing to do: set the fragments as well as possible, and keep them in place. I applied, this morning, the Scultet bandage, with which you are acquainted, after having made, unsuccessfully, some attempts at reduction.

In a few days I shall renew these attempts, and again once more a few days later. If I should succeed in replacing the upper fragment, I shall add to my bandage anterior compresses intended to keep this fragment in place; if I remain unsuccessful, which is most likely, I shall content myself with the same dressings, and I shall not think for a moment of applying any apparatus for making continuous extension.

I expect consolidation to go on more rapidly than in other fractures of the femur, for two reasons: first, because, ordinarily, the callus forms more rapidly in the spongy than in the compact tissue; and, secondly, because the circumstance of a persistent penetration favours this rapidity.

If, at the end of four or five weeks, I no longer find abnormal mobility, I shall remove the apparatus and leave the limb free. I shall not let the patient get up; for it is probable that the callus, though solid enough for the horizontal position, is not sufficiently so to support the weight of the body. But I shall tell the patient to move his knee a little while lying in bed; I shall, myself, communicate some movements to it every morning, and I hope that this little exercise will prevent the formation of an anchylosis, and favour the restoration of motion. You know that this stiffness after fractures is due partly to traumatic arthritis and partly to prolonged immobility. It is to diminish the influence of the latter that I shall remove the apparatus early, and have recourse immediately to communicated movements. I shall thus leave only the influence of the traumatic lesion, but it is true that this influence is so great that I always fear a notable and definitive loss of part of the normal movements of the articulation.

II. *Fracture, supposed to be supra- and inter-condyloid, of the lower extremity of the left femur.*—Here is a man 59 years old, of rather feeble constitution, who fell three days ago upon his left knee, from a stool upon which he was standing to unhook a curtain. When brought to the hospital, yesterday only, he presented the following symptoms:—

Decubitus upon the back; left leg extended, without rotation outwards; inability to raise the heel from the bed; pain at the knee when he tries to move, when movement is communicated, and when the articulation is pressed upon.

The knee is very swollen, and evidently fluctuating; it seems enlarged, and when, raising the foot, we move the lower part of the leg laterally, we feel a very marked abnormal mobility, the maximum of which is evidently above the line of the articulation. It is difficult to feel the patella, because above and a little in front of it is an abnormal bony prominence which is clearly continuous with the shaft of the femur. There is also shortening of the limb to the amount of 1¼ inches.

You recognize from these symptoms a fracture of the lower extremity of the femur. But here I have every reason to think that the fracture is not only supra-condyloid but at the same time inter-condyloid, that is to say, that in addition to the line of fracture which passes above the condyles, and which, from the projection forwards of the upper fragment, runs obliquely upwards and backwards, there is a vertical line which passes through the inter-condyloid notch, and separates the two condyles from one another.

The only physical sign upon which this diagnosis is based, is the transverse enlargement of the knee, an enlargement which I suppose to be due to a slight separation of the fragments from one another; but I was unable to detect any abnormal mobility by grasping each condyle and trying to move it backwards and forwards. If, as I believe, the condyles are separated, they are still so firmly held, either by the ligaments or by their connections with the upper fragment, that they cannot be moved separately.

But if I have no other physical sign to support my opinion, I find a probability which is very nearly a certainty, first in the age of the patient, and then in the ideas we have gathered from the examination of several pieces, and from our studies upon the mechanism of wedge-shaped or V fractures.

I say the age of the patient; for, in several pieces which I have examined, in one, among others, which I presented to the Société de

Chirurgie, the 21st Nov. 1855,[1] and which I recalled in a report upon the works of M. Lizé in 1858,[2] fracture at the same time supra- and inter-condyloid was observed in patients who, like this one, were more than fifty years old, that is, had reached the period of life in which the spongy tissue of the bone has undergone those modifications which render it more fragile and more liable to split under the influence of violent pressure.

I demonstrated distinctly in these same pieces, by bringing the two condyles together, that there was a depression or loss of substance into which the oblique and more or less pointed extremity of the upper fragment passed. It was sufficient to put the pieces in place to see that, at the moment of the accident, the upper fragment must have penetrated into the lower one, and, acting upon it like a wedge, split it all the more easily because at this point (the inter-condyloid notch) the lower fragment is very short. Pursuing, in a word, the studies upon penetration made by M. Voillemier[3] for the lower extremity of the radius, and by Alph. Robert for the upper extremity of the femur, and those which I had made for V fractures with secondary lines resulting from the pressure of one of the main fragments upon the other, I showed that complex supra-condyloid and inter-condyloid fractures belonged to these varieties (fracture by penetration, wedge fracture), of which our predecessors did not make sufficient mention, and which M. U. Trélat alone had pointed out, without dwelling upon them long enough to make our ideas clear upon this subject. It is to give you precise ideas upon it that I remind you, whenever the occasion presents itself, that this mechanism of penetration is intimately united with that of crushing, that both of them intervene in most fractures of the cancellous extremities in old people, and that the wedge action, the consequence of the penetration and crushing, intervene also in these same conditions, and add the lesion which causes the fracture to communicate with the neighbouring articulation.

To recapitulate then, we have here, in all probability, an articular fracture of the lower extremity of the femur, with projection forwards of the upper fragment, and overriding.

Is this fracture reducible? You saw that in making the manœuvres of extension and counter-extension, I strove in vain against the displacement, and that I was able neither to restore to the limb its length, nor to cause the projection of the upper fragment to disappear. If I meet with the same obstacles in the following days, and it is probable that I shall, I shall find myself once more in presence of an irreducible fracture. Do not be surprised at it, gentlemen; irreducibility is a consequence, I do not say inevitable, but very frequent, of these fractures with penetration and secondary splitting of one of the fragments by the wedge-like action of the other. In certain cases it is due to the fact that the long fragment remains lodged within the short one, and is kept there by a kind of connection for which I find

[1] Gosselin, Bulletin de la Société de Chirurgie, tome vi. p. 262.
[2] Lizé, Bulletin de la Société de Chirurgie, tome ix. p. 148.
[3] Vollemier, Clinique Chirurgicale, Paris, 1861.

no other word than interlocking. This is not exactly the case to-day; for the projecting portion of the upper fragment is so voluminous that it has evidently abandoned, at least in great part, the lower fragment after having split it. It may be, however, that the posterior portion of the first is adherent by some irregular points, and by means of adjoining fragments, and that these prevent reduction. It is probable that the principal obstacle is caused by muscular resistance, as in a certain number of fractures of the shaft of the femur, while the obliquity of the main line of the fracture, and the pulverization and packing of the cancellous tissue of both fragments, favor and render irremediable the shortening produced by this muscular action.

I do not mean to say that all supra- and inter-condyloid fractures are as irreducible as this one is. I say only that it is quite frequent, and that in our present patient it is as marked as possible.

You understand the prognosis: the patient will recover with considerable shortening, and the arthritis will be all the more severe, prolonged, and likely to end in anchylosis, because, on the one hand, the fracture communicates with the articulation, and on the other, the age of the patient predisposes to prolonged arthritis and anchylosis.

As to the treatment, it will consist of repeated attempts to make reduction, and of the application of a Scultet bandage which I shall maintain so long as the abnormal mobility lasts. I fear the consolidation will be slow, because only a small part of the upper fragment is in contact with the lower one, and this disposition is not favourable to the formation of a callus.

III. *Supra- and inter-condyloid fracture with wound and projection of the end of the upper fragment. Amputation of the thigh.*—The patient whom we saw at No. 25, and who is 51 years old, was caught yesterday by the caving in of some earth, and, after a moment's struggle, was overthrown, feeling at the same time severe pain in his left knee, but without knowing how or in what position the knee was injured.

We find the parts in the following condition:—

Through a wound in the anterior portion of the thigh above the patella, projects the upper fragment of the femur, which ends in a hard point. About this wound there is no ecchymosis and no effusion of blood. The articulation is swollen and fluctuating. There is very marked lateral mobility, and an enlargement of the transverse diameter of the knee, with inability to move each condyle separately, backwards and forwards.

We have evidently here, a compound supra-condyloid fracture with issue of the upper fragment. I add, that for the moment this fragment is irreducible, for I have made fruitless attempts to return it to its place. It is also very probable that the fracture is at the same time inter-condyloid, and that consequently the external wound communicates both with the seat of this fracture and the cavity of the articulation. My reasons for thinking so are, the broadening of the knee, the abundant and rapidly formed effusion within the articulation, the form of the upper fragment which is well fitted to penetrate and act like a wedge, and finally the age of the patient. This diagnosis leads to a very serious prognosis.

A large wound like this will inevitably suppurate, and it is also inevitable that the suppuration will extend to the fragments of bone and the articular cavity. Now this suppuration in a hospital, upon a man who is quite old, has every possible chance of terminating in putrid infection during the first few days (grave traumatic fever), or in purulent infection, and in any case by death. Although amputation of the thigh is also dangerous, and although amputation for a traumatic cause especially yields only rare successes, yet I consider that this operation is a little less likely to be followed by death than an attempt to preserve the limb would be. That is why I prefer amputation: the patient accepted it, and we shall now perform it.

This will be an amputation of the kind which M. Hip. Larrey called *primitive*, that is, one which is performed before the development of the traumatic fever. If we should wait until this evening or to-morrow, this fever would undoubtedly be established, and the patient would be in a much less favourable condition.

(We found on examining the piece, that the fracture was inter-condyloid as well as supra-condyloid, and that consequently the wound and the seat of the fracture communicated with the articulation. The patient succumbed on the twelfth day, to a purulent infection which succeeded a very intense traumatic fever.)

LECTURE XXIII.

SPONTANEOUS FRACTURES, AND ITERATIVE FRACTURES OF THE SHAFT OF THE FEMUR.

I. Considerations upon spontaneous fractures—They are due to an abnormal fragility —This is caused sometimes by a cancer, sometimes by a rarefying osteitis, sometimes by premature senile rarefaction—Case of a patient affected with spontaneous sub-trochanteric fracture of the femur—Robert's analogous case—Another case in the Hôpital Cochin. II. Iterative fracture of the left femur, due to not keeping the bed long enough—Means of avoiding this accident.

GENTLEMEN: I. *Spontaneous fractures.*—We have the habit of giving the name *spontaneous* to fractures which are produced so easily that they seem to occur without the intervention of any appreciable cause. Notwithstanding our habit, this designation of spontaneous is not absolutely exact, for in reality we can always attribute the solution of continuity to muscular contraction or the weight of the body. But when it is a question of a bone so voluminous and so strong as the femur, of a bone which serves for the attachment of powerful muscles, and to support the body when standing or walking, you will admit that it is allowable to consider as almost spontaneous fractures which have no other cause than the accomplishment of the functions of this bone.

It is sufficient to consider the physiological resistance of the femur to understand that if in certain exceptional cases it yields so easily, it is because this resistance has been weakened by a modification of its structure.

This is very evident when the fracture is consecutive to an osteosarcoma.

I saw, for example, at the Hôpital Cochin, in 1857, a woman 60 years old, who had been admitted for a tumour, larger than the fist, occupying the entire circumference of the right femur, and which we had recognized as a cancer of this bone. A few weeks after her admission to the hospital, they told me, one morning, that she had complained during the night, after a movement to turn in bed, of a very sharp pain, and that since then the pain had not ceased. On reaching her bed I found her with the foot and leg in outward rotation, and with very marked mobility at the point occupied by the tumour. There was no doubt that the cancer had gradually destroyed the bone, and that at last the femur was no longer strong enough to bear without breaking even a movement in bed.

I saw a similar case at the Hôpital des Cliniques, in 1848, in a man 65 years old, who had broken his left femur while getting out of bed, without any other accident, and in whom the fracture took place at the seat of an old cancerous tumour which occupied the femur and had been indolent up to that time.

But the explanation of the loss of strength by the femur at some point in its length is more difficult to give in cases like the one before us, in No. 10, Ward St. Louis (Hôpital de la Pitié).

The patient, 30 years old, of vigorous appearance, has been under treatment here for more than 80 days, and in another fortnight will leave us to go to Vincennes.[1]

When we first saw him he was in a medical ward where he had been placed because they had no reason to suspect the existence of a surgical lesion. He told us that while walking tranquilly across the Grenelle bridge, and without having made any false step, he felt a sharp pain at the upper part of his left thigh. He then sank down gently, and waited until two passers-by came to help him.

Finding himself unable to walk, he was carried to the Central Bureau, and thence forwarded to a medical service for this pain which was supposed to be rheumatic.

Having been asked to examine him, I found rotation outwards, shortening of the limb to the extent of an inch, and abnormal mobility with crepitation in the upper third of the thigh below the trochanters. The patient was then brought to my ward, later examinations confirmed the first impression, and it became more and more evident that this man (who before this time had not been lame, and had a well-formed limb) had suffered while walking, without falling,

---

[1] A succinct account of this case was published in the Gazette des Hôpitaux, 5th April, 1862, p. 158.

and without having received any external violence, a sub-trochanteric fracture. He assured us, moreover, and those who brought him here confirmed the statement, that he was not intoxicated at the time of the accident, and that he was perfectly aware of all that took place. We were then justified in believing that this was a spontaneous frac-ture. But was not this fracture the consequence of a cancer? We felt no appreciable tumour. If there was a cancer, it was one of those hidden ones of the medullary canal which it is permitted to suspect, but the existence of which can be demonstrated by no physical sign.

Moreover, the age of the patient and his vigorous constitution dis-missed the idea of a cancerous affection. But if it was not a cancer which had weakened the femur, it must have been another lesion; what was it? Search through the records left by our authors does not enable me to give you a precise answer; for they have not at-tempted to explain the cause of the fragility of certain bones, and they were not able to do so, for the simple reason that examples of it are very rare. In those which have been presented, no autopsy has been made; it was necessary to be satisfied with the clinical fact which, in itself alone, as in our present case, did not clear up the pathogenic question.

Malgaigne spoke of a peculiar osteitis which causes fragility of the bones, and explains these fractures which are so easily produced. But, as I shall have occasion to tell you when speaking of other fractures by muscular contraction, I would believe in the interven-tion of this osteitis if our patient had suffered for any length of time. Malgaigne appears to have observed these spontaneous fractures in patients who had had these sufferings, and that is what justifies the expression of the opinion. I was able to attribute the fracture to an osteitis in the case of a patient of whom Alph. Robert spoke in his lectures,[1] and whom I treated at the Hôpital Cochin, because this patient had had for two years continual pains in his lower limbs.

But when, as in our present patient, there has been no pain of this kind, must we admit, nevertheless, rarefying osteitis? I think not. For if I understand rarefaction of bony tissue coinciding with an osteitis, I also understand, very well, rarefaction without osteitis, and by a peculiar vice of nutrition analogous to that caused by age, whence the name *premature senile rarefaction* or *alteration* which you have heard me use quite often.

Is there not, at least in this patient, some constitutional cause which might explain the rarefaction? I know none. I have given par-ticular attention to the possibility of constitutional syphilis. Now, on the one hand, it is claimed by nobody that syphilis causes fra-gility of the bony tissue; on the contrary, it rather increases their solidity by producing hyperostosis and exostosis; on the other hand, our patient shows no trace of syphilis, and says he has never had it. It was the same with the case at the Hôpital Cochin. It is true that I gave him the iodide of potassium; but I administered it as a forti-

---

[1] Robert, Conférences de Clinique Chirurgicale, 1860, p. 498.

fying and not as an antisyphilitic measure.   It was the same in Robert's case.

I call your attention to another point.

This fracture occupies the upper third of the shaft, and deserves the name of sub-trochanteric.

It occupied the same place in my patient at the Hôpital Cochin, and also in Robert's patient.   Has the upper portion of the shaft of the femur a special predisposition to this singular alteration of nutrition which causes fragility?   Three cases are not enough to give us any certainty upon this point, but it is allowable, at least, to mention the peculiarity.

Prognosis.—When I began the treatment, I did not know if we should get consolidation.   For if the fragility had been due to a hidden cancer, the callus undoubtedly would not have formed, and in case of premature senile alteration, there was also reason to fear that materials for the callus would not be furnished, or would not be properly elaborated at this affected portion of the skeleton.

Still, as the callus had formed in my patient at the Hôpital Cochin and in Robert's, and as this patient was of a vigorous constitution, I had no reason to despair.

The fact is that the consolidation was obtained in the ordinary length of time, and that to-day, three months afterwards, not only do I no longer find abnormal mobility, but I feel a large strong callus, which makes me think that at the place occupied by the bony alteration, the traumatic inflammation excited a nutritive movement, and restored, perhaps even in excess, the normal strength of the bone,[1] that is, notwithstanding the presumed pre-existing rarefaction, this traumatic osteitis has taken on the condensing form which we see so often after fractures of the long bones.

The fears which I might have had on the subject of non-consolidation have been justified by the case of a patient whom I have since seen at the Hôpital de la Charité.

It was a woman 52 years old, much more feeble and broken down than is usual at that age.   A few months before her admission to the hospital she had broken her right humerus by a very simple fall from a standing posture, and had recovered; a little later she had broken the shaft of the left femur below the trochanters, as in the three patients of whom I have spoken, and so easily that she did not know exactly to what accident to attribute it.   For she had fallen three months before in her room while walking slowly towards the window, and a few weeks afterwards, while turning in bed, she had felt very sharp pain in her thigh, and she was unable to say whether it had been broken by this latter movement or by the antecedent fall. However that may be, the thigh presented shortening, rotation outwards, and very marked abnormal mobility, symptoms either of a fracture still too recent to have become consolidated, or of an old non-consolidated fracture.   This woman died of exhaustion in May, 1868.

---

[1] This patient came to see us two months afterwards at the consultation; he walked with a cane and still had a very solid callus.

We found at the autopsy, below the trochanters, a false articulation, consisting of a fibrous sleeve, quite thick but not ossified, in the cavity of which the two fragments were found at a certain distance from one another. It is evident that the fracture dated from the first accident of which she had told us, and that it had not consolidated. Above and below the vacuoli of the cancellous tissue of the femur were very notably enlarged, the compact tissue was thinned, and a moderate pressure was sufficient to split the bone which was remarkably fragile in consequence of the absorption of a part of its bony substance. There was no trace of cancer of the bone. The right humerus, which had a solid callus with obliteration of the medullary canal, was nevertheless very fragile below the fracture.

We had then, in this case, the example of two almost spontaneous fractures ; one of the humerus which had been followed by consolidation ; the other of the femur which was not consolidated ; hence the conclusion that in cases of this kind consolidation is possible, but may also fail.

II. *Iterative fracture of the left femur.*—I called your attention to No. 2, a young man 19 years old, who has been under treatment here for 50 days, for fracture of the shaft of the femur below its centre. As the callus seemed to be very solid on the 45th day, and as I no longer found any abnormal mobility, and as, furthermore, I did not wish to keep his knee immovable for too long a time, I removed the Scultet bandage. But I had expressly told the patient not to get up, intending to keep him in bed until the 70th or 75th day, and then to make him begin with crutches. But this is what happened : the day before yesterday, the 48th day since the accident, he got up and walked a short distance, supporting himself on the adjoining beds. He slipped, fell, and broke the callus. The next morning we found abnormal mobility and crepitation as at the beginning, and the patient was again unable to raise his heel from the bed. I reapplied the Scultet bandage, prescribed 30 grains of the phosphate of lime to be taken twice a day, and told the patient he would have to remain in bed for three months.

This is not the first time I have seen this rupture of the callus, or iterative fracture ; I saw two other examples of it a few years ago ; one at Cochin, the other at Beaujon, and both of them were young men whose apparatuses I had removed about the 50th day, forbidding them to leave the bed, but both had disobeyed and had fallen in the wards.

The first thing to be remembered from these facts is that the callus may acquire by the 45th to the 55th day, sufficient solidity to prevent communication by our hands of the movements which are pathognomonic of the persistence of the fracture, but nevertheless not be solid enough to bear either the weight of the body or an inflection during a fall.

For you observe that I do not know if, in my three patients, the fracture was produced by the fall, or if the fall was the consequence of the rupture of the callus under the influence of the weight of the body. However that may be, the practical conclusion is that the patients must not be allowed to get up as soon as we find immobility, and we must wait for at least the 70th day before allowing them to leave the bed. Until that time, the callus, although it no longer shows abnormal mobility, is still too fibrous or too little bony to resist an unexpected impulse or inflection. For it is only peripheral and not interfragmentary.

Let us remember another fact, that these iterative fractures are to be feared, especially in young people (and it would undoubtedly be the same for children). The callus certainly forms a little more rapidly at this age than in adults, but it needs, none the less, from eight to twelve weeks to obtain the solidity necessary for walking. Now, we can easily persuade an adult to remain in bed a fortnight after the apparatus has been taken off. During this time, we use friction, massage, and communicated movements, to correct the stiffness of the knee and foot.

But it is much more difficult to keep a young man in bed after he has been relieved of the restraint of his apparatus, and you must not expect them to obey your instructions upon this point. Consequently the wisest plan in their case is to leave the apparatus in place until the 65th or 70th day, while in adults upon whose reasonableness you can place more reliance, you may remove the apparatus from the 50th to the 60th day, and let them walk a fortnight afterwards. The disadvantage of the more prolonged immobility in young people is compensated for by their lesser aptitude for anchylosis and the prolonged stiffness of the concomitant traumatic arthritis.

In children, until the age of fifteen years, I advise you not to leave the apparatus on longer than the 45th day, because consolidation goes on more rapidly ; but it is still prudent, in order to avoid iterative fracture, not to let them walk, even upon crutches, before the 60th day.

You will not often have occasion to see the callus break a second and a third time, because, warned by the first rupture, you will take care to recommend sufficient rest in bed and phosphate of lime, which will ensure a solid recovery. If, however, the patient does not obey your instructions, the fracture of the femur may be reproduced three or four times.

I was consulted in 1864 by a young man from Saint-Pierre-Calais, 25 years old, who had broken his left femur six times in the course of twenty months. A remarkable fact in the case was that the fracture did not occur when he began to walk, but from the 8th to the 15th day afterwards, and generally in consequence of a slight effort, either to save himself from falling, or to run. Once, indeed, the fracture took place while he was dancing. Each time the patient had been allowed to get up on the 45th day. He had reached the 40th day of his sixth and last accident, when his father came to Paris to consult me upon the means of preventing these iterative fractures. I told him to keep on the Scultet apparatus, which had been applied, for two entire months, and not to allow the young man to leave his bed until the end of the third month, and to give phosphate of lime during the whole time. These prescriptions were followed and the fracture was not repeated.

I saw the young man himself in November, 1869, at Saint-Pierre, where I had been called to see another patient. He had remained perfectly well, but with a shortening of $2_\frac{1}{4}$ inches, a limp, and the necessity of using a cane, all of which did not prevent him from walking a great deal, even for several leagues at a time, without difficulty.

LECTURE XXIV.

FRACTURES OF THE LOWER EXTREMITY OF THE RADIUS.

Consecutive and late phenomena. I. First patient on the fiftieth day of the fracture —Study of the shape and functions—Rigidity of the articular synovial membranes, due to arthritis by proximity in the wrist, and arthritis by immobility in the fingers—Rigidity of the tendinous synovial membranes. II. Another patient (woman 69 years old, ninetieth day)—Slower and perhaps impossible recovery from the same rigidities on account of her advanced age.

GENTLEMEN: I have brought to the amphitheatre, that you may all see them better, two patients who have been treated in our wards for fractures of the lower extremity of the radius. One of them is a man 38 years old, the other a woman 69 years old.

I. The first has reached the fiftieth day of his accident. I treated him for five days with poultices, and at the end of that time applied Malgaigne's apparatus, which you often see me use, with a cotton cushion upon the posterior part of the lower fragment, and another upon the anterior portion of the upper fragment; over these a graduated compress, and a splint upon the palmar surface of the forearm and hand, and graduated compress and splint upon the dorsal surface; the whole kept in place by means of three bands of diachylon a yard and a quarter long and an inch wide. Of course before applying this apparatus I had done my best to make reduction by the manœuvres of extension, counter-extension, and coaptation. You remember the bandage was removed a fortnight after its application, that is, the twenty-first day after the accident, and that the patient left us three or four days afterwards.

He returns to-day, the fiftieth day after the fall, to consult us for persistent trouble in the hand. I call your attention to two principal points; the shape and the functions.

1. *The shape of the wrist and forearm.*—At the wrist our eyes detect no irregularity and no trace of the characteristic silver-fork deformity which existed at the beginning. But by comparing this region with that of the other side, we find it is a little larger, and if we then feel

13

of it, so as to better appreciate the difference, we find under the skin a superficial and general induration which can be due to nothing else than the swollen radius. We have then here another example of that variety of bone lesion which so often follows suppurative or non-suppurative osteitis, and which we find especially in non-scrofulous subjects, that is, hyperostosis. I next compare the relative positions of the two styloid processes, and find them the same upon both sides. I therefore infer that the styloid process of the radius, which underwent a slight ascension at the time of the accident, has been restored to its place by our manœuvres to make reduction, and has remained there. I am pleased with this result; for in many cases, after fracture of the lower extremity of the radius, the styloid process remains higher up the arm, so that its point is upon the same transverse line with that of the ulnar. The reason of this is that, the fracture being with penetration, the two fragments cannot be separated from one another at the moment of reduction, or else that, reduction having been made, absorption of that part of the spongy tissue which was most crushed at the time of the accident has taken place between the fragments before consolidation. I suppose that in our patient, who is still young, the spongy tissue had not undergone before the accident the rarefaction which predisposes both to reciprocal penetration in cases of fracture and to considerable attrition. That is why the radius has recovered almost its normal length. I find in this condition of affairs the advantage that the articular surfaces of the lower radio-ulnar articulation are not so much deformed as when there is permanent ascension of the lower fragment and diminution of the length of the radius. This condition is favourable to the ultimate restoration of the movements of this articulation.

Finally, to finish with the shape, I ask you to compare the volume of the two forearms. The left one is a little smaller than the right, and the difference is due to the smaller size of the muscles. This then is another example of the slight and unimportant, but still real, muscular atrophy which follows almost all fractures of the long bones, and of which I so often have occasion to speak.

2. *The functions.*—As for the functions, you see that this man can execute without pain the movements of flexion and extension of the wrist and fingers. But you also see that these movements, especially those of flexion, are more limited than in the normal condition, and that in this respect they are far from being what we desire. The patient also says that he has but little strength in his hand, can carry nothing with it, and uses it very little, even in dressing himself. I now ask him to make the rotary movements which give pronation and supination, and you see that they are incomplete, that they scarcely take place at all in the lower radio-ulnar articulation, and that they are executed almost exclusively at the shoulder.

How can we explain this diminution of the movements and the weakness of the limb which is the consequence? It is not due to the insufficiency of the muscles; for, on the one hand, the atrophy of which I have spoken is slight, and, on the other, we often see atrophy of this kind, and we know that it does not diminish the extent of the movements, since the muscular fibres continue to receive from their nerves, which have remained intact, the impulse necessary for their contraction. That which explains this functional trouble is especially the rigidity and the insufficient extensibility of the articular and tendinous synovial membranes. As for the first, those placed near the seat of the fracture have participated in the inflammatory process, and have lost, in consequence of the traumatic inflammation of which they have become the seat, a part of their extensibility and suppleness. These are the radio-carpal, the carpal, and lower radio-ulnar synovial membranes. The others, placed further from the fracture (I refer to those of the fingers), have not been inflamed in consequence of their proximity; but we have the right to believe that they have become altered and modified as a result of their immobility. You remember that M. Teissier, of Lyons,[1] published a work upon the effects of prolonged immobility of the joints. But he did not make a distinction between the large and small articulations. Now, the first may remain immovable for several weeks, and even for several months, without losing the natural suppleness and extensibility of their synovial membranes. Notice patients who have had a fracture of the leg or of the thigh: the knee-joint in the first, and the hip in the other have remained immovable for a long time, and yet the moment you cease the treatment you can communicate extended movements to them, and without finding much resistance. The large articulations become rigid only when consecutive inflammation has invaded them, as takes place quite often in the tibio-tarsal articulations after fractures of the leg, and always in those of the knee after fractures of the thigh.

It is not the same for the small articulations of the fingers. They are too far from the radius (and, moreover, the same thing follows fracture of the shaft of the forearm or of the humerus) for us to admit the propagation to them of the phlegmasia developed at the seat of the fracture. If they become rigid, it is the immobility alone which is the cause. In consequence of their inaction, their synovial membranes have become dry and shrunken, and have lost their suppleness. That is why they oppose flexion of the fingers; and if a little force is used, the stretching to which they are subjected causes pain.

As for the other synovial membranes, those of the tendons, it is probable that that of the extensor tendons behind, and the great carpal one of the flexors in front, have been attacked in consequence of their proximity to, and by propagation of the phlegmasia which is developed at the fracture, and that, consequently, they have become rigid. I do not deny that the immobility may have contributed to a certain extent to this result. But basing the opinion upon the fact that immobility alone does not cause rigidity of the large tendinous synovial membranes when a centre of irritation, like a fracture or dislocation, is not near them, I am inclined to believe that most of the rigidity is due to synovites by propagation.

Do not be surprised at these results, gentlemen; they are very com-

---

[1] Teissier, Gazette Médicale, 1841.

mon, and you will often meet with them in practice; indeed, you must even take care to forewarn your patients of them, that they may know that the difficult movements of which they will have to complain for a long time after fracture of the lower extremity of the radius, are not due to insufficient or unskilful treatment, but are a consequence of the disease itself.

Moreover, I tell them not to worry, for all these functional troubles will disappear in time. The articular and tendinous synovials will recover their polish and then their suppleness by use, and it is very probable, if I may judge by the facts of the same kind which I have observed, that in three or four months the movements will have recovered their natural extent and ease. Those of pronation and supination will be the slowest to return, but I expect their perfect return all the more confidently, because the radio-ulnar articular surfaces are not notably deformed. This relatively favourable prognosis is further justified by the fact that the patient is young and not rheumatic; you remember that those are favourable conditions.

As for therapeutical advice, I shall tell the patient to communicate moderate movements with the other hand to the fingers and wrist, and to apply friction every morning and evening with pure lard, or lard mixed with alcohol, and to take two sulphur baths every week.

II. The other patient is a woman 69 years old. Her fracture was received three months ago, and you can see that notwithstanding the length of time that has elapsed, the shape and functions leave much more to be desired than in the preceding case.

First, the silver-fork deformity is still quite marked, although at the time of the accident I made the manœuvres of extension, counter-extension, and coaptation, and employed the same apparatus as for the other. Moreover, the styloid process of the radius is higher than it should be. Its summit is on the same transverse line as that of the styloid process of the ulna. What is the reason of this faulty conformation? It is due to two causes: first, to this that the age of the patient having caused rarefaction of the cancellous tissue of the lower extremity of the radius, this tissue was crushed by a fall upon the hand, and then, as described in the excellent study of this accident by M. Voillemier,[1] the fragments penetrated one another, and became so interlocked, that my efforts were powerless to change their reciprocal positions. Second, it is probable that part of the crushed bony tissue was afterwards reabsorbed, which would diminish the chances of a permanent return of the lower fragment to its proper place. Consolidation, nevertheless, took place, because, as I have often told you, consolidation goes on well and rapidly in the cancellous tissue of most long bones (I except intra-capsular fracture of the neck of the femur); but the callus has remained irregular for the reasons which I have just given.

As for the functions, you heard this woman complain of pains which she feels when at rest, and which increase when she tries to move the wrist and the fingers. Voluntary movements are very

[1] Voillemier, Archives Générales de Médecine, 1842, tome xiii. p. 261.

limited, as much on account of the pain which they provoke as by insufficiency of the muscles. I try to communicate movements, and I find that they have but little extent, and are stopped by an obstacle which cannot be overcome. It is very probable that' this obstacle is the painful rigidity of the articular and tendinous fibro-synovial tissues. This is already very marked in the radio-carpal articulation, and is still more so in the phalangeal and metacarpo-phalangeal articulations. Pronation and supination are also much hindered. In short, this patient cannot use her hand for any of the ordinary purposes, although it is evident that the muscles are not paralyzed.

Why this powerlessness? How long will it last? What can we do to suppress or diminish it?

I have already given the explanation. There has been arthritis of the radio-carpal and inferior radio-ulnar articulations near the fracture. This arthritis has passed to the chronic condition, leading to the retraction of the synovial membrane and of the surrounding fibrous tissues, retraction which is the consequence of most prolonged arthritis when they do not take on the fungous form or white swelling. The articulations of the fingers have become inflamed and rigid, in consequence of prolonged immobility. Two causes which did not exist in the preceding patient have contributed in this one, not to the development, but to the long duration of these arthrites; these are her advanced age, and the rheumatism from which she has been suffering for many years.

This union of disadvantageous conditions—the traumatism, immobility, age, and rheumatism—makes me fear that the powerlessness will last much longer than in the man. I advise the same treatment, friction, massage, and sulphur baths. But I am not sure that they will lead to a complete recovery. The movements will undoubtedly recover a little of the extent which they have lost, but will never recover it entirely, and there will always remain some pain. In a word, the condition which you see, instead of being temporary as in the other patient, will undoubtedly be permanent, and will constitute an infirmity.

LECTURE XXV.

FRACTURES OF THE LOWER EXTREMITY OF THE RADIUS—Continued.

I. Early phenomena and symptoms of recent fracture—Study of the mechanism—
Inflection, tearing off, crushing, and penetration—Treatment—Immediate reduction—Restraining apparatus the sixth day—Necessity for great watchfulness if
it is applied sooner. II. Immediate reduction—Simple retention with Robert's
apparatus. III. Recent fracture in a young man 18 years old—Absence of
crushing and penetration—Probability of a cure without deformity and with
prompt return of the functions.

GENTLEMEN: We have at this moment in our wards three patients
affected with recent fracture of the lower extremity of the radius.
I. The first is the one in whom the symptoms are the most marked.
He is a man 58 years old who slipped on the ice yesterday morning
and fell. While falling he threw both hands forwards, and the
weight of his body was received principally upon the palm of his
right hand. No crack was heard, but sharp pain was immediately
felt in the corresponding wrist, and the patient, on looking at it, was
struck to find it sensibly deformed. He was not able to use it, and
saw at once the necessity of coming to the hospital.

You notice the deformity of the wrist. It is perfectly characteristic,
and is sufficient in itself alone to establish the diagnosis. Without
going into many details, which would tell you less than the simple
sight of it, I call your attention only to three things:—

1st. An exaggerated projection backwards immediately above the
articulation of the wrist, with a smaller projection upon the palmar
surface, below which is a slight depression corresponding to the prominence on the dorsal surface; these prominences and depressions together constituting what Velpeau called *talon de fourchette*.[1]

2d. The level of the styloid processes. That of the radius instead
of having its point one-third of an inch lower than that of the ulnar,
as in the normal condition, is exactly on the same level, that is, it
has been carried up the arm. This symptom, to which I attach
great value, was pointed out by Professor Laugier.

3d. If, while the wrist is flexed, you press upon the dorsal surface
of the forearm immediately above the prominence I mentioned, you
feel first the depression, and then in front of it, and deeper, a sort of
tense elastic cord, formed by the tendons of the radial muscles (exten-
sores carpi radiales longior and brevior) which have been removed
from their normal position by the projection of the lower fragment
backwards. This sign also was indicated by Velpeau, who gave it
the name of the cord of the radials.

---

[1] Silver-fork fracture of the English writers.—TRANS.

The hand is very slightly inclined towards its ulnar border, and consequently has not been drawn outwards, as occurs in certain exceptional cases which undoubtedly were seen quite often by Dupuytren, and led this great surgeon to use a curved metallic ulnar splint, with external convexity, along which he bound the cubital border of the hand so as to correct the deviation outwards.

I have made very little search for crepitation and mobility. The patient suffered a great deal and I did not need these symptoms to complete my diagnosis. The deformity was sufficient, for it could not be explained otherwise than by a fracture of the lower extremity of the radius, a lesion which offers this clinical peculiarity that it can be recognized in many cases by the deformity alone. There is, how-ever, a circumstance which might lead us into error, I mean a coutusion or a sprain occurring in a wrist which remained deformed after an old fracture of the radius. The patient would then present himself to us with the characteristic deformity due to the anterior fracture, and in addition the pain and difficult movements caused by the recent injury. It would then be quite natural to think of a recent fracture. To avoid this error I questioned the patient. I asked him if he had ever had his wrist broken, and it was after having received an absolutely negative answer that I admitted without the slightest hesitation the existence of a recent fracture.

Let us see, before going any further, 1st, by what mechanism the fracture has been produced; 2d, the cause of the characteristic deformity.

1st. As for the mechanism, I have to tell you that in this fracture, as in most others, the information furnished by the questioning and examination of the patient does not solve the problem.

We find indicated in our authors three principal modes according to which the lower extremity of the radius may be broken.

According to most of them, to speak only of contemporaneous ones, the radius is caught, at the moment of a fall upon the palm of the hand, between two opposing forces, the resistance of the ground and the weight of the body transmitted through the arm and forearm to the ball of the hand. The lower extremity of the radius tends to bend backwards under this double pressure. If the movement is carried too far, it breaks, and the more easily if the cancellous tissue has been rendered more fragile by the spontaneous rarefaction which is the consequence of age, which arrives more or less early according to the subjects, and indeed in certain persons is really premature. I do not claim that this theory of inflection has been presented in an absolute and exclusive manner, but it has at least been formulated as one of the conditions of the mechanism in certain works and nota-bly in those of Foucher,[1] Am. Bonnet, and Philippeaux.[2]

Others, and especially Nélaton[3] and Voillemier,[4] insisted upon this circumstance, that in the fall upon the palm of the hand the

[1] Foucher, Bulletin de la Société Anatomique, 1852.
[2] Philippeaux, Bulletin de Thérapeutique, 1850, p. 207.
[3] Nélaton, Éléments de Pathologie, tome 1er.
[4] Voillemier, loc. cit.

radius might be broken by the pressure to which its cancellous tissue is subjected. I regret that they did not use more explicitly the word *crushing*, which would have made the idea more easily comprehended. But, if the word is not at all or not sufficiently accentuated, the fact certainly is, and it was the theory of crushing which led M. Voillemier to study penetration which is only a consequence of crushing.

More recently M. O. Lecomte, in a long and interesting work,[1] has opposed the theory of crushing, which he makes the mistake of not designating by its real name, and which he calls the *theory of the direct transmission of the shock to the radius*, and, developing a theory which had already been advanced with reserve by Voillemier and Foucher, maintains that in falls upon the palm of the hand the wrist draws backwards and stretches the anterior ligaments of the radio-carpal articulation, that these ligaments exert traction upon the anterior portion of the lower extremity and detach it by a mechanism which is that of tearing.

'Here then are three theories—forced inflection, crushing, and tearing. Which must we adopt for this patient? Which must I advise you to adopt for most cases? Neither one exclusively, and all three together, with predominance of one or the other of them according to the age of the subject.

For, as I told you a moment ago, the clinical documents do not furnish any peremptory reason in favour of the intervention of one of these mechanisms rather than of another; and, on the other hand, I do not feel disposed to apply to this patient, any more than to all others, the results of experiments upon the cadaver. I know that some surgeons, especially Nélaton, Voillemier, and O. Lecomte, have tried to clear up the question by experiments of this kind. But there are two conditions which cannot be reproduced upon the cadaver, and which contribute greatly to the production of the lesion upon the living subject.

The first is muscular contraction. I would not go so far as to admit with Pouteau[2] fracture of the lower extremity by muscular contraction, and especially by that of the long supinator, but I do not the less admit that in a fall upon the palm of the hand, the contraction of all the muscles of the forearm, excited by emotion and the instinctive desire to avoid danger, ought to draw the ball of the hand upwards and increase the pressure of the bones of the carpus against the articular facet of the radius, a pressure which favours crushing.

The second condition is this peculiar fragility induced by senile rarefaction. It varies much according to the subjects, and it was not noted if it existed or to what degree it existed in the cadavers used for the experiments.

If, for these reasons, I cannot tell you with absolute certainty what took place in our patient at the moment of the accident, I can at least offer you well-founded presumptions. Now, there is one condition which exists in him as in most of those who have passed the age of

---

[1] Lecomte, Archives de Médecine, 1860, tomes xvi. and xvii.
[2] Pouteau, Œuvres posthumes, tome ii. p. 251.

fifty years, that is, the rarefaction of the spongy tissue and the fragility which results from it. Notice that everybody falls, while walking, upon the palm of the hand, that everybody in so simple a fall does not break the radius, and that especially young people, and adults up to the age of 45 or 50 years, escape this injury. To be produced in them it needs a more energetic cause, such as a fall while running or from a high place.

What is there then peculiar in old people that can explain this lesion? It is not the weight of the body nor the rapidity of the fall which accounts for the easy production of the fracture. It is and can be nothing else than the fragility in question. Now this fragility is put to the proof especially by the crushing, that is, by the pressure from above downwards and from below upwards, to which the radius is subjected in a very simple fall, and the intervention of this mechanism has the advantage of explaining equally well the fractures after a fall upon the palm and those upon the back of the hand. I admit that in a fall upon the palm inflection backwards and tearing intervene to a certain extent, and that the anterior portion of the solution of continuity may be produced principally by them, but the crushing of the posterior portion is always the principal and even initial phenomenon.

I said that in the second place we had to explain the deformity. It is the consequence of what we know of the mechanism. At the moment of the fall the lower fragment is forced backwards by the pressure of the ball of the hand against it, undergoing, as Foucher pointed out, a slight movement of rotation about its transverse axis. Sometimes this movement is very slight, or when once produced it corrects itself, and this is what explains fractures without deformity or with a very slight one; sometimes the fragment remains in its new place, fixed there by muscular tonicity or by penetration, and then the deformity persists, being remediable if the muscles are not too energetic, or if the penetration is not accompanied by an insurmountable interlocking, and irremediable, on the contrary, if the opposite conditions exist.

As to the prognosis, remember that we have not to deal here with a serious disease; first, because life is not at all endangered, and then because in all probability consolidation will be soon obtained. In general, 20 to 25 days of immobility and retention suffice. At the end of this time, of course, the functions will not have recovered their integrity, and it will need considerable time for the articulations of the wrist and hand, as well as the neighbouring tendons, to recover their motions and their normal suppleness. But the consolidation will take place by a perfectly bony callus. The callus of course would only remain fibrous in case the patient was still older.

The gravity of the affection lies in the slowness of the return of the functions, slowness of which I have already had occasion to speak, and which will be all the greater here since the patient is nearly sixty years old:

As for the treatment, I remind you of the precept which you often hear me mention for fractures of the upper limb, that of not employing a restraining apparatus at first, and to wait until the inflammatory

period is over to envelop the limb and immobilize the fracture. I
applied flaxseed poultices sprinkled with lead-water or spirits of camphor, and told the patient to stay in bed. To be sure, he might be
allowed to get up, keeping his hand and forearm in a sling; but the
movements would probably cause pain, and it is better to keep quiet.
Before applying the first poultice I made the manœuvre of reduction.
While one assistant held the upper part of the forearm firmly with
both hands, and even drew it slightly backwards, and another grasped
the patient's hand and drew it forward with a certain force, I embraced
the wrist with both hands and exerted the pressure necessary to press
the lower fragment forwards and the upper one backwards, and thus
correct the deformity. I did thus correct it, and you may have seen
that when we laid the arm down, the wrist had recovered its normal
shape. At first I hoped that this result would be maintained, as I
have seen on several occasions, and that then it would be useless to
have recourse afterwards to a restraining apparatus. But my hope
was not realized. In a few moments you saw the deformity reappear,
and you must have concluded, as I did, that if we wished to suppress
it definitively it was necessary to maintain, by means of a restraining
apparatus, the result obtained by the reduction.

Now for what reason did I decide to wait a few days before applying this restraining apparatus? Because in certain cases the apparatus, if applied immediately, is found to be too tight and causes pain,
eschars, and even complete gangrene of the hand and forearm. Do
not forget these two things; in fractures of the lower extremity of
the radius, as in all others, there is, during the first five to eight days,
an inflammatory period, during which the limb swells. Then you
have here two quite superficial arteries, circulation through which is
easily diminished or checked by the compression exerted by the apparatus. If, then, you apply too tight a bandage, you may thereby
stop the circulation and cause the accidents I mentioned. If you
apply one which is not too tight at first, it may happen that, inflammatory swelling of the forearm occurring, the apparatus may exert
at the end of twenty-four or forty-eight hours a constriction upon the
tumefied limb which it did not at the beginning. I am far from
wishing to exaggerate the danger. Certainly you may apply an apparatus early if you are sure of not making it too tight, and especially
if you are able and willing to see the patient twice a day, and to
loosen or even remove the bandage in case pain or purple swelling of
the fingers warns you that the circulation is troubled.

Beware of the first of the symptoms, the pain. I know the lament-
able history of a woman, 70 years old, whose surgeon applied the first
day a roller bandage for a fracture of the lower extremity of the right
radius. A distance of two leagues separated the patient and the surgeon. It was agreed that the latter should be sent for if rather severe pain should be felt, but that otherwise he should come only at
the end of six days. The patient did not suffer, or suffered too little
to send for the surgeon, and when he arrived he found the hand and
forearm gangrenous. A very unpleasant litigation resulted.

It is to avoid a complication of this kind that I advise you not to apply an early apparatus unless you are sure of being able to watch it, and it is still better to apply only poultices during the first five or six days. These recommendations, which are good for all subjects, are especially applicable to children, women, and old people, that is, to all feeble subjects whose circulation is easily checked by compression of the radial and ulnar arteries. It is for those especially that I recommend you not to place an apparatus upon the broken forearm before the fifth day, whether it is a fracture of the extremities or of the shaft. You may reserve, if you choose, immediate application for vigorous adults, but always on condition of exercising a very close watch over it.

At the hospital you see that I reject in all cases the immediate use of the constricting bandage, because, on the one hand, I wish to fix in your minds the possible dangers of its use, and because, on the other hand, this action does not affect disadvantageously the after-treatment and the consequences of the injury. I see only one inconvenience in it for the patient—that of being compelled to remain in bed; for the simple envelopment in a poultice does not sufficiently immobilize the fracture, and exposes it to painful jars if the patient leaves his bed and walks about.

The treatment for this patient will be as follows :—

Poultices sprinkled with spirits of camphor will be kept on for five days, and on the sixth I shall apply the restraining apparatus which I have already described (see page 193), the one which I borrow from Malgaigne, and by means of which pressure is made upon the dorsal and palmar prominences. It is completed by graduated compresses and splints kept in place by three strips of diachylon plaster four feet long and two inches wide, so as to form what I call an open apparatus, by means of which the parts can be watched between the pieces of the apparatus, and relieved by loosening the bands if it is found that, in spite of the late application, the constriction has become too great.

The bands will be removed at the end of a week, the forearm carefully examined, and a new attempt at reduction made if it is found that the shape is not all that could be desired. The apparatus will then be reapplied as at first, and left in place until the twenty-first day, counting from the time of the accident. I advise you never to leave bandages for fracture of the lower extremity of the radius in place beyond this time; first, because twenty-one days are sufficient to obtain consolidation, and then because a more prolonged immobility would increase the painful stiffness of the fingers which I have pointed out as one of the consequences of the immobility caused by apparatuses for fracture of the upper limb.

Finally, after the bandage shall have been removed, I shall prescribe communicated movements, friction, massage, and sulphur baths, so as to shorten as much as possible the duration of the powerlessness to which the patients are condemned for a longer or shorter time, according to their age, in consequence of these fractures of the wrist.

II. The second patient of whom I have to speak interests you especially from a therapeutical point of view.

He is 57 years old and has already been in our wards for a fortnight. You remember that on the first day I made reduction in
the preceding case. The attempt was successful, the characteristic
deformity ceased, and, differing in this respect from the preceding one
and from most of those in which I make the same attempt, the result
was maintained, the displacement was not reproduced. Seeing that
the reduction persisted, I did not apply the open apparatus which I
habitually use, but contented myself with placing the forearm upon
a long bag filled with chaff and a splint, and fixing it with a roller
bandage. The cushion and the splint did not extend beyond the
wrist, so that the hand was left free and flexed. This very simple
apparatus, which was proposed by Robert, has the advantage of
neither compressing nor immobilizing the hand too much, and it also
diminishes the duration of the consecutive stiffness of the fingers. I
removed it this morning, and you saw that the shape of the wrist was
good, and that the functions, that is, the movements, although still
very imperfect, were much less limited than in patients upon whom
the ordinary restraining apparatus has been left for twenty-one days.
I recommend this mode of treatment. It will not do for those patients in whom a first or second well-made reduction is not maintained. But it is excellent for those in whom the reduction maintains itself without retention. The immobility which it supplies is
sufficient for the accomplishment of the consolidation, and it has the
great advantage of diminishing the duration of the painful stiffness
and immobility which, as you know, are the principal inconveniences
of fractures of the lower extremity of the radius.

III. The last patient of whom I have to speak is a young man 18
years old, who fell from a ladder, a distance of about ten feet, striking upon the palm of his left hand.

We found upon him the first day the characteristic antero-posterior
deformity, without marked inclination of the hand towards the radial
or the ulnar side. In addition I easily felt mobility and crepitation,
and I was able at once to make reduction, which, however, did not
remain. Nothing in the way in which the accident was produced
enlightened us upon the mechanism of the fracture; but in taking account of the age which authorizes us to believe in the existence of a
non-rarefied and still very solid cancellous tissue, and of the facility
with which I was able to move the lower fragment and feel crepitation, I think that the mechanism of crushing has not intervened,
that the cancellous tissue has not broken into multiple fragments as
is often the case in old people, that reciprocal penetration of the fragments has not taken place, and that finally the lower fragment has
not split down to the radio-carpal articulation, as it does quite often
in people advanced in age.

From all of this I conclude that the regular shape obtained by reduction and by the restraining apparatus which I applied the sixth
day will be maintained, and that we shall not have consecutive deformity due to the disappearance, by absorption, of part of the cancellous tissue, as is sometimes observed after fractures by crushing
and penetration.

I hope, furthermore, that the arthritis by proximity will be less severe and of shorter duration, for this arthritis, which takes place in almost all cases, is necessarily more marked in those it which the fracture invades the articular surfaces, than in those in which it does not. Finally, this is a young man who has never had rheumatism, and you remember that these conditions of age and health are favourable to the termination by resolution of traumatic arthritis.

I might have discussed the question of diagnosis, and asked if, instead of a fracture, I should not consider this a tearing off of the epiphysis. I do not think so, and for these reasons: the simple tearing off of an epiphysis is rare, and when solution of continuity takes place at the point occupied by an epiphysary cartilage, anatomical observation has shown that it is produced almost always partly upon the cartilage and partly upon the bone, so that a real fracture coincides habitually with rupture of the cartilage. Moreover, an epiphysary separation adds absolutely nothing to the results, nor, consequently, to the prognosis or treatment. All the clinical interest of the lesion, in such a case, lies in this peculiarity, that the spongy tissue is solid, not rarefied; that it must have escaped crushing, penetration, and multiple fragmentation, and that finally the age predisposes to the prompt return of the suppleness and polish of the articular and tendinous synovial membranes which have been consecutively inflamed. We have only reached the twelfth day, but I hope, if the patient consents to come back and see us two or three weeks after he leaves us, to be able to show you how much more rapid and indolent the restoration of the movements has been than in the older patients.

LECTURE XXVI.

FRACTURE OF THE CLAVICLE BY MUSCULAR ACTION.

Considerations upon the mode of production of fractures of this bone—Case of a fracture by muscular action—The fracture is without rupture of the periosteum and without displacement, as in children—Examination and criticism of apparatus invented for fracture of the clavicle—Preference given to the sling—Substitution of the double sling for Mayor's simple one.

GENTLEMEN: We have at this moment at No. 43, Ward Sainte-Vierge, a man, 40 years old, affected with fracture of the clavicle, in whom this lesion was produced in an unusual manner.

You know that, strictly speaking, fractures of this bone may be occasioned by direct causes, such as a heavy body falling upon the clavicle, or a violent blow with a stick. But cases of this kind are much the least frequent, and in any case I have not observed the more or less serious concomitant lesions, generally called *complications*, which, in other bones, are produced by the vulnerant bodies which cause the direct fractures: I refer to considerable effusions of blood, phlyctænæ, eschars, and wounds. It is a remarkable fact that fractures of the clavicle are very rarely compound, and that the skin remains almost always intact, even when one of the fragments makes a very pointed and apparently very threatening prominence under it. I attribute this chiefly to the fact that direct causes rarely take part in their production.

The most frequent fractures are those which are produced indirectly by the action of causes which tend to increase the natural curves of the bone, and to make it break at some point of one of these curves, as when one falls upon his shoulder, or even the elbow, and the clavicle is thus subjected to exaggerated pressure between the sternum and the ground.

Another, which is observed quite rarely, is fracture caused exclusively by muscular action. To this category belongs the one of which I shall speak to-day.

On the 12th December, 1868, this man was helping to place upon the shoulder of a comrade a large, heavy piece of marble. At the moment when he lifted it, he felt a slight crack in his right shoulder, and was unable to continue. The next and the following days he was not able to work as usual; nevertheless, he waited a week before coming to the hospital.

As he had received no blow upon the clavicle, and had not fallen upon the shoulder, I did not think at first of a fracture, and I examined the deltoid region and the right scapulo-humeral articulation. Not finding any lesion at these points, I carried my eyes and then my fingers towards the clavicle. I found at the middle of this bone a round, quite uniform swelling. Then by pressing with one finger upon this point, and gently moving the two ends of the clavicle in opposite directions by seizing each one with one hand, I felt very distinctly a fine crepitation and abnormal mobility.

It is evident then that the clavicle was broken, and as there had been intervention neither of a direct blow, nor of the usual indirect cause, we are authorized to say that the fracture was produced by muscular action; that is to say, that the clavicle—drawn powerfully upwards by the sterno-cleido-mastoideus and the trapezius when the effort was made to lift the weight, and drawn downwards at the same time by the contraction of the deltoid and pectoralis magnus, which take their fixed point upon it to move the humerus—was so forcibly pulled in two different directions that it broke at the point where undoubtedly it was weakest.

It is true that if we consider the usual solidity of the bone we have to doubt whether it could be overcome by muscular contraction, and we ask ourselves whether the fracture had not been prepared in this patient by a fragility due to an osteo-sarcoma, or to syphilis, or to the peculiar osteitis which Malgaigne pointed out for other bones, and which must be placed in the category of rarefying osteites.

Now, the commemoratives were entirely opposed to the first opinion, for the patient had not before the present accident any tumour which could be considered as cancerous.

On the other hand, he has not had syphilis. And moreover, I am

by no means convinced, as I have already said when speaking of
spontaneous fracture of the femur, that constitutional syphilis makes
the bones fragile, and for the moment I know of no fact which proves
that syphilitic osteitis sometimes takes on the rarefying form. Undoubtedly it is not impossible, but it has never been proved by observation, while, on the contrary, there is no lack of cases in which
syphilitic periostitis, called also periostosis, has terminated in a permanent increase of size, or hyperostosis, indicating the intervention
of a condensing osteitis.

As for the special osteitis pointed out by Malgaigne as preparing
the way for spontaneous fractures, we have no positive sign which
authorizes us to believe that it has existed in our patient. Rarefying
osteitis of the compact tissue, indeed, is only manifested to us by
physical signs, and the only functional symptom which might cause
it to be admitted is prolonged pain at that part of the limb where
rarefaction takes place. As our patient declares he has had no pain
of this kind, I cannot say that his fracture has had a rarefying osteitis
for predisposing cause.

Notice two things here: first, it may easily be that the slow and
prolonged osteitis which terminates by rarefaction and fragility was
indolent. Second, it is not impossible, as I have already explained,
that the fragility may be due to a rarefaction independent of the inflammatory condition, rarefaction comparable to that which senility
leads to in the cancellous tissue of many long bones and which is produced without pain. I there touch upon a question which has been
but little studied. Our anatomo-pathological studies have made us
acquainted with senile rarefaction of the cancellous tissue; but they
have produced nothing yet for the analogous trouble of nutrition of
which the compact tissue becomes the seat as age increases, and even
without senility, or without the influence of a sort of premature senility. I should like to have this question studied; it might enable us
to understand better than we can to-day the facility with which direct
or indirect causes produce fracture of the most voluminous bones,
such as the tibia, the patella. I have long asked myself whether, in
such cases, premature senile rarefaction has not induced a fragility
which has facilitated the production of the fracture by chance causes
apparently quite slight, and it is a subject which I recommend to
your investigations.

But it is not only with respect to its etiology that our fracture is
an unusual one; it is so by its physical symptoms also.

I said that I had found a little mobility and fine crepitation; but I
did not speak of a projection upwards of the inner fragment, nor of a
lower prominence formed by the end of the outer fragment pulled
downwards and pressed under the other. In other words, I have
not spoken of the prominences and deformities which are most frequently found in fractures of the clavicle in adults. Why? Because these prominences and this deformity do not exist here. We
see only a round tumour, rather voluminous, but regular and without
inequalities. The fracture then is without displacement, and with a
volume which is explained by the fact that it is a week old; that

during this time the patient has not been treated, and although he
has not been working he has continued to use his arm.
Why this absence of displacement? Because there has been no
rupture of the periosteum, or because the fracture is toothed, and
the points have remained interlocked, and the periosteum has thickened, as it does in our experiments upon animals when the fracture
has been without displacement, and the fragments have been kept end
to end.

This variety is rare in adults, but much more common in children,
where it merits special attention on account of the difficulty of the
diagnosis. I show you from time to time at the hospital consultation
children four, five, or six years old who are brought to us for fracture of
the clavicle without rupture of the periosteum, the principal symptom
of which is a swelling, painful on pressure, at some point of the bone.
Immobilization with a sling for a fortnight is sufficient to reduce the
volume of the tumour and to have it replaced by a solid and scarcely
visible callus.

You saw me employ for this patient the treatment which I use for
almost all cases of fracture of the clavicle. It is a sling similar to
that of Mayor, but which, instead of being a single triangle, is a
double one, or, if you prefer, a piece of cloth, such as a handkerchief,
folded so as to form a triangle with two thicknesses. The forearm
is placed in the fold formed by these two flaps. The extremities of
the base of the double triangle are attached to one another behind the
back; the point of the posterior flap passes in front of the uninjured
shoulder, that of the anterior flap in front of the injured one, and they
are fixed to the ends of a compress looped around the posterior and
horizontal part of the sling, which ends pass over the shoulders to
meet the two points to which they are then pinned or sewed.

This simple bandage has no other object than to keep the shoulder
and the clavicle immovable, and to thus favor the consolidation. In
the present patient there is no other indication to be met. But in
those cases where there is displacement of the fragments, you see me
use the same sling. I only add, when the inner fragment projects
forcibly upwards, compression on it by means of a layer of cotton
and two compresses placed under the junction of the anterior point
of the sling and the compress to which it is fastened.

I do not mean to say that this simple apparatus always gives perfect results, that is, cure without deformity. For fractures of the
clavicle are like those of the leg. Some are without displacement,
like this one and like those which we often see in children, and then
the most simple apparatus is sufficient if it immobilizes. Others have
a displacement which it is easy to reduce and to keep reduced. The
simple apparatus does very well for these also. Others, finally, are
reducible, but very difficult to maintain, because the displacement
is reproduced by the slightest movement. In such cases I claim,
and it is the opinion already expressed by M. Nélaton,[1] that a simple,
well applied sling gives as good results as any of the more or less
complicated apparatuses proposed at different times.

[1] Nélaton, Éléments de Pathologie chirurgicale, tome 1er, p. 721.

In fact, if we study these apparatuses, we see that the principal object of most of them is to meet a proper indication. A great number, for example, from the time of Hippocrates to the end of the eighteenth century, are intended to carry upwards and backwards the outer fragment which is lowered and carried forward. Such especially was the object of those described in the works on surgery under the name of Heister's cross, Brasdor's corset, and Brunninghausen's strap.

At the end of the last century Desault showed that it was necessary to carry the outer fragment not only upwards and backwards, but also and especially outwards. For that purpose he proposed the axillary arrow-head cushion, intended to carry the humerus, and with it the scapula and clavicle, outwards, while a figure-of-8 bandage passed around the elbow of the injured side and the opposite axilla, and crossed over the broken clavicle, and held the shoulder and outer fragment up and back. Boyer's corset was also constructed to meet the same triple indication.

All these apparatuses, one after the other, have had to undergo about the same criticisms.

Desault justly reproached all that had preceded his with not meeting all the indications, with troubling the patients, and often giving a cure with prominence of the inner fragment.

Boyer objected to Desault's bandage because its hard cushion caused pain, because it interfered with respiration, and after all did not always prevent displacement of the fragments.

Boyer's apparatus is open to exactly the same objections, and when Mayor, of Lausanne, in 1834, proposed to suppress the arrow-head cushion and the complicated bands, and to substitute for them a simple sling which would carry the elbow inwards and upwards, and consequently the shoulder and the outer fragment of the clavicle outwards and upwards, he had no difficulty in showing that this bandage, reduced to its most simple expression, gave results not inferior to those of the complicated apparatuses previously used.

I have modified Mayor's sling by making it double instead of single, and thus fixing it more solidly. But I add that the main indication which it meets is that of keeping the clavicle and shoulder immovable.

Before applying it I make as complete reduction as possible by the manœuvre which consists in carrying the elbow inwards and upwards with one hand, while with the other, p a e   at the inner and upper part of the arm, I draw the shoulder further outwards. That having been done, I press the upper fragment downwards, and while the reduction is made I apply the sling as before described; on the following day I raise the anterior point of the sling and renew, if it has become relaxed, the pressure exerted upon the upper fragment by the compresses. But I do not believe, like all of my predecessors and some of my contemporaries, that I can maintain reduction of all fractures with displacement. I maintain some of them, but there are many which are maintained only very imperfectly, and which recover with a slight deformity and shortening. But as the objections made successively to all the methods of treatment prove, to my mind, that these defective results were inevitable and depended upon the condi-

14

tions of the fracture, I accept them as such, and do not claim to be able to avoid them. These irregular calluses, moreover, cause very little inconvenience; on the one hand, they do not interfere in any way with the functions of the limb, and on the other hand, they diminish with time because the point of the upper fragment is absorbed little by little. That which remains would be disagreeable only in case the patient were a young lady and compelled to appear in society with bare shoulders.

To avoid criticism, and to protect his responsibility, the surgeon should, in such a case, give the preference to Desault's bandage, the application of which, because it requires minute care, excuses the imperfection of the result. Indeed he might, in imitation of the fact cited by Mayor,[1] propose manual retention, that is, retention with one hand left permanently upon the fracture, as the only means of certainly obtaining a cure without deformity.

I have a last remark to make upon the treatment of fractures of the clavicle. It is not necessary to leave this bone immovable for a long time; twenty to twenty-five days are sufficient for an adult, fifteen to twenty days for a child.

At the end of this time it is necessary to examine carefully the condition of the bone, and allow movement if mobility and crepitation are no longer found. In those cases where the functions of the limb are slow to become re established, it is due most often to this, that, the apparatus having been kept on too long, the articulations, and especially the small ones of the hand, have taken on, in consequence of the immobility, a greater rigidity than they would otherwise have done.

[1] Mayor, Chirurgie simplifiée, tome ii.

PART III.

TRAUMATIC OSTEITIS AND NECROSIS.

LECTURE XXVII.

TRAUMATIC OSTEITIS OF LONG BONES.

Exposed wounds of the bones—Acute osteo-myelitis, suppurating, and putrid—Its relations with septicæmia (traumatic fever and purulent infection)—Its anatomical characteristics—Its coincidence with simple phlebitis and putrid phlebitis.

GENTLEMEN: I gladly take the opportunity which is offered to-day to show you the pieces coming from three patients who have succumbed, one of them to traumatic fever, the other two to purulent infection, after injuries which had placed the bones in contact with the air and had exposed them to suppurating traumatic osteitis.

I shall speak to you on some other occasion[1] of the relation which exists between acute suppurating osteitis and these two dangerous diseases which it often engenders: traumatic fever and purulent infection or pyæmia.

To-day I leave the latter aside to call your attention solely to the first, the osteitis, which you will not find described in our classical authors with all the details which it deserves.

I. Notice first these two tibias : they belong to that one of our patients who was admitted six days ago for fracture of the middle portion of the right leg complicated by a quite large contused wound. The skin was not gangrenous, the wound was covered with blood clots, exudations, and small superficial eschars, which are seldom lacking in the first period, that during which suppuration of the contused wound is preparing. At the same time an abundant and fetid liquid escaped from the superficial and deep layers. Twenty-four hours after the admission of the patient a burning fever came on, with 125 to 140 pulsations, the temperature rising to 105° in the evening, and varying between 103° and 104° in the morning. Then, after two days, delirium set in, so that the patient had to be tied in his bed; then the abdomen swelled, and at the end of six days, during which the leg had notably increased in size, and the wound had not ceased to furnish an abundant and reddish fetid discharge of which I shall speak in a moment, death occurred.

The fever was not preceded by a chill.

[1] See Lecture xxix.

At the autopsy we found none of the visceral lesions of purulent infection. Furthermore, we found no appreciable lesion, either of the brain, or of the throax or abdomen. The only thing which attracted our attention was the enlargement and friability of the spleen, and the same distension of the intestines which we had remarked during the last days of the patient's life. It is evident, then, that the patient has succumbed to one of these febrile affections without appreciable lesion, upon which we can discuss for a long time without coming to a conclusion, or at least without convincing those who demand visible, material demonstrations in support of the explanation of the death. Without spending any time in this discussion I shall content myself with telling you that in my opinion, according to the negative results of the autopsy, the patient succumbed to what we have called, since Dupuytren,[1] *intense traumatic fever*, and to what we can consider as one of the varieties of traumatic septicæmia, that is, acute and primitive septicæmia.

But let us return to the examination of the bones. This is the tibia of the uninjured side. Externally it shows nothing peculiar. But I have broken it with a hammer to see the inside; you there find the medullary substance of the shaft and that of the cancellous tissue of the extremities with its reddish-yellow colour. Its injection is more marked than in many subjects, and might be considered hyperæmic. But you must remember that nothing varies in different subjects so much as do the proportions of the vascular and fatty parts of the marrow of the bones. Here, the vascular element is greatly developed; but you find nevertheless the yellow colour of the fat which crushes easily under the finger, but is not fluid; when rubbed upon paper, as I rub it now, it leaves large greasy spots. Its appearance is the same throughout; you find in it no effusions of blood, no plastic deposits, and, above all, you do not find the fetid odour which recalls that of putrefaction or maceration of the bones.

Compare this with the other tibia, the one which has been broken, and broken by an indirect cause (the patient had fallen while running, and the upper fragment had pierced the skin). Between the two principal fragments, for the fracture is slightly comminuted, you see softened blood clots which break under the fingers and give a very fetid odour; in the medullary canal of these fragments you find a substance which is much darker than that of the opposite side, is softer, and, above all, has a fetid odour. This substance shows in only a few small places the yellow colour of fat, and it greases the paper much less. At two points you find whitish deposits which are also fetid, and are composed of inflammatory products. These lesions extend about an inch beyond the solution of continuity, and on the upper fragment are continued as far as the cancellous tissue of the extremity.

If you saw the marrow of this side alone you might fail, as happened to many of our predecessors, to appreciate what I consider the very considerable morbid condition which exists. But if you

---

[1] Dupuytren, Leçons orales, tome vi.

notice the differences between it and the opposite side, you see that this medullary substance is profoundly altered, and that its alterations consist especially in the intimate combination of the fat and the albuminoid substance with blood poured out by the torn vessels, a disappearance, either by absorption or by escape to the outside, of a part of this fat, and finally a putrid decomposition, as well of the infiltrated blood as of the marrow itself and the exudated products. Something has taken place here which is analogous to that which occurs in a wound of the soft parts, and which always takes place in the first period of contused wounds which are preparing to suppurate. The tissues exposed to the air by the accident inflame, become partly gangrenous and putrid. But here the putrefaction has attacked the fatty parts at the same time with the blood inclosed in an almost incompressible cavity, into which the air penetrated easily as soon as a part of the liquid contents escaped. Notice, on the one hand, that this putridity has invaded that one of the fatty tissues of the body which is normally the best protected and most hidden, and which, for this reason perhaps, supports less easily than any other the consequences of exposure to the air.

Even if it should not be admitted that this lesion has the gravity which I attribute to it in considering it the starting-point of the putrid absorption which causes the septicæmia, you will admit that this decomposition of fat and blood at the bottom of a bony cavity ought to be mentioned.

Our predecessors paid no attention to it, and the modern writers who have the merit of having attached their names to the description of osteo-myelitis, especially Raynaud,[1] Chassaignac,[2] Th. Vallette,[3] and Jules Roux,[4] omitted to describe the first period of this osteomyelitis.

They spoke especially of the period of suppuration. It is true that they said that before the suppuration there was hyperæmia with exudations, but they did not describe this form, at the same time exudative and putrid, which is not yet gangrene, but is very near it, and is even sometimes gangrene in places. It is the possible but not inevitable consequence of compound fractures, and I consider it as one of the forms of osteo-myelitis. I call it *putrid osteo myelitis* preceding suppuration, or primitive. Taking into account the propagation of the medullitis along the medullary canal, I might even call it *putrid and diffuse osteo-myelitis.*

I looked to see if the neighbouring veins were affected. I could find nothing in the nutritive vein at its point of emergence from the nutritive foramen. But the posterior tibial and the popliteal veins were obliterated by clots, without admixture of serosity or of pus, and without the fluidity and the bad odour of coagulated blood. I did not

[1] Raynaud; De l'Inflammation du Tissu médullaire des Os longs (Archives Générales de Médecine, 1831, tome xxvi. p. 161).

[2] Chassaignac; Mémoire sur l'Ostéo-myélite (Gazette Médicale, 1854).

[3] Th. Vallette; Gazette des Hôpitaux, 1855, p. 594.

[4] J. Roux; De l'Ostéo-myélite et des Amputations secondaires à la suite des coups de feu. (Mém. de l'Acad. de Médecine, 1860, tome xxiv. p. 539, avec plate.)

find the internal membrane of the vein thickened, and I cannot say that this vein was actually inflamed; I might then use the term spontaneous coagulation or thrombosis, accompanying putrid osteo-myelitis. I shall often have occasion to point out to you the frequency of the coincidence of these venous lesions with osteo-myelitis, and to discuss the nature of the first. To-day, I content myself with telling you that if it is allowable to doubt, in this and in similar cases, the reality of the inflammation of the surface of the vein, there are, on the other hand, reasons to admit this inflammation; and, as the blood contained in the veins thus affected presents capital differences, according to whether it has retained or lost its chemical qualities by decomposition, according also to whether it alone fills the vein or is mixed with pus, which can be attributed to nothing else than a phlebitis, I continue to admit phlebitis in cases of this kind. I only say that here the phlebitis is coagulating and not putrid.

II. Examine now this upper half of a right femur.

It comes from a patient 32 years old, whose thigh I amputated eighteen days ago, for a white swelling of the knee. He was carried off by a purulent infection, of which the first chill occurred on the tenth day, and which had been preceded by an intense traumatic fever.

You know that we found metastatic abscesses in both lungs, but to-day I wish you to study especially the lesions of this femur.

You notice, first, that the periosteum has entirely disappeared for a distance of about an inch. What has become of it? Has it been destroyed by gangrene? Has it been absorbed? It is very difficult to give a satisfactory answer to these questions, because we do not see the succession of the phenomena upon the living patient. We perform an operation; we leave the bone covered by the soft parts; and we carefully avoid raising the latter every day to see what is taking place upon the former. And, when we have the opportunity to examine it, either during life or after death, we no longer find the periosteal covering, and we cannot know how it disappeared; but remember that Reynaud[1] has pointed out the remarkable peculiarity that, in such cases, the marrow inflames and suppurates to a height which is about the same as that of the destruction of the periosteum.

We have broken the femur and found the marrow altered a little higher than the periosteum. The alteration consists, as you see, in a diminution of volume, which has left a gap and, consequently, a place for the air; a grayish putrilaginous softening; and an absolute impossibility to discover the normal anatomical characteristics of the medullary substance; here and there very fluid pus; but above all, a fetid odour, as well of the putrilaginous as of the liquid part. I look to see if the Haversian canaliculi also include this broken-down matter and fetid pus; it is not very certain, but that is undoubtedly due to the smallness of the parts; for, by using a glass, I can see in the small open cavity of the canaliculi, a grayish liquid which looks like serous pus; and I do not find the reddish colour which indicates

---

[1] Reynaud; loc. cit.

the presence of bloodvessels.   Most of these vessels seem to have disappeared, and, as the different sections of the compact tissue are less red than those of the other femur, I conclude that this one, although still living, had nevertheless lost a part of its means of nutrition, and, calling to mind those patients who, after suppuration of the bone, have had consecutive necrosis, I find here the first period of a necrosis which would inevitably have taken place if the fatal pyæmia had not intervened.

The chief point in this specimen is the profound alteration of the marrow, its transformation into dirty broken-down matter, and its fetid suppuration; lesions which are doubtless due, in part, to the nature of the inflammation, and mainly to the decomposing influence upon this inflamed marrow of the outer air within the gaping cavity of the medullary canal; and, as the walls of the Haversian canaliculi are also rigid and gaping, I find in it another reason for believing that putrid suppuration in them coincides with that which takes place in the central canal.

However that may be, I see there the second degree of the disease of which I showed you the first degree upon the preceding specimen. It is still a putrid osteo-myelitis, but the putridity no longer affects the infiltrated and effused blood; it is that of the pus and of the remains of the profoundly altered marrow.   It is, in a word, consecutive putrid osteo-myelitis, or, if you prefer, putrid suppurative osteo-myelitis.

Remember this fact and its coincidence with purulent infection, for, when I shall discuss the pathogeny of the latter in your presence, I shall refer to it in support of the opinion which I shall then express.

A final remark: the crural vein, which I here show you, is filled with softened clots, and here and there contains fetid pus.   Its internal membrane is slightly thickened and friable; its cellular coat is also thickened.   These are certainly the anatomical characteristics of phlebitis, and since the matter contained in the vessel has undergone putrid decomposition, like that of the marrow, I conclude that this is a putrid phlebitis.   I look in vain for direct vascular communication between the marrow and the crural vein.   On the one hand, the amputation having been made above the nutritive foramen, I cannot find the nutritive vein, the only one large enough to be easily dissected out.   On the other hand, the other veins, which might perhaps have established the communication, are too small to be perceived, and many of them have doubtless disappeared in consequence of the beginning of the mortification of which the marrow and the compact substance itself were the seat.

You see that I am again, as I was a moment ago, struck with the coincidence of the osteo-myelitis and the phlebitis; I am preoccupied with the possibility of a pathogenic relation between them; I should like to know if the suppurative phlebitis is developed independently, or if it owes its origin to the passage into the veins of putrid matter coming from the marrow through the veinules leading from the bones.   But I have no proof, and can only insist upon the coincidence of the putrid phlebitis with the putrid osteo myelitis.

I do not claim that these two things always coexist. I showed you, a moment ago, a primitive putrid osteo-myelitis with a non-putrid phlebitis. I shall show you, in other cases, putrid suppurative osteo-myelitis without any apparent phlebitis. The coincidence is nevertheless very frequent, and ought to be considered when the mode of development of purulent infection is discussed.

III. The third piece is the skullcap of a patient in whom we recognized the existence of a fracture of the parietal bone, together with a contused wound of the right side of the head.

Suppurative inflammation had invaded both the external wound and the bone, the parietal bone became denuded by one of those rapid disappearances of the periosteum which occur in acute suppurating osteitis, and the mechanism of which is not yet well known. On the 13th day chills commenced, then followed the cortege of the symptoms of purulent infection, and the patient died on the twenty-second day after the accident.

You know how frequent this kind of death is after compound fractures of the top of the skull. You will read of cases of abscess of the liver occurring after wounds of this kind, and the insufficient theories offered in explanation by J. L. Petit, Bertrandi, Quesnay.[1] Your books will show you that afterwards, according to the valuable works of Dance[2] upon suppurative phlebitis, and those of Breschet[3] upon the large venous canals of the diploë, the opinion was produced that the abscesses of the liver are the consequence of a consecutive infection or mixture of the blood with pus formed in the large bony veins of which I have just spoken. The latter become inflamed and suppurate, as do those of the soft parts, and allow a part of the pus, which is formed by the phlebitis in their interior, to enter into the circulation.

In this specimen you recognize the exactitude of the fact. One of the fragments into which I broke the bone with a hammer shows us an open vein of the diploë. This vein contains serous pus. Undoubtedly here was a suppurative phlebitis. Moreover we followed a veinule leading from the inner surface of the skull to the superior longitudinal sinus. This veinule and the sinus itself inclosed clots without apparent pus, so that we have a suppurative phlebitis of the diploë with a non-suppurative and simply adhesive phlebitis of the veins external to the bone. But I beg you to again notice here, two anatomo-physiological characteristics which escaped the attention of our predecessors. First, this pus which is in the vein of the diploë is serous, of a bad aspect and fetid odour. Secondly, it is not the vein alone which is suppurating; it is the entire diploë of the parietal bone. It is true that you do not see the pus flow; it is not abundant enough for that. But look more closely at this diploë, and compare it with that of the other parietal which I have also broken. The

[1] Mémoires et prix de l'Académie de Chirurgie, Paris, 1747-1797.
[2] Dance, Sur la Phlébite externe et la Phlébite en général. (Archives de Médecine, tome xviii. p. 286.)
[3] Breschet, Recherches Anatomiques, Physiologiques et Pathologiques, sur le Système Veineux, Paris, 1827-29, in folio.

Colour is not the same; it is a dirty-gray in the first, and pink in the second. Nor are the contents of the cells the same; yellowish in many points, and blackish in others in the first, where it is composed of pus mixed here and there with blood; it is more purely red in the second, where it is composed of blood and fat. Nor is the odour the same. That of the first comes much nearer putrefaction than does that of the second. In short, here too is suppuration not only of the bony vein but of the whole diploë, and as the contents of the diploë are really analogous, in the normal state, to those of the medullary canal and of all the cavities of the long bones, I consider this also an acute suppurative osteo-myelitis; and on the other hand, as the pus is of bad quality and putrid, and as a fatal infection followed the diploic suppuration, I consider that this suppurative osteo-myelitis is putrid, and, for reasons which I shall hereafter give you, I place in this serious lesion the origin of the purulent infection which carried off the patient.

LECTURE XXVIII.

NECROSIS OF THE LONG BONES.

Its origin is most often traumatic in adults, spontaneous in children and adolescents—Obscurity of former descriptions—Too ready belief in a period of repair—Necrosis is a result of suppurative condensing osteitis, like the hyperostosis which accompanies it—Account of a necrosis of the humerus with invaginated sequestrum—Operation—Persistence of a long cavity in the humerus.

GENTLEMEN: I have often had occasion to show you patients upon whose limbs were fistulæ with longer or shorter suppurating tracts, which ended at denuded portions of the long bones, some of which portions were still immovable, others movable and about to be expelled. You have not forgotten, especially, the femurs, tibias, and humeruses which had been broken by balls, and which, after having been attacked by general suppurative osteitis, lost at different times mortified fragments, which we called *splinters* when they were small, *sequestra* when they were rather large. Nor have you forgotten those adolescents in whom I showed you the elimination of similar splinters and sequestra after spontaneous epiphysary osteitis. Finally, you know that we gave the name *necrosis* to the condition of mortified parts of the skeleton which are destined to be expelled. But you understood and have remembered that necrosis is an incident superadded to suppurating osteitis, when the latter is not putrid and fatal, and especially to general suppurating osteitis, that which occupies at the same time the periosteum, the parenchyma, and the deep parts of the bone, that is, the medullary canal, and the whole thickness of the cancellous tissue, when it is the extremity that is affected. Our authors, in describing necrosis, made a mistake in isolating this deep

suppurative osteitis, or osteo-myelitis, and making of it a special
pathological entity. That is true and proper for the very thin flat
bones, such as those of the palatal arch, and the turbinated bones.
For them the phenomena of the suppurating osteitis are so slight, and
the consequences of the loss of substance of the bone, which, moreover, are generally inseparable, are so predominant, that I understand
the importance given to the phenomena mortification and elimination
by a description which is confined almost exclusively to the necrosis.

But you may have noticed in the shaft of the long bones, in the
cases of which I have just reminded you, that a great anatomo-
physiological and clinical phenomenon, non-putrid suppurating osteitis,
precedes the necrosis, and that another phenomenon, hyperostosis,
accompanies and follows it. The necrosis consequently is a consecutive lesion, and, as it were, superadded to two others, suppuration and
hypertrophy; and it belongs to a variety of osteitis which, to be
well characterized, ought to be called *condensing and necrotic suppurating osteitis.* This connection of course is not sufficient for us to
give up absolutely the description of necrosis. On the contrary, I
consider this description necessary for those cases in which the disease
has reached a period at which, the suppuration and hypertrophy no
longer having any gravity or clinical interest, the mortification and
elimination constitute the morbid condition, and alone call for the
attention and intervention of the surgeon. But this too ready belief
in the entity *necrosis* is based upon a physiological error which has
greatly obscured the descriptions, and which it is time to correct.
This error consisted in subordinating all the phenomena of the disease to a reparatory effort preceded by a destructive one. Read the
works of Troja, Weidmann, Boyer, and all the contemporaneous
French treatises upon this subject, you will see that their main object
is to show how the bone is renewed, and to present its excess of volume
as the result of a reparatory process supposed to be produced sometimes by the periosteum, sometimes by the marrow.

This opinion was based upon experiments made by Troja and
Weidmann, experiments which consisted in destroying the periosteum,
the marrow, or the nutritive artery of an animal's tibia, and noticing
the anatomical phenomena which followed these lesions. These
authors found that, after a certain length of time, the central part of
the bone, which had been deprived of its nutritive materials, became
mortified and surrounded by a bone which they supposed to be new,
and to have been furnished by the uninjured periosteum. But to
protect this interpretation from criticism, the destruction of the
marrow should have been followed by the mortification of the whole
thickness of the bone in those animals in which they found central
necrosis. Now, this has not been observed, and it is very possible
that a part of the thickness nourished by the periosteal and muscular
vessels may have escaped the destruction, and that the new bone may
have been furnished by this portion of preserved bone, and not by the
periosteum. On the other hand, in the experiments in which they
destroyed the periosteum, the mortification did not necessarily extend
to the marrow, and they were not authorized to say that in such cases

it was this organ that had produced the new bone; for, as in the other case, it might have come from the part of the bone which remained alive.

I have never understood why they have so readily and so generally admitted the reproduction of the bones, either by a pretended medullary membrane, the non-existence of which I long ago demonstrated, or by the periosteum, and why they have had so much difficulty to admit that the bone itself, by its compact as well as by its cancellous tissue, should be able to grow, to vegetate, to produce, in a word, new ossification. In my opinion, it is sufficient to observe the clinical course of osteites, and a few specimens of pathological anatomy, in order to be convinced of two things: 1st. That bones can complete and repair themselves after spontaneous lesions, as I told you took place after fractures, by an augmentation of the nutritive movement in their frame itself, as well as by the hyperactivity of their envelope; 2d. That, moreover, in osteitis in man things take place differently than in experiments upon animals, and that observation of the facts, far from showing a period of repair consecutive to a period of elimination, tended rather to show that destruction was a salutary effort to rid of superfluous matter the bone, which had become too voluminous as a result of the hypertrophy and the osteitis which produced it.

To convince you of the correctness of these ideas, let me remind you of two pieces which I had occasion to show you last year, and which had been taken from two patients who had had for a long time before their death, the one a spontaneous osteitis of the femur, the other an osteitis consecutive to a fracture and the formation of a callus. I insisted upon the capital fact that, in one as in the other, there had been no bony suppuration. The osteitis had remained plastic, to use an expression which I have often employed; the periosteum and the medullary organ had been neither thinned nor hypertrophied. But I showed you in the sawn bone a compact tissue twice as thick as in the normal condition, and much more dense, and a cancellous tissue with smaller cells and stouter trabeculæ than usual. An excess of bony substance had evidently formed, and had increased the volume and the weight of the bone, and the object of this excess had not been to repair a loss of substance, for none had taken place. It was a simple product of the disease, that is, of the osteitis, and I showed you how just and useful was the expression of condensing osteitis invented by Gerdy. But in the cases of which I speak, the condensing osteitis had taken place without suppuration, it had been the plastic condensing osteitis.

Let us now return to the traumatic suppurating osteitis of adults, to the acute spontaneous suppurating osteitis of adolescents. What has the clinical and anatomo-pathological study of them shown us? The clinical study has shown us four things in the succession of observable phenomena.

1st. The destruction of the periosteum to a certain extent.

2d. Suppuration invading the surface, the whole thickness, and the medullary canal of the bone, taking, in short, the extension which it has in the acute suppurating esteo-myelitis of adolescents, and accompanied, furthermore, by similar febrile phenomena.

3d. The increase of volume, quite similar to that which we found in the simple plastic and condensing osteitis.

4th. Afterwards, and long after this hypertrophy, an elimination of the necrosed portions, a single elimination in some patients, and a repeated one in others, with numerous variations in the volume of the sequestra and the interval of the eliminations, while the disease is prolonged for several months, and often for several years.

The anatomo-pathological study of the few pieces which I have had occasion to show you has shown us:—

1st. A first period, characterized by an injection of the periosteum at the points where it had not been destroyed, by a concomitant hyperæmia of the medullary organ, and finally by the dilatation of the Haversian canaliculi of the compact tissue which may be considered as a hyperæmia or injection of the compact tissue.

2d. A second period, in which the vascularized bone suppurates and increases notably in volume. Suppuration is found in the medullary canal and in all the canaliculi of the compact substance, canaliculi which are the principal theatre of the appreciable anatomical phenomena of inflammation of the bone. But at the same time certain points of the compact tissue, previously hypertrophied, lose the vascularization of which I spoke, and take a more or less eburnated aspect which is explained by a diminution of vitality following the augmentation which was indicated by the enlargement of the vascular canaliculi.

3d. A third period, in which the mortified portions are separated from the rest of the bone by a groove, at the bottom of which lies the pus whose formation coincides with the destruction of the bony tissue which is intermediate between that which is necrosed and that which remains alive. This period is more or less prolonged according as the sequestra are or are not invaginated, that is, surrounded by living bone, and according as the portions destined to die are more or less numerous, and succeed one another more or less rapidly.

4th. Finally, a fourth period, which always appears late, and which is characterized by the cicatrization of the fistulous openings, their adherence to the bone, and the preservation by the latter of a greater volume than normal.

What is to be remarked in this evolution is the formation, from the beginning and before the mortification is realized, of a hyperostosis exactly similar to that which takes place in the cases of non-suppurating osteitis, and in which the parenchyma of the compact tissue shares as well as the periosteum and the marrow. Now I cannot see in the increase of size a reparatory process destined to replace the mortified portions, since it commences before the necrosis, properly so-called. Between plastic condensing osteitis of the long bones and suppurating condensing osteitis, I find this difference, that the former takes place without necrosis, and that the second is easily accompanied by necrosis.

Why and how is this difference? The explanation is easy. I suppose that in suppurating osteitis of the compact tissue the inflammation is severe, and is followed by the obliteration of a certain number of vascular canaliculi by the deposit of too abundant bony layers, that this obliteration may produce mortification at the points where it takes place, and that the latter occurs particularly at the points where the periosteum has been destroyed by the excess of the inflammatory process, the bone being deprived at these points of a part of its means of nutrition, while at the same time those which remain are compressed and afterwards obliterated by the diminution of the calibre of their protecting canals. I do not know if my supposition is correct, but in any case, no one can give in the present state of the science an irreproachable explanation of necrosis in acute suppurating osteitis. The important thing, clinically speaking, is to recognize the phenomena, and not to allow ourselves to be turned from observation of them by the acceptation of theories which themselves are only presumptions, but which, instead of being accepted as such, pass, by being often repeated, for demonstrated truths.

In order not to obscure your ideas upon this subject I must add three more considerations:—

The first is, that, if suppurating osteitis of the long bones is often accompanied by necrosis, yet it is not inevitable, and you will sometimes see the first without the other.

The second is that the necrosis, that is, the mortified part, may be external or invaginated. The external one is unquestionably the most frequent, doubtless because, as I explained it, the previous destruction of the periosteum by an inflammatory or a gangrenous process contributes to the mortification. The invaginated form is found when, the periosteum not having been destroyed, chance or circumstances with which we are not acquainted cause the mortification to take place in the centre of the compact tissue or very near to the medullary canal. It is the custom to say in such cases that the old bone, or a part of the old bone, is inclosed in new bone. That is true in some exceptional cases, in those, for example, in which after an amputation the purulent osteo-myelitis has been followed by the mortification of the whole thickness of the bone to a certain height, and in which the remaining periosteum has furnished, under the influence of its excessive vitality, a new bony substance which forms in fact a real new bone. In most of the other cases the invaginated sequestrum is surrounded, not by a new bone, but by the part of the old bone which has not mortified, which is hypertrophied, and of which the hypertrophy, moreover, is not produced by the periosteum, since the latter is habitually destroyed over a certain extent. Nor is it produced by the marrow, for that too is sometimes destroyed, sometimes invaded itself by ossification, and because also it is too far from the sequestrum for us to admit the formation by it of such a thickness of bone as is sometimes seen.

In short, it is the same with the hypertrophy of necrotic suppurating osteitis as with that which accompanies the non-suppurating osteitis of adolescents. Strictly speaking it is not the result of a special reparatory process. It is due to the nature of the inflammation in the compact tissue. This nature doubtless intervenes when there is repair, as in the case of fracture. But its intervention is no more a benefit than is an erysipelas or a phlegmon in the cicatrization of a wound. I consider this augmentation of volume a superfluity, a complication, and I consider it even as being one of the causes of necrosis in long bones.

My third remark relates to the anterior condition of the constitution of those who have, with or without suppuration, hyperostoses consecutive to osteitis. In most of them the health was originally good. You will often hear it said that suppuration of the bones is due to scrofula; that is true of the suppurating osteites of the cancellous tissue of the short bones, or of the extremity of the long bones, and I will show you, at the proper time and place, that this suppurating osteitis of scrofulous persons is at the same time rarefying, and that if it becomes condensing, it is so only in places, and not over a great extent, as is the case in condensing osteitis of the compact tissue. We might give as an axiom this proposition, that condensation and hypertrophy, during and after osteitis, indicate a good constitution, or at least the absence of the scrofulous diathesis. I do not mean by this that patients do not die of an acute suppurating osteitis, for, on the contrary, I have shown you that this affection sometimes causes death by traumatic fever or by purulent infection; I mean only to say that they do not die of exhaustion and of phthisis, as is so often the case with patients affected with caries, that is, with rarefying suppurating osteitis of the cancellous tissue. Should we go so far as to say that patients affected with necrosis of the compact tissue never become tuberculous or phthisical? Of course not; I admit that they may become so; but it is occasionally, after the deterioration of their health by an abundant and prolonged suppuration, much more than by an original disposition. In a word, if necrosis can give rise to the lesions of the scrofulous diathesis, it is not, generally at least, the scrofulous diathesis which gives rise to necrosis.

The object of these general considerations, gentlemen, was to prepare you to grasp the details concerning a patient affected with necrosis of the humerus, in whom the suppurating osteitis, terminating in mortification, is not of traumatic origin like that of which you have seen so many examples after gunshot wounds. It is of spontaneous origin, and although it began at the age of eighteen years, and although in this respect we have in it another of the so frequent examples of spontaneous suppurating osteitis of adolescence, yet the disease has differed from what it ordinarily is, under these circumstances, by a much less acute, slower, and milder course.

The patient, who is now 32 years old, says his disease began at the age of 18. At that time, however, as I just told you, he did not have the acute or hyperacute form which we see so often in adolescents, and which we see more frequently upon the bones of the lower limb than upon those of the upper one. He knows of no particular cause to which this origin can be referred. He only knows that an abscess formed slowly on the outer side of the right arm, and that this abscess, after having opened spontaneously, remained fistulous. He came to me in 1859, three years after it began, when he was twenty-one years old, and I treated him at the Hôpital Cochin, where I had charge of the surgical service. I felt with a probe a denuded and movable portion of bone at the bottom of the fistulous tract; I made an incision, withdrew the sequestrum, which was superficial and not invaginated, and, with the hope of modifying the vitality of the bone, I cauterized it with the hot iron. Notwithstanding that, the patient left the hospital with the fistulous openings, which he has retained for ten years, and you see them to-day (22 Feb. 1870), five in number, upon the superior external portion of the right arm, for the bony lesion occupies the upper fourth of the shaft of the humerus, without at the same time interesting the head of the bone.

Notwithstanding these fistulæ through which the pus continually flows, the patient is hearty and muscular, and for the last ten years has done, almost without interruption, the heavy work of a mason. But, annoyed by this continued suppuration, he has again come to ask my care.

A probe passed into these fistulæ finds a portion of bone denuded over a certain extent, and giving on percussion the dry sound and the sensation of hardness which necrosis presents. The sensations perceived are very distinct; it is a necrosis, there is no doubt remaining upon that point; but I should like to be enlightened upon two others: If the necrosed portion is movable, and if it is or is not invaginated. You understand the important bearing of these questions upon the method of operation. For, if the sequestrum is invaginated, it will be necessary, in order to remove it, to open all that portion of the still living bone which surrounds it. I made in your presence the examination needed to clear up this point. You saw that it gave me certain results only at the end. I felt at the beginning indistinct mobility of the denuded and sonorous portion, but I did not know if I ought to regard that mobility as real, or attribute the sensation to the bending of the probe. To remove this chance of error I abandoned the probes, and made use of grooved directors. I introduced two of them by different orifices, and leaving one of them loose in the fistula, I tried with the other, which I held in my right hand, to move the bone in which I suspected mobility. I at once saw the loose director move freely, and these movements could have been given to it only by the portion of bone upon which the other director was pressed, and proved clearly that this portion was movable.

The mobility of the sequestrum being recognized, it remained, as I told you, to know whether it was invaginated or external; I inclined towards the latter opinion, but in view of the possible existence of invagination I prepared the instruments necessary to hollow out the bone.

The patient was anæsthetized with ether; I made an incision over the deltoid; uncovered the sequestrum, the mobility of which became still more evident when my finger touched it; then seizing it with strong forceps I drew it out. It was about an inch long, and three-quarters of an inch wide. Then introducing my finger into the wound to see if there were other sequestra, I felt none at first, and found only a large gutter in the humerus. It had been occupied by the sequestrum I had just removed, and its very smooth walls were covered by a pyogenic membrane. But at the lower part I felt a movable piece of bone, which projected through an opening at the bottom of this gutter, and seemed to occupy the interior of the humerus. I seized it with a pair of dressing forceps, and drew out a sequestrum much longer and larger than the first. It was invaginated, and occupied in the thickness of the bone a canal which opened at the top into the gutter of which I have just spoken. The opening had been large enough to allow the fragment to pass. I again explored the different hollows of the wound, and withdrew two more splinters; I could feel no others, but, notwithstanding the care with which I sought for them, I cannot affirm that none remain.

Will this operation suffice to bring about a radical cure? I do not dare to hope so, for these affections are extremely long, and pass many times through the same phases before getting well. As I told you, there are splinters which may escape notice, and, on the other hand, new portions of bone may subsequently mortify and cause fresh inflammation. In children, these osteites with suppuration and necrosis disappear generally at the end of three or four years, leaving only the hyperostosis behind them. In adolescents, they last habitually until adult life, that is, until the age of twenty-five or twenty-six years. In this respect our patient is exceptional, for he has retained his bony suppuration and necrosis until he has reached the thirty-second year of his age; perhaps that is due to the fact that the disease was not very acute at the beginning.

Before going further, let me show you what there is peculiar and difficult in the etiology and pathogeny of this necrosis, and also in the anatomical form which it presents.

As to the etiology, I shall say nothing more about the absence of a known occasional cause. I tell you only that, although resembling traumatic necrosis, such as we see after gunshot wounds and compound fractures, it is spontaneous, and commenced at the period of adolescence, but without presenting the acute or hyper-acute form which we sometimes see at that period of life. I will remind you also that this patient has neither commemorative nor present signs of scrofula, that nothing in him indicates tuberculosis, and that if there has been intervention of an internal cause, as I am willing to admit, it remains unknown to us, and belongs to none of those which characterize the generally accepted diatheses.

As to the pathogeny, the mortification which occupies the compact tissue of the upper part of the shaft of the humerus coincides, as you may have discovered by comparing the size of the two arms, with a notable augmentation of the volume of the humerus, so that you have here another example of that triple lesson of which I spoke a moment ago: suppuration of the bone, its necrosis, and its hypertrophy.

As for the anatomical form we had, at first, an external sequestrum, the one which I first withdrew, then an invaginated sequestrum, the second one withdrawn. It happened that the opening in the living portion of the bone was large enough to allow me to reach and withdraw the invaginated piece through it.

Remember that it is not always thus, and that when the opening is too small, we are obliged to enlarge it with a gouge and mallet. I shall tell you in a moment that, so far as the consequences are concerned, it is better not to have thus attacked the surrounding bone. But is this surrounding bone of new formation, or is it formed of the original bone which has remained alive and has become hypertrophied in its superficial layers? Certainly, I cannot give you in this case a rigorous demonstration; but, if you remember the considerations which I presented at the beginning, you will admit hypertrophy of the original bone as at least possible and even probable, and you will not admit as proven (for nothing proves it) that it is a new bone formed by the periosteum. Finally, you will see in the bony hypertrophy a result of the suppurating osteitis and not a salutary effort, just as mortification at certain points of the same bone has been another result which is neither more nor less salutary than the former.

Let us now examine the prognosis. Well, I admit that I do not fear the consequences of the operation. You will perhaps think that I am too bold in saying that, for this morning the suppuration was fetid, and you know that fetid suppuration of bone may lead to dangerous septicæmia. But what reassures me is, that I have made no fresh solution of continuity in the humerus with the gouge and mallet. Experience has taught me that dangerous traumatic fever and purulent infection are consecutive especially to osteo-myelitis caused by a recent solution of continuity, and the putrid form of osteo-myelitis does not occur when, as in the present case, the bone has been spared.

I do not, however, shut my eyes to the fact that this preservation of the integrity of the humerus has its disadvantage, the existence in the interior of the bone of a canal closed below and open at the top. It will be difficult to prevent the pus from collecting in this canal, and it may become necessary to make a counter-opening with a drill so as to prevent stagnation of the liquids, and thus cause that bleeding solution of continuity which predisposes to pyæmia.

But, on the other hand, it is possible that the bony canal may become filled by the continuation of the hypertrophic process, and that the formation of pus may cease without having caused any accidents. However that may be, there is, in the persistence of this canal, which is about an inch long, a disadvantageous condition which may keep up suppuration and hecticity, and prolong the affection. This condition does not exist when the sequestra have been superficial, and in this respect the prognosis has a greater gravity in this patient than if the necrosis had not been invaginated.

(The patient affected with necrosis of the humerus had no fever and presented no complication. The wound made by the operation suppurated, the bone itself continued to suppurate, the pus flowed with difficulty from the canal in which the sequestrum had been lodged. We made injections of a weak solution of carbolic acid every morning and evening, by passing a gum catheter attached to the canula of the syringe into the bony canal. The patient wished to return home, and we showed him how to make the injections.

15

I am still unwilling to propose a counter-opening, because this operation might have unfortunate results, and because I hope the canal will dry up or fill by the addition of new bony layers. If this does not take place, if the suppuration continues, if it becomes more fetid, if the patient is unable to work, he will return to us, and then, recognizing the inability of nature to complete the cure, I shall make a large opening at the bottom of the accidental canal so as to prevent the stagnation of the pus.)

PART IV.

TRAUMATIC FEVER, PYÆMIA, AND SEPTICÆMIA.

LECTURE XXIX.

TRAUMATIC FEVER.

Gunshot wound of the right elbow—Resection followed promptly by death from traumatic fever—Considerations upon grave traumatic fever following compound fractures.

GENTLEMEN: We lost yesterday a patient who was struck at the battle of Montretout by a ball which passed through his right elbow, causing a comminuted fracture of the three bones forming the articulation. He was brought to the hospital the next day, and on the following morning, thirty-six hours after the accident and while the fever of the first period was still moderate, I resected the elbow. You remember that the bones were so shattered that I found it very difficult to remove all the fragments, since most of them were still adherent and had to be separated one by one from the muscular and aponeurotic fibres. I made a T-shaped incision, the vertical portion of which was on the outer side of the arm and forearm, and the horizontal portion posterior, passing above the olecranon. This incision is similar to that adopted by Roux,[1] but differs from it in this: that in the latter the vertical incision is on the inner side, while in the one which I used and which belongs to M. Nélaton, it is on the outer side. This enables the operator to reach the radius immediately and resect it, and then, having thereby opened the articulation freely, to isolate and remove, while avoiding the ulnar nerve, first the upper extremity of the ulna and then the lower extremity of the humerus. In this case the operation was not as regular as it would be under many other circumstances, for after having made the external incisions, I came upon a mass of splinters which I removed without knowing to which bone each belonged, and then I sawed off the end of each bone so as to substitute a regular and uniform surface for the irregular and jagged one due to the injury. You remember that I then brought the edges of the solution of continuity together with four points of metallic suture, rather with the view of giving them a good position and immobilizing them than in the hope of obtaining immediate union. Indeed the latter is very difficult to obtain, and

---

[1] Thore, Résection du Coude, Inaugural Thesis, 1843.

experience has taught us that immediate union after large operations almost always fails, and fails in the same way, that is, because if by chance it takes place in the outer or superficial layers it does not in the deeper ones, where the fetid pus accumulates and is retained more easily in consequence of the union of the edges of the wound and the formation of a cavity behind them. Now this retention of fetid pus behind a closed wound favors that absorption of putrid substances which is the starting point of infectious fevers. My intention then was not to seek an immediate union, which from the moment it became impossible would have offered only disadvantages, and the same principle guides me after amputations, as I have had and shall doubtless again have occasion to show you.

After putting in the sutures I placed the limb in a wire splint properly lined with cotton batting and oiled silk. You know that this splint is a recent improvement which we owe to those skilful manufacturers, Messrs. Robert & Colin. It has on the outer side a movable piece attached to the rest by straps and buckles, which can be removed and replaced at will. We removed it morning and evening to dress and clean the wound, which was done without communicating any movements to the limb and without causing any pain. The dressing was completed by means of a double compress soaked in a mixture of alcohol and water and renewed every morning and evening.

You remember what followed. The next day the pulse was 130; the skin hot; the thirst intense. The patient had no appetite; had not slept; complained of headache, and was very anxious about himself. The wound and the adjoining parts were very painful; the lower half of the arm and the entire forearm were considerably swollen. I removed the compress wet with alcohol and substituted poultices; prescribed a potion containing one and a half ounces of the syrup of the acetate of morphia to be taken by spoonfuls, and an opium pill at night.

The following day the conditions were the same. The abdomen became tympanitic. The wound yielded an abundant sero-sanguinolent discharge, and was covered with a grayish diphtheritic pulp.

The third day the fever still persisted ; the pulse was 130; temperature in the axilla 104° (Fah.); tongue slightly dry; sub-delirium at times; increase of the local swelling. The sero-sanguinolent discharge had given place during the night to a hemorrhage, en nappe, which evidently came from the capillaries. As it was not possible to apply a ligature, the flow had been arrested by means of charpie wet with dilute perchloride of iron and a band which included the splint in its folds.

The fourth day still worse. Fresh hemorrhage during the night; the wound covered with pulp and sloughs; the swelling of the deep diffuse phlegmon in the arm and forearm had become enormous.

The following days the general and local conditions grew worse; the tongue became drier; the abdomen more and more tympanitic; the delirium continuous, and finally death took place at the beginning of the seventh day.

We had in this case, gentlemen, an exaggeration of the phenomena which we often observe in the first period of large wounds which, if the patients survive, suppurate and granulate before cicatrization. You remember that in gunshot wounds involving only the soft parts, I have applied the term *preparatory to suppuration* to this period which most of our authors have called *inflammatory*. It is true that when the bones are not involved the suppuration is always preceded by local phenomena of inflammation: slight swelling, heat, moderate pain; but ordinarily the general symptoms, especially the fever, are absent. On the other hand, when the skeleton, as well as the soft parts, is injured, this period preparatory to suppuration is almost always marked by general and febrile as well as local symptoms, so that it more than ever deserves the name of inflammatory period. I say almost always and not always, because the general symptoms are sometimes lacking, and that occurs in the fortunate cases in which the skeleton itself, the bones, and the synovial cavity, when a joint is involved, do not suppurate. I have had occasion to call your attention to cases of this kind, and as the result of observation of such I offer this formula: intense fever appears in the first period of compound fractures where suppuration is preparing in the bones themselves, and it is lacking when the bones are destined not to suppurate.

Have we now any special names to designate this group of local and general symptoms? If you often hear me ask this question of nomenclature it is because the words are associated with ideas and theoretical explanations with which we ought to be acquainted and from which we have even to choose when these ideas and those explanations lead to therapeutic or prophylactic measures. I have told you before that the term *hospital gangrene* has sometimes been applied to wounds in this condition, and also that I did not approve of it. Let us seek one that is more appropriate.

After Hunter's and Broussais's works on inflammation the denomination of *inflammatory period*, which I have just mentioned, was adopted. By this was meant that the suppuration depended upon a peculiar condition of the wound and of the entire organism called inflammation. When the fever was lacking, or was not very high, they said the inflammation was moderate; when the fever was very marked, it was explained by the intensity of the inflammation.

A little later, about 1840, surgeons began to express some doubts of the sufficiency of this explanation of the symptoms which precede and seem to prepare the way for suppuration. Without giving any reasons, they adopted new terms which seemed to indicate another, but still vague and indefinite, theory.

This is seen in an article published in 1848 by an English surgeon, Fenwick, in which the causes of death after amputation are discussed; deaths occurring during the first ten days instead of being charged to a too intense or malignant inflammation are attributed by this author, some to nervous complications, the others to gangrene of the stump. Fenwick has certainly included under this head of *nervous complication* those cases in which the patients were delirious, and under that of gangrene those in which the wounds presented in a very marked degree the sloughs and pulp which you saw on our patient. Moreover, as Fenwick's statistics were taken from the records of different hospitals, and were of patients whom he himself had not treated, he had to take as the causes of death those assigned by the surgeons in charge, and they wrote the words *nervous complications* or *gangrene* according as their attention was attracted more by the delirium or by the sloughs. That meant that in their opinion death was due to a concomitant cerebral affection, or to gangrene, but they did not explain the intervention of this as a cause of death.

Since that time we have had other American and English statistics which still attributed the deaths of this first period of capital operations to one or the other of these two causes.

Still later, about 1850, and still without giving any positive explanation, the German surgeons, and Billroth in particular, made use of the term *traumatic fever*, and attributed to this fever that which in France we had first attributed to inflammation, and that which Fenwick and the English had afterwards attributed to nervous complications and to gangrene of the stump.

Then came the experiments of Otto Weber, those of Billroth himself,[1] and Panum's. These experiments consisted in the injection under the skin of different animals of sanious and putrid discharges coming from patients whose suppuration was of bad character, and then in watching the subsequent condition of the animal by means of the thermometer. It was found that in almost all cases the temperature rose several degrees, that some of the animals died, and the others recovered after having been sick for several days. The experimenters inferred that the passage of putrid substances into the blood can cause fever, and they explained by this passage the so-called traumatic fever, so that at last this term came to convey the idea of an infectious fever due to the absorption by the lymphatics and bloodvessels of the wound of the putrid materials found upon the surface of the latter.

Before the experiments of the German authors were made, I had worked out the same solution of the problem, and I said in the paper which I read in 1855 before the Société de Chirurgie that the fever which sets in during the early days of a large wound was due to an infection, that is, to the passage into the blood of putrid materials having their origin in the decomposition, by contact with the air, of the sanguinolent, serous, and sero-purulent liquids poured out during the first hours, before the complete establishment of suppuration, and absorbed by the vessels of this wound. I was led to this opinion by two series of experiments. The first were made upon human beings by applying the iodide of potassium to wounds with the view of studying their power of absorption. I found this power was very marked, and as, on the other hand, I often found putrid liquids during the preparatory period, I did not hesitate to infer that these liquids might be absorbed, and, passing into the economy, produce fever.[2]

[1] Billroth, Arch. Générales de Médecine, 1865, 6 series. tome vi.
[2] Gosselin, Mémories de la Société de Chirurgie, tome v. p. 147.

The others were made upon animals; the skin was incised, and sanguinolent and fetid pus, procured from fresh amputation wounds, was introduced below it and retained by three or four points of suture. I did not take the temperature, but I found that the animals (dogs) became ill and died promptly, while others inoculated in the same way with phlegmonous pus, that is, pus not coming from an acute osteitis, survived, and, indeed, were scarcely affected at all.

I admit then that the German experiments have been of service to this new theory, because they were more numerous, and more widely published than mine. But I may be allowed to repeat what I said in the Académie de Médecine,[1] that, so far as I am concerned, I did not wait for the results of foreign work before expressing my opinion upon this subject.

To-day, adopting the word *septicæmia* for all the febrile conditions which we are authorized to explain by the passage of putrid substance into the blood, we say that traumatic fever is a septicæmia, the traumatic septicæmia of the first few days, as distinguished from the purulent infection which occurs a little later.

Two questions arise here:—

Are all the symptoms observed during the first period of wounds which are destined to suppurate due to septicæmia?

What is the origin of the putrid poison the absorption of which gives rise to traumatic fever or primitive septicæmia?

1. We must distinguish three varieties among the symptoms of this initial period of wounds.

The first, which we find especially in the cases in which the solution of continuity involves only the soft parts, is that in which the symptoms remain local and are not accompanied by fever.

The second is that in which, while the local symptoms remain quite moderate and the surface of the wound especially does not become gangrenous, a certain amount of fever is nevertheless present. This is what I call *mild or benign traumatic fever;* it is seen in some cases of very extensive wounds interesting the soft parts alone, and in some of those in which the bones are involved and are destined to share in the acute suppuration, but without putridity.

The third is that in which, the bones being involved and about to become the seat of acute suppurative osteitis, the surface of the wound becomes gangrenous, a deep-seated, fetid, diffuse phlegmon is developed, and fever sets in and takes on a very serious form. To this I give the name *grave traumatic ʃfever or essentially malignant primitive septicæmia.*

I do not wish to affirm that septicæmia really exists in the first variety; indeed I am inclined to think that it does not, and that the local symptoms should be attributed to a group of local anatomical conditions or modifications which are necessary to the establishment of the pyogenic membrane and the suppuration, a group to which we can give no other name than the one by which it is now known in

¹ Discussion sur l'Infection purulente. (Bull. de l'Acad. de Médecine, 23d March, 1671, vol. xxxi. p. 182.)

pathology, that of inflammation. I will say then that in such a case suppuration is preceded by a purely inflammatory period.

In the second variety where there is fever, but a mild one, I am more ready to admit a certain degree of septicæmia. It is true that local inflammation exists, but it is not sufficient, I think, to account for the fever, and when I see this coexisting with the presence of more or less putrid substances upon an absorbing surface, I am disposed to consider it due to absorption, and consequently to septicæmia.

As for the third variety, I do not hesitate a moment. The intense and dangerous fever coincides with extreme putridity of the wound; the symptoms observed accord with those furnished by experiments upon animals. The absorption seems no more doubtful to me than the septicæmia which is the consequence of it. It would remain to determine whether the gangrene of the soft parts, which would then have to be attributed to a bad character of the inflammation, precedes the septicæmia and is the cause of its gravity, or whether it is the intensity of the septicæmia which reacts upon the wound and leads to gangrene.

We here touch upon questions which can be answered only by hypotheses supported neither by experiments nor by analogy. For that reason I shall offer you no definitive solution, wishing simply to leave you with this impression that grave traumatic fever owes its gravity to the extreme malignity of the putrid poisons formed upon the surface of a wound in a certain number of cases where these wounds are complicated by the imminent appearance of acute suppurative osteitis.

2. I asked a second question: What is the origin of the supposed poison which gives rise to the septicæmia of traumatic fever?

The authors who first spoke of putrid absorption, and who prepared the doctrine of septicæmia, confined themselves on this point to generalities, saying that the poison was formed by the decomposition in the presence of air of the serosity and blood exuded from the surface of the wound during the first few days, and they spoke of the poison as if it might be formed, and with the same facility, on the surface of every wound.

Now, if my idea has been properly expressed, you must have understood that, if I admit the existence of inflammation during the first period of all wounds, I am far from admitting septicæmia in all, and that, if I admit it for some, I make a distinction between benign septicæmia or mild traumatic fever, which is never fatal, and grave septicæmia, which often causes death. You must also have understood that grave septicæmia is rarely seen in cases where the skeleton is not involved. We see it especially when there is fracture of a large bone at the bottom of a wound caused by a gunshot or by some bruising body, and when this bone is about to take on acute suppurative inflammation of all its constituent parts (periosteum, bony substance, medullary tissue, or marrow), or when a large articulation is widely opened and becomes the seat of acute suppurative synovitis. So that in my opinion the problem is restricted to this: What is then

the origin of the supposed poison in the cases of osteitis and traumatic synovitis, which, together with the coexisting wound, are to
pass through acute suppuration?

A. As for the cases of osteitis, I have often explained to you the
opinion which I first expressed in 1855,[1] that the medullary fat is
probably the origin of the poison. When a bone takes on acute
osteitis, the marrow shares in the inflammation, to which I am always
obliged to concede a certain part in the evolution of the symptoms
preceding the establishment of suppuration. This marrow becomes
hyperæmic, infiltrated with blood which escapes from its congested
vessels, and with plastic matter exuded by these same vessels; part
of the fat and of the albuminoid substances which form the marrow
escapes and mingles with the serosity, the clots, and the exudations.
All this decomposes as the result both of the admixture and of an action
of the air similar to that which produces putrefaction. I wish I could
help you to see and touch this peculiar alteration of the fatty substance
of the bone; but I cannot do so, for chemistry has not yet given a final
opinion upon the subject. I have, however, read an article by M.
Klose of Breslau,[2] in which he speaks of the special alteration of the
fat of inflamed bones and of the putrid principles to which it gives
rise. I admit that I have no positive demonstration to offer you,
but how are we otherwise to account for the frequency, and above
all, the gravity of septicæmia in those cases in which the bones suppurate? I know that fat is to be found in the soft parts, and that
it would seem as if this fat ought to change in the same way as in
the cases where the bones are involved. But the fat of the soft parts
has not the same composition, that is, it is not combined with the
same albuminoid or gelatinous substance, the presence of which
perhaps renders the decomposition of the fat of the bones easier and
more deleterious; moreover, I have told you that traumatic fever
sometimes occurs also during the first period of wounds of the soft
parts. It may be because their fat does not furnish such pernicious
substances that this fever is rarer and more generally mild. But it
is none the less allowable to explain it also by a certain degree of
septicæmia, admitting that the organic poison supplied by the altered
fat of the soft parts is a little different, or, if it is the same, that it is
formed and absorbed in less quantity.

In 1855 I ventured another supposition, that, the poison being the
same in the traumatic fever following lesion of the soft parts as in
that following lesion of the bones, its greater gravity in the latter was
the result of a more ready and more abundant absorption, due either
to the fact that the solution of continuity of the bone increased the
extent of the absorbing surface, or that perhaps the marrow itself
possessed a very great power of absorption. I published the results
of several experiments upon dogs, in which I trepanned the shaft of
the femur, and injected through a syringe a preparation of iodine into
the medullary canal, results which showed that the marrow possesses
the power of absorption, although not to a greater degree than other
parts of the organism.

<hr />

[1] Gosselin, loc. cit.   [2] Klose, Gazette Médicale.

The results of recent experiments communicated by M. Demarquay to the Académie de Médecine in October, 1871,[1] are more favorable than mine were to the opinion that a rapid and easy absorption takes place within the medullary canal. These experiments consisted in the injection of fuchsine by means of an Anel syringe through a hole made between the condyles of a rabbit's femur.

B. As for the cases of synovitis, I shall first make a distinction between those in which the penetrating wound of the articulation is complicated by fracture, as in gunshot wounds, and those in which fracture does not coexist. Intense traumatic fever is rarely absent in the first case; but it can be explained, in part at least, by the acute suppuration of the fragments. It is not so intense nor so grave in the second, but it nevertheless exists, and is more marked than is ordinary wounds of the soft parts.

Whence comes the poison then? Probably from the altered fat of the synovia; but perhaps the extent of the absorbing surface must be considered, especially when a large articulation is involved. I may add that liquids are retained and stagnate easily within the cavity of an articulation, and that consequently when once formed the poison is brought into contact for a longer time, and more freely with the large absorbing surface.

Etiology, Prophylaxis.—We have discussed the pathogeny, the ultimate mechanism, that which is so difficult to grasp in all diseases, and I wish now, returning to the practical standpoint, to speak of the etiology, of the appreciable causes of traumatic fever. And yet I should tell you at once that I have very little to say. You know that the principal cause of this affection is a solution of continuity involving the soft parts and the bones. But all persons who receive wounds of this kind are not sure to have the fever, and among those who are attacked by it, some are but slightly affected, and others so severely that they die speedily. Do we know the reasons of these differences? Very slightly.

I can again tell you that traumatic fever is absent, or is moderate, in the rare cases in which the bones do not take part in the suppuration. We have had several examples of this, and I have discussed it sufficiently on other occasions. But I do not know what are the causes which favour this suppuration, and make it inevitable in most cases. However that may be, acute purulent osteo-myelitis having been set up, the causes which aggravate traumatic septicæmia are probably all those which may have deteriorated the constitution shortly before the wound was received, such as fatigue, privation, bad food, loss of sleep, forced marches, moral emotions, chagrin, all those circumstances, in a word, which affect the soldier, and give a special gravity to gunshot wounds of the large bones. I believe, however, that bad domiciliary conditions in the hospitals, and notably the hygiene of the wards, exert but little influence. After the battles about Paris, I so often saw grave traumatic fever make its appearance in large rooms, or in

¹ Demarquay, Recherches sur la Perméabilité des Os dans ses rapports sur l'Ostéo-myélité et l'Iufection purulente.   (Bull. de l'Acad. de Médecine, Octobre, 1871, tome xxxvi, p. 877.)

well-ventilated and not crowded military hospitals, that I cannot admit that bad atmospherical conditions have any influence in producing it, at least not so certainly as they have in purulent infection. In addition to the nature of the wound, and all the individual conditions which I have enumerated, we can only invoke, to explain the intensity of the traumatic septicæmia, as we do for so many other diseases, an idiosyncrasy, that occult cause of which I have spoken so often, in consequence of which certain persons are more apt to supply, from the liquids of their organism altered by contact with the air, or by the consequences of a violent inflammatory process, the quantity and quality of septic poison necessary to compromise life.

From what has been said I wish to draw the conclusion that, in the present state of our knowledge, we possess no real prophylactic measures to be employed against grave traumatic fever.

The best plan, when a patient has received a compound fracture, is to do everything that may prevent suppuration of the bone. To obtain this result in gunshot fractures, we can do little beyond immobilizing the limb and the fragments, and taking the special precautions which are necessary during the removal of the patient from the field to a more or less distant place.

As for the constitutional conditions of which I have spoken, and which predispose to dangerous suppuration, it is plain that we can do nothing against them, and that no prophylactic measures could oppose their influence.

It is always well, especially in view of purulent infection, which, next to grave traumatic fever, threatens the patient most—it is well, I repeat, that he should be placed in as pure an atmosphere as possible which can be renewed easily and without chilling, and if possible, in a room which contains no other wounded patient. From what I have said, you may have comprehended that this precaution is not so necessary against traumatic fever as against purulent infection, but so long as isolation is a precious prophylactic measure against the latter, it will inevitably be used against the former. I have returned to this subject in order to leave this idea in your minds, that, if we are authorized in our statistics to attribute the mortality caused by purulent infection to bad atmospherical conditions, yet we must not attribute that caused by traumatic fever to the same cause, since it is due rather to individual than to external conditions.

There is, indeed, a prophylactic measure to be found in a mode of dressing which we should always bear in mind when we wish to prevent a suppuration, the consequences of which may be serious. I refer to the occlusive dressing, which I have often had occasion to mention, and which you have seen me use successfully. Its result may be either to suppress all suppuration or only that which is dangerous, suppuration of the bones, by favouring the union of the deep parts and allowing suppuration of the superficial parts alone. But, although this dressing succeeds perfectly when the wound is small and when it has been made by an ordinary instrument, it is of no use when the wound is so large and contused as it is when caused by a gunshot. Consequently you have never seen me use it in cases

of this kind, and I have shown you that when patients have occasionally escaped suppuration of the bone after gunshot wounds; this
fortunate result could not be attributed to our method of dressing
the wound, but was due simply to the idiosyncrasy of the patient,
the immobilization of the limb, and abstention from irritating explorations.

Finally, do not be surprised that I do not speak of curative treatment; there is none that has much influence upon this dangerous
affection. Derivation towards the alimentary canal by means of laxa-
tives is always indicated, also alcoholic stimulation, and even sulphate
of quinine and tannin as antiseptics. You have seen me employ
these, but your observations and mine have shown that they were not
very efficacious.

LECTURE XXX.

PURULENT INFECTION OR PYÆMIA.

Two cases of purulent infection or pyæmia, one following gunshot fracture of the
thigh, the other, gunshot fracture of the leg—Anatomical characters and pathogeny of this disease.

GENTLEMEN: We have recently lost two of our patients who were
suffering from gunshot wounds. One had had the femur, the other
the tibia broken by a ball. In each case the fracture was near the
middle of the bone and moderately comminuted. They suppurated;
the patients, who were both young but much broken by exposure to
cold, forced marches, and loss of sleep, had intense traumatic fever
from the beginning, and, in one case on the ninth, in the other on the
eleventh day, had an initial violent chill which lasted twenty or thirty
minutes, and was followed by great acceleration of the pulse. The
tongue became dry, the skin clayey, and then subicteric in color. The
chill was repeated once or twice each day at irregular intervals, the
strength grew less, slight delirium, diarrhœa, and abdominal tympa-
nites set in. Meanwhile, the suppuration diminished, the pus became
thinner, and had that fetid odor which you have heard me compare
to that of a mouse. Finally, death took place on the twelfth day in
one case, on the fifteenth in the other.

The autopsies were made, and I now show you some of the specimens taken from the bodies.

. I. The principal lesions were found in the chest, abdomen, some of
the joints, and the broken bones.

A. *In the chest*, each pleural cavity contained a notable quantity
of serosity, together with soft false membranes lining the parietal
pleura and the lungs, especially at the base and the lower lobes.

After having taken out the lungs and removed the false membranes, I examined the upper and middle lobes, without finding anything worth mention in them. Then, taking hold of the lower lobes, in which lesions are most frequently found in cases of this kind, I felt, in the tissue of the lung along the outline of the base and behind, several hard lumps about as large as peas, over some of which the surface of the lung was of a deeper colour than elsewhere, whilst over others the colour was yellowish. On cutting into these different points, we found different appearances. I here show you two of them, in which the surface of section is black, and from which I can scrape or squeeze a thick sticky liquid which is nothing but blood. But this blood does not flow away freely; after the scraping and squeezing there is still enough left to keep the colour dark and to give the pulmonary parenchyma a firmer consistency at these points than elsewhere.

Here are two other spots, in which you find the centre of the section yellow and the outer part of the same deeper colour as before. The yellow centres yield, when pressed and scraped, a small quantity of liquid which to the naked eye seems to be pus, and in which the microscope shows us purulent globules; but this pus does not flow away in sufficient quantity to leave a cavity behind. In addition to this rather scanty infiltrated liquid, there is a yellow substance, pro-bably plastic matter, united very intimately with the parenchyma of the lung.

Lastly, I show you three other spots over which the surface itself of the lung was yellow. On cutting into them you see real pus flow, yellow and creamy like wholesome pus. After its escape there remains a cavity, here as large as a large pea, there as large as a hazel-nut, the inner surface of which is still lined with a rather adhe-rent yellowish exudation. But the red and yellow centres have dis-appeared, and with them all that remained of the parenchyma.

You see there, gentlemen, the three stages of what are called metastatic abscesses of the lungs; the brown foci belong to the first, those that are gray in the centre and brown at the periphery to the second, and the purulent collections to the third. The anatomical characters during the first two stages differ from those of ordinary phlegmonous abscesses. In the first, for example, instead of a simple hyperæmia with infiltration of serosity, it seems that we have an ecchymosis, that is, a flow of blood from torn capillaries, and at the same time a thickening of this blood and an intimate union of its coagulum with the infiltrated portion of the parenchyma of the lung.

Dance[1] and Cruveilhier,[2] however, explained these brown foci in another way. They attributed them to small blood clots formed within the capillaries of the lungs in consequence of the development of a capillary phlebitis.

Virchow[3] and the German authors afterwards adopted this explana-

[1] Dance, Article Absces metastatiques, in the Dict. de Méd., in 30 vols. Paris, 1832.
[2] Cruveilhier, Article Phlébite in the Dict. de Médecine et Chirurgie pratiques, in 15 volumes.
[3] Virchow, Pathologie Cellulaire, Paris, 1868, 3d edition.

tion of the formation of the brown foci by clots, but they added that these clots, instead of being formed locally, as Dance and Cruveilhier thought, came from a distance; that they were embolic clots formed in the affected veins near the wound, swept along in the current of the circulation, and stopped in the capillaries of the lungs; and they invented the word infarctus, which bears the signification of an obstruction of the capillaries by fixed, but imported, clots.

I wish I could show you which of these two theories, that of ecchymotic infiltration, or that of embolic clot, is the right one; but I cannot do so.

I see the thick blood intimately mingled with the parenchyma of the lungs, but I cannot make out whether it is contained within the capillaries or whether it is outside of them, and seductive as the theory of embolism may be, I do not find evidence sufficient to make me consider it irrefutable, as most authors do.

I can understand as easily the possibility of an ecchymosis analogous to that which we see formed in the lungs after the ingestion of narcotic and narcotico-acrid poisons. I shall tell you in a moment that I consider purulent infection as a septicæmia, as a poisoning; it is possible that the poison acts upon the lungs like those I have just mentioned, that is, that it gives the blood qualities which are irritating and corrosive for certain vascular walls, hence its escape and infiltration. It is certainly difficult to understand why this corrosive action should be exerted upon the lungs and liver more than upon the other organs, why in the lungs themselves the vessels of the base and those of the superficial layers of this base are more often and more easily torn than those of the upper lobe and of the deep portions of the lung.

This difficulty is, moreover, only the prelude of many others which the study of this singular affection will offer us. You will see at every moment that I shall be at a loss how to explain the various phenomena which characterize it.

Look, for example, at these yellow foci of the second stage. By what are they formed? Probably by an exudation of plastic matter at the centre of the red spot. But whence comes this exudation? Is it, as the name would indicate, a new formation substituted for the blood, which, originally arrested, would then be reabsorbed? Is it not rather a transformation of this blood? I cannot give you a satisfactory solution of this question.

And then these cavities of the third stage, how are they formed? Is it again by a new formation, which would presuppose the absorption of the exudation just as its deposit presupposed the absorption of the blood; or might it perchance be a transformation of the original exudation into pus? These are obscure questions, which I ask and do not answer, although I do not hide from you that I incline rather towards the theory of substitution than towards that of transformation.

B. *In the abdomen*, we found the spleen larger and more friable than usual, and filled with very thick black blood. On the convex surface of the liver we found two yellow spots of about the size of a dime;

on cutting them they proved to be formed of a concrete semi-solid substance, resembling that of the second stage of pulmonary metastatic abscesses, and which seemed to us to be likewise formed of plastic material mingled intimately with the tissue of the liver. Furthermore, on cutting more deeply, we found two cavities within its parenchyma, containing thick, yellow, creamy pus. Were these abscesses preceded by a plastic deposit analogous to that which we found on the surface of the liver? It is very probable, although in cases of pyæmia we find metastatic abscesses of the liver more often in the condition of collection than in that of infiltration. You notice here what is generally the case, that there are no brown spots similar to those which, in the lungs, characterize the first stage of metastatic abscesses. The infiltration of blood, if it precedes, must then disappear very rapidly. But as I have never met with it, even in cases in which death took place very early, I believe that it is ordinarily absent, as is also the case in the muscular interstices and the articulations, and that consequently the embolic clots to which so much importance is attached in Virchow's theory must not be considered as inevitably preceding the formation of pus in abscesses of this kind. So long as we do not find sanguinolent foci in the liver we are not justified in believing in a preliminary morbid condition, with or without rupture, of a certain number of capillaries.

C. We opened the right scapulo-humeral articulation of the first patient, who had complained of pain there, and we found in it a considerable amount of pus. I called upon you to notice: 1st. That this pus also was thick, creamy, and presented, consequently, the characteristics of what we term wholesome or laudable pus; 2d. That the synovial membrane, notwithstanding this abundance of pus, presented neither ecchymoses similar to those which we found in the lungs nor the infiltrations, nor even the redness, nor the thickening which in articular abscesses of different origin indicate the existence of a synovitis ending in suppuration. In like manner, as you saw no traces of hepatitis below and about the abscesses in the liver, so you see here no traces of synovitis.

The same thing is seen in the cases in which we find metastatic abscesses among the muscles. There are collections of pus, but about them we find neither injection nor serous infiltration, nor any of the anatomical characters which belong to a phlegmon preceding an abscess.

In a word, purulent collections without preliminary inflammation; that is the most striking point in these so-called metastatic abscesses of purulent infection; for I cannot consider as belonging to inflammation, properly so-called, the lesions of the first two stages of the pulmonary metastatic abscess. These lesions are unusual, bizarre, if you choose, but they are not those of an ordinary phlegmasia.

D. Here now are the femur and the tibia, which were broken by the balls. Both offer the multiple fragments of comminuted fractures, and these fragments lay in the fetid and blackish pus which communicated with the exterior by the openings of the perforating course followed by the projectile. The periosteum still remains on some of the fragments, but is lacking for about an inch on the two principal ones, the upper and lower pieces.

If you examine the outer surface of the compact tissue of these fragments, you will find there a little reddening, and that enlargement of the Haversian canals which was pointed out by Gerdy[1] as one of the characters of osteitis of the compact tissue. Neither upon this outer face, nor upon the fractured surfaces of the fragments, nor upon what remains of the periosteum, do we find any appearance of the process of consolidation. It is evident that the purulent secretion has taken the place of the secretion and subsequent transformations of the plastic lymph, which, at the stage of injury, if there had been no suppurating wound, would have supplied the cartilaginous callus. If the patient had lived, the granulations of all the surfaces of fracture would have undergone this transformation, as I have previously had occasion to explain it to you (see p. 76 et seq.).

I call your attention particularly to the condition of the medullary tissue of the two bones. In order to understand it properly, I have had recourse to two measures: I have broken the upper and lower fragments of each of the fractured bones with a hammer, and I have taken out and broken in the same way the corresponding bones (femur and tibia) of the other side. I wished to show you the interior of the medullary canals, and to enable you to compare the appearance of the healthy with that of the affected side. What do you see on the healthy side? The medullary canal, and the meshes of the spongy tissue which are continuous with it at the ends of the bone, are filled with rather firm fat, very yellow in one case, pinkish, and at the same time a little more diffluent, in the other. The predominant fact, notwithstanding the differences in appearance and consistency (differences which are very common, and by no means imply an abnormal condition),[2] is the fat. Look now at the fractured bones: at the line of division there is no longer any fatty marrow; in its place is a substance red in some places, gray in others, blackish here and there, rather firm, with a fetid odour, not looking at all like fat, hardly greasing paper when rubbed upon it, and apparently composed of an exudation mingled with what remains of the marrow. Scraping it with a scalpel removes a puriform substance. At a little distance from the line of division, we find here and there collections of pus, instead of the thick substance infiltrated with pus of which I have just spoken, and that continues for about one and a half inches beyond the point of fracture. It is only after reaching the spongy tissue near the extremities that we find normal medullary fat without admixture of pus. There is then in the medullary canal a mixture of plastic deposits, of purulent infiltration and collections, and of gangrene here and there, with diminution and total disappearance in places of the normal fat. This is somewhat similar to diffuse phlegmon with sloughs of the soft parts.

[1] Gerdy. Maladies des Organes du Mouvement, p. 155, Paris, 1855.
[2] The marrow of the bones is always more vascular and more diffluent in the child and adolescent than in the adult and aged, and, in this respect, there are many individual varieties among adults; sometimes the marrow is more, sometimes less, vascular, and these differences are not due to appreciable pathological causes.

The lesion which you find here is that which on other occasions I have shown you under the name of putrid and diffuse osteo-myelitis (see p. 215 et seq.).

E. *Veins.*—We examined the femoral vein near the point of fracture of the femur, and found it filled with black uncoagulated blood, without any sign of pus, and without the changes in the lining membrane which we often see in phlebitis. We also examined the nutrient vein at the nutritious foramen, and found that it also contained no pus and no blood clot. Consequently, in this case, the purulent infection could not be attributed to a suppurative phlebitis. We examined the tibial veins in the other case; one of them contained soft and badly smelling blood clots without pus; the others were permeable. In this also there was no suppurative phlebitis.

II. I am naturally led by what has preceded to ask the.pathogenic question: What is the cause of purulent infection, and what relations exist between these visceral, articular, and muscular abscesses, and the suppurating wound which preceded and doubtless caused them? That is a question which has occupied surgeons since the end of the last century, and upon the answer to which they have not been able to agree, for the very simple reason that, in this malady, as in many others, such as most of the contagious diseases, a moment comes when appreciable phenomena are wanting, and when we are obliged to substitute an hypothesis for them, which some are willing to accept, but which the others criticize or reject, asking for a demonstration which no one can give them. The best plan, perhaps, in the presence of this difficulty would be to adopt no theory, and to wait until we should possess one established upon solid bases.

I am not quite ready to adopt this plan, for a reason which I gave to the Académie de Médecine at the time of the discussion on purulent infection,[1] that is, because we have efforts to make to preserve the wounded and those upon whom we operate from this dangerous affection, and it is very difficult to advance safely in the search for prophylactic measures if we are not guided by some idea of the pathogeny.

We can group in three main classes the opinions which have been held upon the mode of development of purulent infection.

1st. *Metastasis and Absorption of Pus.*—The authors who first noticed the connection between internal abscesses and external suppurations, especially Van Swieten, J. L. Petit, and Morgagni, spoke of the transfer of the pus from the wound to the viscera, but without explaining the manner in which this transfer was effected.

Afterwards Velpeau[2] and Marechal[3] were more explicit, and expressed the opinion that the pus of a wound could be absorbed by the open veins, pass thus into the circulation, be deposited in certain viscera, and there form the abscesses known as metastatic. This doctrine rested upon two incontestable facts: the presence of pus in the

---

[1] Discussion sur l'Infection purulente (Bulletin de l'Académie de Médecine, March 27th and August 16th, 1871, tome xxxvi. pp. 182 and 620).

[2] Velpeau, Graduation Thesis, 1823, and several articles in the Archives Générales de Médecine, in 1824, 1826, and 1827.

[3] Maréchal, Graduation Thesis, 1828.

veins adjoining the wound in many cases of amputation, and the presence of pus in the parenchyma of the lung, liver, and brain. But the absorption of pus by venous trunks opening on the surface of a wound was a pure hypothesis. That venous capillaries are able to absorb liquid substances in contact with them is incontestable, but it was difficult to make a cautious physiologist admit that divided, gaping vessels could do the same. Again, by admitting for the formation of metastatic abscesses the transfer and the deposit of pus in the internal organs, they placed themselves in contradiction with the facts, since we have a first and even a second stage in which is found, at the place which would afterwards be occupied by the abscess, an infiltration first of blood and then of plastic material. Nevertheless the theory was accepted, and reigned for a certain number of years under the name, which you still hear from the mouth of old physicians, of purulent absorption.

2d. *Theory of Phlebitis.*—Dance[1] taught, and after him Cruveilhier, Blandin, and P. Bérard developed, another doctrine, in which the mixture of pus with the blood still appeared as the main explanation of the disease, but in which phlebitis was made to play a great part, as well in the origin of the pus as in the mode of formation of the metastatic abscesses. Dance had discovered in many puerperal women this fact, recognized afterwards by surgeons in patients who had undergone amputation, that the venous trunks of the affected parts, we may say of the wound, were inflamed and suppurating, and that the pus often extended to the neighbourhood of a collateral branch opening into the affected vein. He inferred that the stream of blood through this collateral might carry away the pus and pour it into the general circulation. This pus once in the blood would mingle with it so thoroughly that it could not afterwards be separated from it. But it would alter it and render it so irritating that its passage into certain capillaries, notably those of the viscera, would lead to new phlebites (capillary phlebitis) characterized first by the formation of small clots, and then by the production of pus which would be the consequence of the irritation caused by the clots.

Although based upon an undeniable fact, the presence of pus in the veins, yet this theory was frequently found in contradiction with the facts, and still left a large part to hypothesis. It first supposed that in every case the veins corresponding to the wound which was the starting point of the infection had suppurated; but Darcet, Sedillot, Tessier, in works which I shall presently mention, had been led to modify Dance's and Blandin's theory, because they had often sought for pus in the veins without finding it.

I myself, when examining the bodies of patients who had died of purulent infection, have often carefully dissected the veins of the region of the injury or operation, within which the disease must certainly have had its origin, and I have found no pus in them. The theory of phlebitis supposed moreover that this pus found an easy

[1] Dance, De la Phlébite uterine et de la Phlébite en Général (Archives Générales de Médecine, 1828-29).

passage into the neighbouring veins. But Tessier[1] proved clearly that the inflamed veins contained blood clots as well as pus, and that in many cases these clots lay above the pus, and were so adherent that they must have opposed its migration.

Finally, this theory would lead us to expect that the pus globules that had passed into the blood could be detected in it by the aid of the microscope. But examination of the blood of pyæmic patients has shown that it does not contain more than the usual number of leucocytes.

As for a capillary phlebitis preceding the formation of the metastatic abscesses, that might possibly be admitted for the lungs, but it could not for the liver, the synovial membranes, or the muscular interstices, in which we do not find the purulent collections preceded by those blood clots which may be attributed to coagulation in the veinules.

To these serious objections it must be added that the theory of phlebitis had the disadvantage of leading to no prophylactic measures. Admitting that the disease is engendered by pus in the veins, we can suggest nothing to prevent the production of this result. Surgeons could only bow and wait. You will see that the final theory of which I have yet to speak, the one which I have long accepted, purely hypothetical as it still may be, has the advantage of inviting and justifying prophylactic measures the efficaciousness of which has been proved by experience.

3d. *Doctrine of Septicæmia.*—It was after the objections made by Tessier to the doctrine of phlebitis as the starting point of purulent infection, that the first works appeared in France upon this theory, which in the beginning received no special name, and to which we have since given that of *septicæmia.* This theory explains purulent infection by the absorption and introduction into the blood of invisible and intangible putrid or septic materials produced by the blood, serosity, gangrenous tissues, and mortified inflammatory exudations which are found on the surface of wounds during the early weeks of suppuration and sometimes later.

This theory, generally attributed, even by French authors, to German physicians, had in reality its origin among us. To assure yourselves of this fact you have only to follow the chronological sequence of works published upon this subject.

Darcet is the first, so far as I know, who, without using the word *septicæmia,* formulated in France the doctrine in question. But his work was based upon facts and ideas which were related not to purulent infection itself, but to other diseases which are closely allied to it by their nature and gravity, and which, in fact, belong to the great morbid group now called septicæmia.

Thus Gaspard and Magendie published, in 1823,[2] a series of experiments showing that the injection of putrid matter, notably of pus and urine, into the veins of animals produced artificial fevers similar to putrid and typhoid fevers.

---

[1] J. P. Tessier, Journal l'Experience, 1838.
[2] Gaspard and Magendie, Journal de Physiologie de Magendie, 1823.

Bouillaud also, in a very remarkable article upon phlebitis, published in 1825,[1] pointed out the frequent coincidence in human beings of phlebitis with symptoms analogous to those of putrid or typhoid fever. He recalled Gaspard and Magendie's experiments, and spoke of pus formed by phlebitis and poured into the general circulation. But on the one hand he occupied himself especially with putrefied pus as the cause of the trouble, and assimilated it to the putrid matter used by Gaspard and Magendie, and, on the other hand, he explained the development of fevers by the passage of deleterious substances into the blood, without paying special attention to the one which has since been known as purulent infection.

Thus, too, Bonnet of Lyons, in 1837,[2] studying the changes of pus due to contact with the air, showed that in consequence of the habitual presence of sulphur in pus the usual products of its decomposition were sulphuretted hydrogen and sulphydrate of ammonia, and that these essentially deleterious substances, when once formed, could be absorbed by wounds and give rise to febrile complications, to which he gave no special name.

Lastly, Prof. Bérard also, long before the publication of his masterly article in the *Dictionnaire* in 30 volumes,[3] taught that a distinction was to be made between purulent infection, which he attributed, as did Dance and Blandin, to the passage of pus into the blood, and another variety of poisoning which occurred later, and which was due to the passage into the blood of the materials formed by the decomposition of the pus, which had been so well studied by Bonnet. Bérard gave the name of *putrid infection* to this malady, similar in its origin to purulent infection, but differing from it by the later period of its development, by its symptoms, its anatomical lesions, and its prognosis. If P. Bérard had applied the same opinion to the development of traumatic fever, and if he had employed the expression septicæmia to indicate these various morbid conditions due to the absorption of deleterious substances differing themselves according to the moment of their formation, he would have completed the edifice whose entire construction has been very improperly attributed to our German contemporaries.

The ground had thus been prepared by previous works when Félix Darcet,[4] leaving the rather vague generalities in which Gaspard, Magendie, and Mons. Bouillaud had remained, and leaving aside also P. Bérard's putrid infection, came to give an explanation, analogous to that of the others, of purulent infection properly so called.

This author reported a series of experiments which showed, according to him, that the decomposition of pus in contact with the air gave rise to two products: the one a subtile intangible poison, which, after having been absorbed, and thus distributed over the entire economy, would produce the phenomena of fever; the other less toxic, solid,

---

[1] Bouillaud, Sur la Phlébite (Revue Médicale, 1825).

[2] Bonnet, Mémoire sur la Composition et l'Absorption du Pus (Gazette Médicale, 1837, p. 593).

[3] P. Bérard, Dictionnaire de Médecine, article Pus, 1842.

[4] Darcet, Recherches sur les Abcès Multiples et sur les Accidents qu' Amène la Présence du Pus dans le Système Vasculaire (Inaugural Thesis, Paris, 1842).

divided into very fine particles, which could pass through vessels of a certain size, but were promptly stopped in the capillaries, especially in those of the lungs, and might, by acting as irritating foreign bodies there, lead to the formation of metastatic abscesses.

I am glad to recall this opinion, for you see in it the germ of the one uttered by Virchow fifteen years afterwards. The latter author attributes metastatic abscesses to the arrest in the pulmonary capillaries of small so-called embolic clots coming from the veins of the injured region. According to Darcet, also, fibrinous particles were arrested in the capillaries, but he supposed them to come from the pus and not from the blood.

After Darcet, M. Sédillot[1] wrote that purulent infection was not due simply to the passage of pus as such into the blood, but to the passage of putrid substances absorbed from the surface of a wound, and resulting from the ulcerative and gangrenous destruction of the parts in which suppuration was impending. According to this eminent surgeon, in short, the deleterious principles which cause the disease come especially from the mortified and sloughing portion, which we always find upon wounds at the beginning of suppuration.

Then M. Alphonse Guérin,[2] in 1847, likewise opposed Dance's theory, and sought to prove the correctness of the opinion which he afterwards defended warmly before the Académie de Médecine in 1871,[3] that purulent infection is due to the passage into the blood of special miasms scattered through the air, which fall upon wounds and are absorbed through them. According to M. A. Guérin the miasms in question are found especially in hospital wards, in those in which cases of purulent infection are already present, and in all crowded, badly ventilated places, and thus he explains the greater frequency of the disease in hospitals than in private practice, in the city than in the country.

Notice in passing, that this theory, without being strictly proved, had at least the advantage of causing the adoption of the great prophylactic measure, free ventilation and renewal of the air about those who have been wounded or operated upon.

Similar ideas, so far at least as the explanation of the disease by a sort of poisoning is concerned, were maintained by Jules Guérin[4] and Maisonneuve, who, admitting like Darcet and Sédillot the decomposition of the pus, blood, and mortified tissues on the surface of a wound, explained purulent infection by the absorption of these deleterious substances, whose passage into the blood may take place with the pus, but also without it.

I myself had been familiar for several years with these ideas. The autopsies of a certain number of wounded and amputated whom it was my lot to treat in one of the services of St. Louis Hospital, in

[1] Sédillot, De l'Infection Purulente (Annales de la Chirurgie Française et Etrangère, 1843, tome vii. p. 128), and De l'Infection Purulente ou Pyoémie, Paris, 1849.
[2] Alph. Guérin, Thèses de Paris, 1847.
[3] Alph. Guérin, Discours sur l'Infection Purulente (Bull. de l'Académie de Médecine, 1871, tome xxxvi. pp. 202 and 307).
[4] J. Guérin, Bull. de l'Acad. de Médecine, 1871, tome xxxvi. p. 332.

charge of which I had been placed at the beginning of my surgical career, after the bloody outbreak in June, 1848, proved to me that suppurative phlebitis was absent much more often in patients affected with purulent infection than the works of Dance, Cruveilhier, and P. Bérard had led me to believe. And by suppurative phlebitis I mean that of the large veins which run through the soft parts of a limb that has been amputated, or has received a comminuted fracture. On examining the bones of those who had succumbed after multiple suppurations of the skeleton and soft parts, I found, it is true, suppuration and putrid changes in the medullary substance, and I at first supposed that, according to the theory warmly taught by Blandin, the pus, instead of forming in the large veins just mentioned, had started in those of the marrow, and that thus a phlebitis of the bones had been the starting point of the purulent infection.

Seeking next upon the cadaver for the proof of this phlebitis of the bones, I found in many cases the nutrient vein filled with pus. But in many others I found nothing of the kind. I was unable to isolate the veinules of the marrow itself sufficiently to determine the presence of the pus which would demonstrate the existence of phlebitis.

I was, therefore, forced to recognize that if phlebitis of the bones may in certain cases, and when phlebitis of the large veins of the soft parts is absent, be invoked as the cause of purulent infection it cannot be demonstrated anatomically.

But while making these searches, I was struck with the profound alteration of the medullary substance, in which I vainly sought for suppurating veins. I saw that it was gangrenous, mixed with altered blood and decomposed pus, and that it had the odour of putrefaction. I then began to ask myself if these products of putrid osteo-myelitis of which I have already spoken to you (page 214) might not pass into the circulation without being carried there by the pus.

For such a thing to be possible, it was necessary that the surface of the wound and that of the bone should be capable of absorption. Bonnet of Lyons[1] had admitted the first. The teachings of physiology also justified the belief. Nevertheless, I studied this question by experiments upon men and living animals. In 1854 and 1855, I placed a great many times pads soaked with a ten per cent. solution of the iodide of potassium upon wounds at different periods of their course, and half an hour or an hour afterwards I easily detected the iodine in the urine or salivæ by the aid of starch, the mixture of which with these liquids gave the blue colour of the iodide of starch. I have already spoken to you (page 228) of these experiments, and of another which I made upon dogs three different times, and which consisted in forcing into the medullary canal of the femur, by means of a syringe and a tube provided with a screw, which I fixed in one of the walls of this canal, a little of the same solution of iodine. A faucet placed at one of the ends of the tube enabled me to retain the liquid, and to keep it from spreading over the soft parts. In each case I found the iodine in the animal's urine about three-quarters of an hour afterwards.

---

[1] Bonnet, loc. cit.

In my opinion, therefore, it could not be doubted that the surface of a wound and that of the medullary canal were capable of absorption. A new demonstration of the former has likewise been furnished by M. Demarquay in a paper read before the Académie de Médecine in 1867,[1] and upon which I made a report.[2]

Having acquired these two facts, the presence of putrid substances upon wounds and in the medullary canal, and the possibility of absorption, I continued to examine the large veins in the bodies of those who died of purulent infection, and the interior of the bones which had been attacked by acute suppuration, and I felt more and more convinced that it was not simply the passage of the pus of suppurating veins into the blood which occasioned the infection in question, that if this passage took place consecutively to phlebitis, the pus of the veins probably swept along with itself putrid matter, coming either from the wound or from the bone, and that finally the passage of these putrid substances might take place and cause the affection without the veins sharing in the suppuration, and without the pus serving as vehicle. I developed this opinion in my work upon V-shaped fractures [3]

But I did not stop at purulent infection. In the same article, as I have already told you (see page 229), I did not hesitate to assign a poisoning as the cause of grave traumatic fever; and as that occurs especially in cases in which the large bones are the seat of suppurative inflammation together with a concomitant wound, I thought that the poison in such a case also was formed out of the medullary substance exposed to the air, and seriously inflamed in consequence of the accident. I further expressed the opinion that other febrile surgical affections, "such for example as that seen after the opening of an abscess by congestion,"[4] after incisions and operations upon the urethra, after the opening of hæmatoceles with thickened walls, that which characterizes erysipelas, and lastly, that called puerperal fever" can be explained by an analogous poisoning.

You see, gentlemen, I also lacked only the word *septicæmia* to sum up and make intelligible my conception of the pathogeny of purulent infection, as well as of the other forms of febrile affections that may complicate wounds at the different stages of their evolution. I admit that I was wrong in not making use of this word which has the advantage of expressing very well the general doctrine I adopted, but I did not think of it.

Since that time I have not failed to expound in my pathological and clinical lectures these ideas of the method of development of traumatic fever and purulent infection, and some years afterwards I saw with satisfaction the confirmation by German authors, by means of experiments upon animals, of the views which I had uttered re-

---

[1] Demarquay, De l'Absorption sur les Plaies (Bull. de l'Académie de Médecine, Paris, 1866–67, tome xxxii. p. 157, and Mémoires de l'Acad. de Méd. 1867–68, tome xxviii. p. 424.)

[2] Gosselin, Bull. de l'Acad. de Méd. 1866–1867, tome xxxii. p. 930.

[3] Gosselin, loc. cit.

[4] A collection of pus which has migrated under the influence of gravity or other mechanical cause from the point at which it was formed.—TRANS.

garding traumatic fever, and those which my compatriots and myself had held upon purulent infection properly so-called. These authors did not quote us, and seemed to think that they were the sole inventors of the doctrine of septicæmia. They fell into this error, doubtless, because they were not familiar with what had been done here. The thing which astonishes me, that against which I protested before the Académie de Médecine,[1] the 27th of March, 1871, is the readiness with which French authors, forgetting in their turn what has been done amongst us to establish this doctrine, have not feared to give it the name of German doctrine. According to what I have just told you the Germans did not invent this doctrine, they only strengthened it, fortified it, and popularized it. Neither did they invent the word septicæmia, which for more than twenty years has had a place in the nomenclature of our learned compatriot Piorry.

And now, gentlemen, after all the researches I have made, after the fresh study of the subject into which I was necessarily led by the long discussion in the Académie de Médecine, I adopt and I offer you the following theory in explanation of purulent infection. This grave disease is composed mainly of two things:—

1st. A set of clinical symptoms which we can classify under the name of fever.

2d. Multiple anatomical lesions the chief of which are the so-called metastatic abscesses.

Let us examine these two points successively.

1st. I consider the fever as the result of a poisoning by toxic materials formed on the surface and especially in the deep parts of wounds.

These toxic materials are often transported by the large veins, within which they are mixed either with pus or with blood. I do not believe that simple non-putrid pus causes the disease in question. If the pus passes into the blood it produces it only because it is mingled with deleterious substances formed either by the decomposition of the pus within a vein which has become the seat of a putrid suppurative phlebitis, or by the decomposition of other parts of the wound, the products of this decomposition being capable of causing suppuration by their passage into the large veins, at the same time that they infect the organism. In my opinion thus there are several gates by which the toxic substances which cause the infection can enter: first the large veins containing altered pus and communicating with the general circulation by some collateral branch, the flow through which has not been obstructed by a clot; next, the veinules which absorb and transport putrid materials without their being arrested in the large veins and mixed there with pus or coagulated blood; and lastly the lymphatics which may likewise convey these poisons without themselves receiving any injury or any irritation from contact with them which might make them suppurate as the veins do. For, notice it well, gentlemen, the lymphatics and the veins act in three ways in the development of purulent infection:

---

[1] Bull. de l'Académie de Médecine, 1871, tome xxxvi. p. 182.

sometimes they are merely passages and undergo no change, sometimes their internal surface inflames and suppurates in consequence
of the contact of the poisons which pass over it; sometimes they take
on suppurative inflammation before this passage and as a result of
their participation in the inflammatory process which invades all the
constituent parts of the solution of continuity, and the pus which has
formed within them becoming putrid furnishes the deleterious material which the collateral branches then carry into the general circulation. Thus we explain all the facts which occur since we have
recognized the relation between phlebitis and purulent infection, to
wit: sometimes the coincidence of the suppurative phlebitis with
this disease, sometimes, and more rarely, the coincidence of suppurative lymphangitis, sometimes, on the contrary, the absence of pus in
these same vessels, or at least in those of them which anatomical
investigation allows us to trace and to observe.

Now, whence came the poisons and how are they formed? I have
told you that possibly they may come from pus previously formed
within the veins and the lymphatics, and changed either by contact
with the air or by the unwholesome nature of the morbid process
which gave rise to it. But they often come from the suppurating
wound and are carried into the lymphatic and venous trunks by the
capillary vessels which have absorbed them on its surface. Their
origin then is either in the decomposition of the pus, or of the blood,
or of the suppurating and gangrenous medullary substance, or of the
gangrenous and broken-down soft parts, or several of these together.
This decomposition is still the consequence either of contact with the
air, or of the malignity of the suppurative inflammation; but the
conditions in which the disease is most frequently developed compel
us to attribute most influence to the air. For you know, gentlemen,
that the suppurating wounds which are most often complicated with
pyæmia are the deep ones, that is, they are those in which, notwithstanding the surgeon's efforts, the pus is retained between the muscular
layers, in which, furthermore, the sloughs of the aponeuroses, tendons,
and muscles are slow to be eliminated, and remain so long as their
separation has not taken place in the depths of the wound.

This forced sojourn of poorly vitalized or quite dead tissues in the
midst of soft parts which at the same time admit the air, leads to the
decay—that is, a putrid or septic decomposition similar to putrefaction in the open air—of the soft parts which are entirely separated
from the organism. You see how much more favourably constituted
in this respect superficial wounds are; the pus flows away easily, the
eschars are thin and quickly eliminated, and, if necessary, we can
ourselves remove them. The prolonged sojourn which is favourable
to decay and to the formation of toxic substances does not exist here.

And let us not forget that among the deep wounds the ones which
give rise most often to this affection are those at the bottom of which
large bones take part in the suppuration.

In fact, before the development of suppurative inflammation, and
during the first few days which follow it, something analogous to
what we see upon the soft parts takes place within the bones. In

the former there is no suppuration without a certain amount of alteration of the blood remaining on the surface of the wound, and without
the production of eschars and of exudations likewise destined to mortification and elimination. When the wound is deep these phenomena appear throughout its whole extent, consequently within the
medullary canal, and probably also in the canaliculi of the bone.
Suppuration is preceded and accompanied within these canals by
gangrene and exudations whose products are altered by contact with
the air which has penetrated and become confined there.

Putrid and toxic products, therefore, are formed in every suppurating wound. But when the wound is superficial they are less abundant and remain for a shorter time, and consequently are less liable
to be absorbed than when it is deep, or where a broken or divided
bone lying at its bottom takes part in the suppuration. In this latter
case there are moreover the toxic products formed by the medullary
fat, products which may be dangerous in themselves, but which are
rendered especially so by their prolonged retention in an open cavity.
This, I think, explains why purulent infection is much more common
when suppuration of the soft parts is accompanied by suppuration of
a bone than when it is not so accompanied.

In short, gentlemen, according to the theory which I propound to
you the dangerous alteration of the blood which produces the disease is not due exclusively to pus; it is due to numerous putrid substances, of which some have their origin in the pus, and the others in
the decomposed blood, the eschars, and the exudative detritus of the
putrid and gangrenous marrow.

But here three objections are made. I do not hesitate to meet and
answer them.

They say to me: You attribute a rôle to gangrene and to the detritus which it furnishes for absorption, and yet you are the first to
recognize, and you often teach, that destruction of soft parts (normal
tissues and tumours) by caustics which produce eschars is almost never
followed by purulent infection. That is true, but notice the differences: when we use caustics their first effect is to destroy the lymphatics and bloodvessels, and to cause their obliteration by the coagulation of the blood and lymph, and by primitive adhesion by means
of plastic lymph; the eschar is produced immediately, or at least is
completed very rapidly, and when decomposition sets in, when suppuration and elimination begin, all communication has long since
ceased between the mortified part and the adjoining living tissue.
Moreover there is no blood to putrefy, no exudation deprived of vitality, no serosity liable to decomposition; in a word, there are none
of the many sources of poison which we find in wounds. The eschars
of the latter form much more slowly; during several days they have
still enough vitality to carry on exchanges with the living parts, and
to communicate to them the putrid substances they have produced;
the adjoining vessels are not yet obliterated, they too share in the
unhealthy inflammation which invades the entire solution of continuity; and, lastly, there are, together with the eschars, those other

liquid and fatty products which suffer change by contact with the air, and which are not found upon parts destroyed rapidly by caustics. The second objection is this : You regard as one of the factors the suppuration of the bone and especially of the marrow, and yet you show us every day patients suffering with suppurative osteitis, in the affections generally known as *caries* and *necrosis*, who are not attacked by purulent infection. They live months or years with this suppuration of the bones and die from other diseases. That is all very true ; but notice again that it is not the suppuration alone that I regard as a factor, but also the destructions and mortifications that accompany its beginning, and which you do not have when the osteitis advances slowly towards suppuration and when the latter is not carried on in contact with the air. When these ossifluent abscesses of caries and necrosis open and the air penetrates into the cavity, it finds pus and nothing but pus there. It may still cause this pus to putrefy. When the cavity is deep and extensive, as in abscess by congestion, this putrefaction may become the cause of another variety of septicæmia, that known by the names of putrid infection, hecticity, hectic fever. But the air does not meet, as it does in wounds, with those mutiple elements of which I have spoken, blood, fat, mortified exudations; now, it is this multiplicity of elements which gives rise to the septic products capable of engendering pyæmia. In short, a great distinction must be drawn, in this respect, between acute suppurative osteitis and chronic suppurative osteitis. The first produces, together with pus, putrid substances which the latter does not.

Furthermore, we must draw a distinction between the acute suppurative osteitis which is set up without preliminary solution of continuity, and that which occurs after such solution of continuity. The former sometimes causes purulent infection, as I told you when speaking of the spontaneous acute osteitis of adolescents; but the latter is much more liable to do so, though not always and inevitably.

Remember that the essential condition of the production of purulent infection is that the acute suppurative osteo-myelitis should become putrid. Now this does not always happen, and, as I have often told you, our treatment should be directed towards, and should sometimes succeed in, reventing it.

The third objection is as follows : You speak to us of poisons coming from the blood, from serosities, exudations, pus, eschars, and mortified marrow ; but now which one of all these furnishes the real poison of purulent infection ? And furthermore, when you explain traumatic fever you still take your poisons from the same sources. Are they then the same in both cases ? On this point, gentlemen, I do not conceal my embarrassment and my doubts. If I could isolate the organic poisons of a wounded patient, if I could watch their formation, I would tell you exactly where they arise, whether they result from the union of molecules coming from all the altered parts of the wound, or whether they come mainly from certain ones of them. I would tell you also in what the pathogeny of traumatic fever differs from that of purulent infection. But none of these points can be made out by me. I see an important effect produced—a dangerous

fever. I see, as a plausible explanation of this effect, putrid substances and their absorption. But I can go no further, and that is why
I told you at the beginning that, whatever we might do, we always
brought up in this research against something that was inexplicable
and hypothetical.

I presume that the poison of purulent infection has a complex
origin, and that the molecules furnished by the putrescent marrow of
the bones play a large part in it. I presume that the poison formed
during the first few days, that which occasions traumatic fever, is different from that which is developed later and which gives rise to purulent infection. I recognize that according as the symptoms of the
presence of the former have been more marked, so is the latter more
likely to be produced. I understand how distinguished surgeons,
M. Billroth, in Germany, M. Verneuil, in France, seeing so often
grave traumatic fever precede and in some sort prepare the way for
purulent infection, have been led to think that these two affections
are but one and the same, and that pyæmia is the second degree of a
septicæmia of which traumatic fever is the first. But upon this point
we are all unable to prove anything. We are obliged to confine ourselves to suppositions, to ask indulgence for our theory in consideration of the excellent points it furnishes for prophylaxis as I shall try
to show you in another lecture.

2d. Let us now see how the multiple suppurations, often internal,
sometimes external, the so-called metastatic abscesses, can be explained by the theory of septicæmia.

Here again I shall be compelled to admit that a rigorous explanation is nearly impossible.

I have already spoken of the original theory, the deposit in all
parts of the body of pus taken up or absorbed from the surface of the
wound; and you know the reasons why we could not adopt it.

The first was that it is difficult to believe in an absorption sufficiently abundant to supply the numerous and sometimes large collections which we find, especially those which form within the synovial
and serous cavities.

Next, the theory being true, the microscope ought to show large
quantities of leucocytes in the blood of pyæmic patients; but, as I
told you, the blood contains only the usual number. And finally,
since the facts have led us to the opinion that it is not pus but invisible
and intangible poisons which cause the infection, we cannot admit
that the pus is all formed in the blood and has only to be deposited
in the organs.

I spoke also of the suppurative capillary phlebitis admitted by
Dance and Cruveilhier as a means in the formation of metastatic abscesses. These authors thought that the blood, by admixture with
pus, became irritant, phlogogenic, as it is termed to-day, and that,
passing into the venous-capillaries of certain viscera, especially those
of the liver and lung, it produced in them a suppurative inflammation similar to that caused by mercury and other foreign bodies
when injected into the veins, as in Cruveilhier's and Darcet's experiments.

I should be willing to accept this interpretation if the metastatic abscess developed everywhere in the same manner, that is, if it passed everywhere through a first stage characterized by the black spot resembling an ecchymosis, and which might possibly be attributed to the stoppage of clots in the inflamed veins. But this first stage is seen only in the lungs, sometimes in the spleen. We do not find it in the liver, where the abscess seems to begin by a yellow spot which is not blood, and which is not pus either. Still less do we find it in the serous and synovial membranes and the muscular interstices, where the pus forms very rapidly without being preceded by any appreciable lesion.

The same objections can be made to Darcet's fibrinous and Virchow's sanguineous embolus. You may possibly accept it for the lung, but you need another explanation for the liver, the serous and synovial membranes, and the muscular interstices.

In presence of these varieties in formation, as shown by anatomical investigation, there is only one thing to be said, and that is that as soon as the blood has become altered by its infection, and the fever has declared itself, the whole economy becomes apt for suppuration. So long as there is no poisoning, the suppuration remains local, and all the efforts of the organism are turned to the process of repair, of which the regular secretion of pus is an essential condition. As soon as poisoning has occurred, the pyogenic aptitude is disarranged; it becomes generalized, and the organism makes pus, at the expense of the altered blood, everywhere except at the point where it first prepared to make it.

LECTURE XXXI.

ETIOLOGY OF SURGICAL SEPTICÆMIA.

General etiology of traumatic fever and purulent infection. 1st. Local or anatomical causes. 2d. Individual general causes—Influence of age, sex, temperament, alcoholic habits, moral emotions, physical suffering. 3d. Atmospheric general causes, vitiation of the air by crowding—Possible absorption of miasms by the wound and by the respiratory organs.

GENTLEMEN: I gave you in a former lecture my opinion upon the mode of development of purulent infection. But that lesson would remain sterile if I did not try to show you how, on the one side, the tangible causes of the disease accord with this pathogeny; and how, on the other, the knowledge which we have of the relations between the etiology and the pathogeny leads to therapeutical and prophylactic notions. But, as a close connection exists between traumatic fever and purulent infection, and since the prophylactic measures employed against the one are equally suited for the other, I prefer now to unite them under the name of *septicæmia*, or, as M. John Guérin has styled it, of *purulent intoxication*, and to apply to both the considerations which I have to present you.

I warn you, moreover, that these considerations apply not only to gunshot fractures but to all wounds and operations which expose to surgical septicæmia.

Etiology.—Purulent poisoning (and by this term it is understood that we mean that which starts from a wound in which suppuration is impending, as well as from one which has begun to suppurate) recognizes three kinds of causes: local or anatomical causes, individual general causes, and atmospherical general causes. Let us see how these causes accord with the pathogeny I laid before you.

1st. *Local or Anatomical Causes.*—We know them; they may be summed up as follows: formation upon the wound of putrid substances or septic poisons, and possible absorption either before or after the establishment of the suppuration. We know that deep wounds, especially those in which the bones inflame and take on putrid osteo-myelitis, are more likely than any others to cause it.

Do not lose sight of the fact, that, if decomposition of the pus is one of the sources of the formation of the poisons, it is not the only one, —it is not even the most important. In fact, if putrefaction does not occur upon the surface and in the deep parts of the wound during the first few days, and if the pus alone appears there, poisoning is rare. Next, when the wound has passed this period of twenty or twenty-five days, during which putrid substances are formed upon and remain in it, and when there is no longer anything but pus, poisoning again becomes more difficult and rarer. If then I have retained the name of purulent infection, it is in order to conform to general usage, and also because the formation of the poisons coincides with the beginning of the formation of the pus. Do not forget, on the other hand, that this formation of putrid substances upon wounds is the consequeuce of a process of destruction which follows the traumatism and precedes the definitive establishment of the process of repair. Certainly it would be much better if things took place differently; but the fact is none the less true, that a large wound, before it becomes lined with a red and freely suppurating membrane which is the indication of properly advancing repair, covers itself with sloughs more or less deep, useless exudations, and blood clots, and that all these products exposed to the air may there undergo putrid changes.

This preliminary destruction is more or less marked. It is accompanied by a more or less considerable putrefaction. There lies the explanation of the differences which we see in practice, certain subjects being much more exposed to putrefaction and its consequences than others. The study of the general causes will also show us the same thing.

2d. *Individual General Causes.*—It has been correctly said that persons of every age, of both sexes, of every temperament may be attacked by septicæmia. But with respect to frequency there are individual variations which we must recognize in practice.

Let us first consider age.

Beyond all question, children may have both kinds of poisoning. But traumatic fever, violent enough to be fatal, is quite exceptional among them, and it is undeniable that of one hundred children who have suffered amputation or have received gunshot fractures, the number attacked by purulent infection is much less than is the case with adults. I wish I could indicate this proportion by figures, but I cannot, since it has been my lot to treat only a few children. I make this statement in accordance with the general impression left by my personal experience, limited though it may be, and with the results furnished me by surgeons of hospitals for children. This diminished frequency can be easily understood. The constitution of a child has not been exhausted by the general causes just mentioned: bodily fatigue, moral impressions, alcoholisms, syphilis; furthermore the marrow of their bones is less abundant, less fatty, more vascular, less liable to putrefy; lastly the vitality of all their tissues is greater. There is then less tendency to destruction, and consequently fewer obstacles to the process of repair than in the adult; it is more diffi-cult for the phlebitis and osteo-myelitis to take on a putrid character.

Let us now consider sex.

It seems to me that women are rather less exposed than men to purulent infection. This is both the result of a general impression and of my own statistics. In the paper which I read before the Medical Congress of 1867,[1] I reported eight cases of amputation of the thigh or leg, in women, with three deaths, two of which were by purulent infection and one by hecticity. I had had these two cases of purulent infection out of eight operations, a proportion of twenty-five per cent. The same operations performed upon men have given me, on the contrary, the proportion of about forty per cent. of the same affection. Again, I recall the cases of women treated by me after the civil war in 1871, for gunshot wounds involving important parts of the skeleton. They are not numerous: a fracture of the shoulder, a fracture of the humerus, two fractures of the leg, a frac-ture of the superior and inferior maxilla. None of them had purulent infection, none died, and yet all had at first acute and then chronic suppurative osteo-myelitis. But the osteo-myelitis was not putrid, or was so to so slight a degree that poisoning did not follow. Three of them had traumatic fever, but it was moderate and, as happens in such cases, did not lead to the fever of pyæmia. In this respect there is a distinction to be made between traumatic erysipelas and purulent infection in women. They suffer more frequently from the first and less frequently from the second than men do. The explanation is to be found in causes analogous to those favouring childhood. Al-though a woman is more impressionable, her constitution is ordi-narily less broken down by bodily toil, irregular hours, and alcoholism, than a man's is, and this is especially true of the men of the working classes in large cities, those who supply most of our hospital cases.

As for temperament, I know nothing in particular, and I am forced

[1] Actes du Congrès Médical International de 1867, p. 269.

to recognize that the most robust, as well as the most delicate, may be affected in the same proportion as soon as the other causes begin to act.

The facts which came to our notice after our late battles convinced me that fatigue resulting from long marches and loss of sleep, alcoholic habits, exposure to cold prolonged over several hours, especially at night, after receipt of the injury predispose, as essentially debilitating causes, to the spread of the preliminary destructions which are the main source of the poisoning.

Moral emotions—those resulting from the discouragement produced by defeat, those caused by the prospect of a long illness, of a permanent infirmity, by the fear of death, a fear necessarily increased in a hospital ward by the sight of the death of neighbours or comrades wounded on the same day—these emotions are incidental, though not predisposing causes of poisoning. In order that repair shall go on regularly, and that the putrefaction of the preliminary work of destruction shall remain limited, it is necessary for the patient to eat, sleep, and digest. This he does not do, or he does badly, if his mind is preoccupied and saddened, as it often is after severe injuries.

I have spoken elsewhere[1] of the influence of physical suffering, the long duration, or too frequent repetition of which, produces similar results.

3d. *Atmospheric General Causes.*—These are certainly the ones which exert most influence.

Tessier, when opposing Dance's doctrine of the consequences of suppurative phlebitis, was the first to show clearly that purulent infection was due mainly to the crowding of the wards of a hospital with sick and wounded, and that this crowding did not explain the development of venous suppuration and the consequent passage of pus into the blood, and that it certainly acted in another way.

Since then hospital surgeons in large cities have learned from those of their confrères who practise in the country and small towns, and who treat their wounded at home or in hospitals containing few patients, that purulent infection and grave traumatic fever are very rare among them. When Messrs. Topinard[2] and Léon Lefort,[3] after their visits to England, taught us that surgical poisonings were less frequent in the London than in the Paris hospitals, they indicated as principal causes of this difference: 1st, the fact that the English wards were less crowded than the French; 2d, the more complete renewal of the air in the wards by the frequent opening of the windows as well as by an efficient system of ventilation.

Still later American surgeons confirmed these views by the statistics of the wounds and operations which the war of the rebellion gave them the opportunity of observing upon a large scale.

While in France, at the time when Malgaigne published his first and important work upon the results of capital operations in the

[1] Actes du Congrès Médical International de 1867, Paris, 1868.
[2] Topinard, Thèses de Paris, 1860, No. 28.
[3] L. Lefort, De la Résection de la Hanche dans les Cas de Coxalgie et de Plaies par armes à feu (Mém. de l'Acad. de Médecine), 1861, tome xxv. p. 445.

Paris hospitals, the proportion of deaths, almost all of them due to purulent infection, was from 70 to 75 per cent., in these American statistics the proportion was only 30 to 35 per cent. for the same operations. The difference was explained by the two circumstances that in America the patients' beds were widely separated from one another, and, above all, were placed in tents far from other habitations and almost constantly open.

The general impression which resulted from these works,—and which, for my part, I aided to create in France by giving the greatest publicity to M. Lefort's comparative studies upon the English and French hospitals in my report to the Académic,[1] and in the long discussion upon nosocomial hygiene which followed,—the general impression, I repeat, was that vitiation of the air by crowding is the principal cause of surgical poisonings.

In what does this vitiation consist? Is it due simply to the various emanations arising from the presence of too many people in a limited space where the air is not sufficiently renewed? Is it due to special miasms arising in wards occupied by wounded persons from suppurating wounds, or to specific miasms coming from those already affected by surgical poisons? Does it occur in all these ways at once? Thus far our experience has not enabled us to pronounce upon this subject. Everybody admits and ought to admit, for clinical experience proves it most positively, that the crowding of patients vitiates the air, and that this vitiation engenders septicæmia in patients who have deep suppurating wounds. But no one can say positively in what this vitiation consists.

And here another question naturally arises. The air being vitiated by these miasmatic emanations, by what way do they penetrate into the organism of the wounded patients, and how do they act in producing surgical poisoning?

As for the penetration, we have to choose between two routes; that of the wound, and that of the respiratory organs, unless we admit that the poison enters by both.

Our learned colleague, M. Alphonse Guérin, did not hesitate to choose the first. He distinctly maintains the opinion that wounds, being able to absorb, introduce into the general circulation the miasms which the vitiated atmosphere deposits upon them; the first conclusion that he drew was one confirming Tessier's views, that we should prevent, above all, the vitiation of the air by crowding. Afterwards, in 1871, he adopted a second one, the necessity of the occlusive apparatuses of which I shall soon speak.

This theory, which has had the merit of giving a great impulse to the search for and application of prophylactic measures, is certainly very attractive. But I have made and still make this objection to it: all wounds are capable of absorption, the superficial as well as the deep ones, the ossifluent as well as those which do not communicate with the bones, and yet they do not all absorb those atmospherical miasms which are supposed to be able to develop the infection. You

[1] Bulletin de l'Académie de Médecine, 1861–62, tome xxxvii. p. 53.

17

know that patients with superficial wounds are less exposed to it than those with deep wounds, and those with deep wounds, and without osteo-myelitis, much less than those with deep wounds and osteo-myelitis. It is in vain that M. Alphonse Guérin replies that deep and ossifluent wounds have much larger surfaces of absorption. The answer to that is in these enormous solutions of continuity seen in burns and in certain accidental wounds which pass through all their phases without becoming the occasion of purulent infection. More-over, if the infection were caused by the absorption of atmospherical miasms by the wound, why should this absorption take place during the first twenty-five days and not afterwards? The wounds of which we are speaking last for forty, sixty, ninety days. During all this time they are able to absorb, during all this time they are in contact with vitiated air, yet the further we get from their beginning the less is infection to be feared.

I do not deny, if you will, the absorption by the wound of miasms contained in the air. But it is impossible for me, for the reasons I have already given, to believe that this absorption is sufficient by itself to give rise to grave traumatic fever and purulent infection. We can, moreover, explain the local action of the vitiated air other-wise than by the direct penetration of the miasms into the circulation. I have told you that the mortifications and putrid changes in wounds were due to two main causes: a certain quality of the inflammation which depends upon the idiosyncrasy of the patient, and the contact of the air. Now it is possible that air vitiated by these invisible miasms in hospital wards exerts its decomposing influence more easily than perfectly pure air does. Still, I do not hide from you that this is only a presumption, and that I can in no way prove the proposition.

Let us now examine the other route, that of the respiration. If the vitiated air enters the lungs at each inspiration, it is allowable to believe that the deleterious miasms contained in it penetrate into the blood, and that this penetration affects the health in a way that is in-jurious to the progress of a wound. Two serious objections present themselves here: First, this same vitiated air is breathed by other patients who have no wounds. They are not attacked by any fever, and their health does not seem to be affected in any way by this hygienic condition which is so unfavourable to those with serious wounds. Then all those who have wounds do not become poisoned, notwithstanding that they all breathe the same air. How is it then that this vitiated air, if it acts through the respiratory organs, pro-duces upon some what it does not produce upon others?

There is, it is true, a new difficulty in the explanation. But it seems to me capable of removal by the ideas which I propounded upon the conditions of local putridity necessary to the development of surgical poisonings. In order that these putrid substances should not form it is necessary, as I have already told you, that the patient's health should be good, and that all his functions should be regularly performed. It is especially needful that the blood should be properly transformed and purified, and that no foreign element should change it. This condition is necessarily affected by respiration in an atmosphere charged with miasms. If the passage of these latter into the blood does not sensibly affect the health of those who have no open wounds, or have only superficial ones, yet I can understand that it might so affect those who have to undergo deep suppuration, and especially that of osteo-myelitis. In fact it is at the expense of the blood that the exudations necessary for the formation of a good pyo-genic membrane are made. If this blood is not sufficiently pure it produces unhealthy membranes, which mortify; it excites this exces-sive inflammatory process, which leads to the partial death, and ulti-mately to the putrid decomposition of the tissues covering the solution of continuity. In a word, vitiation of the blood by imperfect hæma-tosis acts upon the wound which is about to suppurate in the same way as vitiation caused by fatigue, loss of sleep, moral emotions, alcoholism, and prolonged exposure to cold; and you understand that when all or many of these causes of vitiation act at the same time, the patient has but a slight chance of escaping a grievous poisoning. Happily there are organisms which resist everything, and we see from time to time in our wards patients who, notwithstanding the existence of unfavourable conditions, escape suppuration, or, in whom, if it occurs, it does not assume the putrid character.

I sum up my views upon the influence of unfavourable atmos-pherical conditions in saying that if this influence is local in a certain measure, which I cannot prove, it is also general, in the sense that it gives the blood, through the respiratory organs, certain qualities which predispose it to furnish upon the wound and in the medullary canal products which putrefy easily.

And I express my views upon the general etiology of traumatic poisonings in saying that they depend upon a series of individual and atmospherical causes, each of which acting alone may produce them, but which in all probability unite and act simultaneously; and it is not unlikely that poisons varying in nature and amount may result from the complex intervention, and in different proportions, of all these causes. Thus may, perhaps, be explained both the differences which we see in the more or less rapid course of regular traumatic fever and purulent infection, and those unusual forms of fever which do not appear early enough to belong to primitive septicæmia, and which, on the other hand, not presenting the ordinary symptoms of purulent infection, ought to be considered as intermediary or incom-plete septicæmias, to which the clinic has as yet given no special name.

LECTURE XXXII.

TREATMENT AND PROPHYLAXIS OF SURGICAL SEPTICÆMIA.

Curative treatment of septicæmia almost nil—Prophylactic treatment very useful—Isolation of the wounded in pure air frequently renewed—Different dressings: uniting, occlusive, infrequent, simple, and repeated—Preference given to the infrequent and occlusive cotton batting dressings.

GENTLEMEN: I have little to say on the subject of the curative treatment of surgical poisonings.

In traumatic fever, as I have told you, it is limited to diluent or tonic drinks, a laxative, a few injections, and a dose of opium at night. But we must not deceive ourselves; these measures have but little effect and are almost unmeaning.

In purulent infection the tincture of aconite has been recommended, and I have often prescribed it in a potion or in the tisane, in the dose of two grammes the first day, three grammes the second, and four grammes the following days.[1]

I have also given the sulphate of quinine in moderate doses, say seventy-five centigrammes or a gramme daily, or even in a large dose, as M. Alphonse Guérin advises, say a gramme and a half the first day, and two grammes on the following days, and although our colleague has had some success with this, I have seen it, like the preceding one, fail in most cases.

It is true that I saw one of our patients in May, 1871, with a suppurating gunshot fracture of the right humerus, recover from a purulent infection after having taken for a fortnight the daily dose of two grammes, and even during the last few days of two and a half grammes of sulphate of quinine. But, on the other hand, I saw a wounded man at the Hôpital St. Louis, in 1848, and two at La Pitié, in 1865 and 1866, get well without the help of any medicine.

In short, some fortunate subjects after having shown all the symptoms, especially the repeated chills, of purulent infection, get well. But this has not happened often enough to prove the real efficaciousness of any drug. The few who have recovered after treatment with one or another of them, would probably have done just as well without them.

I do not, however, wish to discourage you, and to advise you to remain inactive spectators of the contest carried on by the organism against the poisons. I advise you to give sulphate of quinine notwithstanding my doubts of its value, to give with it from thirty to sixty grammes (℥i–ij) of brandy daily, pure or mixed, in a potion with from two to four grammes of the extract of cinchona. I wish

---

[1] This is the French tincture. The dose of the *tinctura aconiti radicis* (U. S. Pharm.) is from 5 to 10 drops gradually increased.

only to warn you that recovery is very rare, that the real curative treatment is yet to be found, and that consequently we must first turn our attention to prophylactic measures.

Well, the theory which I have developed before you has, above all others, the advantage of opening the way to every prophylactic endeavour, and that is why I have adopted it, notwithstanding the hypothetical nature of so much of it.

I have told you, that, according to the unanimous opinion of all contemporary surgeons, air vitiated by crowding is one of the main causes of the poisonings, and especially of purulent infection. You see at once the consequences. When you have a patient whose wound exposes him to septicæmia, and especially when, in all probability, acute suppurative osteo-myelitis may set in, you should put him in a room which is not crowded and in which the air can be changed.

Of late years you have heard small hospitals recommended, small wards, and, so far as possible, the erection of hospitals outside of the large cities. As applied indiscriminately to all patients, these precautions are exaggerated and useless.

Speaking only of patients with surgical affections—those who have no wounds and those whose wounds or ulcers are superficial are not exposed in ordinary hospitals to the diseases we are now considering. It is always well to avoid crowding, to have, for example, about 40 cubic metres of air for each bed, to have means of ventilation, to change the air by opening the windows, to have separate rooms for the delirious and those with erysipelas. On these conditions a hospital may be established in a large city and receive without objection 500 or 600 patients.

But these conditions are not sufficient for those whose wounds expose them to traumatic poisoning, nor are they sufficient for puerperal women whose uterine wounds expose them in the same way.

For such patients, in hospital, large isolated rooms with good ventilation are needed, each to contain only three or four persons. These rooms may, if necessary, be in an ordinary building, but the hygienic conditions are best realized by a tent, large enough for four or six beds, placed in a large open space, such as our Paris Administration has already furnished to the Necker, St. Louis, and Cochin hospitals, and such as I have for several years asked for at La Charité, where the small size of the courtyards and gardens renders the plan difficult of accomplishment. And this leads me to say, in passing, to those of you who will be called some day to advise upon the construction of hospitals, that it is necessary above all things to have open spaces large enough to contain, under conditions of proper aeration, warmed tents or huts for patients whom you know to be threatened with acute putrefaction and all its consequences.

Of course, if the patient is in a private house every effort should be made to give him a large room facing to the east or south, with at least one large window, and, if the season is suitable, an open fire heating sufficiently to allow the windows to be opened occasionally without chilling the room.

If the topographical conditions of the hospital or of the home do not allow these indications to be properly and permanently met, you must try to do it temporarily at least by carrying the patient from one place to another. At the St. Louis and Lariboisière hospitals in Paris, for example, I have seen patients suffering from serious wounds and amputations placed in tents during the day and brought back to the wards at night. In case there are no courtyards or gardens, the balconies can be made use of in the same way, as they are large enough to hold several beds, and allow the patients to be brought into the open air, when the weather is suitable, without the inconveniences incidental to carrying them. Balconies, however, are lacking in most of our hospitals. They are an improvement which you may find it well to remember.

In private practice, if there is no courtyard or garden to which the patient can be taken during the day, if moreover the season is not suitable, or if it is too cold for the windows to be opened long enough to effect a renewal of the air, the patient should at least be moved from one room to another in his bed, as I advise and practise in the treatment of erysipelas.[1] When the change has been made, the windows of the room which the patient has just quitted are left open for three or four hours, and then the fire is lighted and the room warmed before he is brought back.

But if the conditions are such that the patient can be isolated neither permanently nor temporarily, if his room cannot be changed, and if, as is too often the case in our hospitals, he has to remain constantly in a more or less crowded ward, our only resource is to secure the renewal of the air, as far as it is possible, by keeping the windows open whenever the weather permits. When the weather is warm the problem is solved easily enough, but when it is cold it is much more difficult and we have to contend against all sorts of opposition. A draught of fresh air is often disagreeable, the patients, the orderlies, the nurses themselves are slightly incommoded by it, infer that it is dangerous, and hasten to close the window. In this respect La Pitié Hospital was better than the others in which I have served. One of the windows in the male ward was so arranged that it could be left open all day and often part of the night without troubling any one. The nurses and servants were not disobedient, and I obtained very good results, better than I obtained elsewhere, which I mentioned in my paper read before the Medical Congress of 1867.

Apropos of ventilation, you often hear managers and architects praise artificial ventilators, like those which have been constructed at Beaujou and Lariboisière hospitals, into the details of which it would be useless to enter here. The principle of these systems is very good, for its object is to renew the air without chilling the room. But the results obtained in the surgical and lying-in wards of these two hospitals have proved that they are not sufficient to prevent traumatic poisoning. It may be that, well arranged as they are, these ventilators renew the air only very imperfectly. They establish only very

---

[1] Article Erysipèle in the Dictionnaire de Médecine et de Chirurgie Pratiques, Paris, 1871, tome xiv. p. 1.

narrow and limited currents instead of the broad ones produced by open windows and fireplaces that draw properly. And then these apparatuses rarely work well. They depend upon a fire which has to be fed constantly, and which, either by negligence or lack of fuel or for any other cause, is allowed to go out. Then the ventilation stops. I am far from proscribing ventilators absolutely; but I consider them insufficient for the object which we now seek, and their use, though it may be advantageous for the mass of patients, does not relieve us from the necessity of using for those now under consideration the measures of isolation and aeration which I have mentioned.

Dressings.—Surgeons have always sought, but especially during the last sixty years, for modes of dressing large wounds which would protect their patients from the complications which now occupy us. The ideas which guided them varied, and were gradually modified by those which were advanced as to the origin of these complications. Not wishing to speak of all kinds of dressings I shall mention only those whose principal aim has been to prevent traumatic fever and purulent infection, and I shall try to show how their mode of action accords with the pathogeny I expounded before you. From this standpoint I shall examine successively: *uniting dressings, infrequent dressings, dressings by aspiration or pneumatic occlusion, occlusive dressings, disinfecting dressings,* and finally *daily, simple, and painless dressings.*

Uniting dressings.—By this name I designate those which keep the edges of the wound near together and, so far as possible, in contact for five or six days by means of strips of diachylon plaster, or of linen dipped in collodion, or of interrupted or quilled sutures. Their object is to obtain what is called *immediate union,* that is, cicatrization of the solution of continuity without suppuration and by prompt transformation into cicatricial tissue of the plastic lymph or blastema which is poured out after the first twenty-four hours on the surface and between the lips of the wound. You see at once how, so far as putrefaction and septicæmia are concerned, this kind of dressing would act. It would prevent suppurative inflammation, and with it the whole train of local symptoms, at the head of which we placed the formation of eschars and the decomposition in contact with the air of all the organic parts deprived of vitality.

Nothing could be better than such a result; but can it be easily obtained? is it often obtained in practice? and, in case of failure, have the measures taken to procure it any disadvantages?

Notice first, gentlemen, that immediate union is impossible in many cases: in those, for example, in which the integuments have suffered a loss of substance; in those in which although there has been no loss of substance the edges are so widely separated that they cannot be brought together; and finally in those of contused and gunshot wounds with such bruising of the edges that mortification and suppuration must take place. We can examine it then with reference only to those cases in which it is possible, and that is mainly those in which amputation has been performed.

As for those, I do not hesitate to tell you that immediate cicatrization is very rarely obtained. I have seen it, and so have other surgeons, succeed in children, in whom, moreover, the attempt if unsuccessful has not the disadvantages of which I shall presently speak. But I have seen it succeed very rarely in adults, and all my colleagues at Paris have had the same experience. A few years ago I heard it said, and I have also read in Serré's *Traité de la Réunion Immédiate*,[1] that they succeeded more often in the south of France, and especially at Montpellier. But I doubt if this assertion has been justified by a sufficient number of facts, for now I hear the contrary asserted, that attempts to obtain immediate union upon adults have no greater success in the south than in the centre and north of France.

I believe myself then justified in saying that in the immense majority of cases suppuration is not prevented by this mode of treatment, and that in your practice hereafter you should use it only if the experience of your predecessors and yourselves has shown that the locality where you practice is exceptional in this respect, and that in it wounds, when their edges are brought together, generally heal without suppurating.

Understand, too, how difficult it is to obtain completely the result sought for by dressings of this kind. In an amputation wound you have to distinguish two things, the integumental edge and the bottom of the wound. The edges are easily kept in contact by the means of reunion, and have a simple structure which allows prompt agglutination without suppuration. But the bottom, that part composed of muscles, tendons, aponeuroses, and bones, cannot be brought together so exactly.

Even when a flap amputation has been made, there are always irregularities of the surface which do not allow all the points to be brought, and especially to be kept, together; how then can we hope that all these parts differing in vitality will be simultaneously protected from that which always threatens in the first period of exposed wounds, that is, the mortification of some of the tissues over which the knife has passed. However perfect may be the coaptation of the edges, is there not reason to fear that a little air may have been imprisoned at the bottom of this wound, and that the blood and the lymph, when poured out, will be subjected to its decomposing influence? Clinical observation, gentlemen, has shown these objections to be well taken. At the beginning of my surgical career I tried, and saw others try, to get immediate union; this was in consequence of what Prof. Ph. J. Roux[2] had told us of the habitual and even exaggerated use of this practice in the English hospitals, and of the views which John Bell's[3] and Richerand's[4] works had popularized among us; and yet I never saw perfect immediate union without any suppuration : that is, in the very exceptional cases in which I got good results, and in the two children upon whom I had to amputate at the thigh, there was suppuration at the surface of the wound, the edges of which had not united immediately, and a little deep suppu-

[1] Serre, of Montpellier, Traité de la Réunion Immédiate, Paris, 1837.
[2] Roux, Relation d'un Voyage fait à Londres en 1814, Paris, 1815, p. 117.
[3] John Bell, Traité des Plaies, Paris, 1825.
[4] Richerand, Nosographie et Thérapeutique Chirurgicales, Paris, 1821.

ration along the ligatures which reached from the bottom of the wound to the surface. This suppuration, however, ceased as soon as the ligatures came away.

The best that I saw and obtained, then, was not a complete avoid-ance of suppuration, but its absence from the bottom of the wound, especially about the bone, and with this so limited suppurative inflam-mation, the absence of the febrile phenomena engendered by acute suppurative osteomyelitis.

This result, rarely obtained as it may be, is so favourable that we should have to continue to employ this mode of dressing if it were not for its disadvantages, which are real and serious when it fails. Immediate union of a part of the edge, or, if you prefer, of the super-ficial portions of the wound, takes place. But the deep parts remain separated, the effused blood and serosity have prevented permanent contact. Air has been inclosed when the dressing was applied, or enters at those points on the surface where union has failed. In short, the blood and the liquids decompose and stagnate in the wound. Their retention causes a painful distension, increases the intensity of the inflammation, causes it to take on the gangrenous form, and ex-poses necessarily to absorption of deleterious substances.

For these reasons immediate union, although excellent in principle, is not now practised; and I repeat that you should have recourse to it only for children and small wounds in adults. Do not use it for the large wounds of adults unless you are practising in a country where wounds rarely take on gangrenous and septicæmic inflamma-tion.

Infrequent dressings.—Under this name we class dressings with which, while seeking, if possible, the same end as with the former, we expect to have suppuration, but we try to avoid the consequences of the inflammation which precedes and produces it by protecting it from contact with the air, and by prolonged rest of the limb.

You will find quoted as being the first, or one of the first, to re-commend infrequent dressings, a writer of the seventeenth century, Cæsar Magatus, an Italian surgeon who managed to write a very large folio volume upon this subject.[1] This author objected to the practice of repeatedly forcing into the wounds tents of charpie, covered with drugs supposed to favour suppuration, growth of the flesh, and drying of the wound, and which they changed according to the stage reached by the wound. Magatus also insisted upon the fol-lowing points:—that in a dressing we must avoid: 1st, The contact of the air, because it irritates the wound; 2d, Movements, because they interfere with agglutination; 3d, The removal of the pus, which, according to him, is a topic which favours repair. With this object in view he recommended that dressings should be simple and rarely renewed—every three, four, or five days. You know, and I shall speak of it presently, that we go further than that, for you have seen me leave the first dressing of an amputated limb untouched until the twenty-second day.

[1] Magatus, De rarâ medicatioue vulnerum, seu vulneribus rarò tractandis, Veni-tiis, 1616.

266 TRAUMATIC FEVER, PYÆMIA, AND SEPTICÆMIA.

We must suppose that Magatus's practices and precepts remained unknown to the French surgeons, or that they were forgotten, or that if followed they did not give good results; for when Belloste published his work at the end of the seventeenth and beginning of the eighteenth century[1] he again protested against the practice which still existed in his time, of uncovering wounds twice each day; and in a chapter entitled, *Why wounds should be dressed infrequently*, he advised that dressings should be renewed only every two or three days. "Repose," he says, "is necessary for all growths. The nitrous parts of the air alter the natural balm or nutrient juice which is intended to act as a glue to reunite the divided parts."

Afterwards, when the precepts of the English surgeons concerning immediate union had been formulated conformably to Hunter's ideas of adhesive inflammation and suppurative inflammation, all those who adopted this plan of dressing followed the recommendations of Magatus and Belloste, for the first part of the treatment at least, and left the first dressing in place for four days. Then J. D. Larrey[2] called for seven, eight, or nine days, and Josse of Amiens[3] advised that the first dressing should be removed on the tenth day, and the subsequent ones only every two or three days.

Up to this time, you see, they hardly went beyond the tenth day. Maréchal, in the cases of amputation of the forearm reported by Sazie,[4] went twelve days. But at the present time, as I have already told you, M. Alphonse Guérin, taking up again this method which hitherto had not yielded results good enough to attract surgeons very strongly, based his action upon the pathogenic theory that purulent infection is due to absorption by the wound of miasms carried by the air. The conclusion was simple. Wounds must be protected from this contact by more suitable apparatuses, and this protection must be provided especially during the first twenty or twenty-five days—that is, for the period during which septicæmia is most to be feared. Indeed, after its second application, the apparatus should again be left in place for about the same length of time; and thus the infrequent dressing should be continued until the end, or near the end of cicatrization.

M. Alphonse Guérin might have used the apparatuses invented by Jules Guérin and Maisonneuve, of which I shall presently speak; but in the first place he wished to avoid the complications of this special arrangement; and, secondly, he wished to add a certain amount of compression to the proposed occlusion, and he justly sought to use common materials, which the surgeon would readily find everywhere. His idea then was to use cotton batting, and to dress amputated limbs with cotton apparatuses, making elastic compression similar to those used by Burggræve[5] in the treatment of white swelling, so that his

[1] Belloste, Chirurgien d'Hôpital, Paris, 1696 ; another edition, 1708.
[2] Larrey, Clinique Chirurgicale, tome i.
[3] Josse, Mélanges de Chirurgie, 1835.
[4] Sazie, Mémoire sur la Réunion Immédiate et la levée tardive du premier appareil des plaies qui succèdent aux grandes opérations. (Archives Générales de Médecine, 2d série, tome ii. p. 153.)
[5] Burggræve, Les Appareils Ouatés, Paris, 1859.

infrequent dressing is at the same time a cotton occlusive one. To make it, the author, who published his method in June, 1871, covers the wound and the limb for a long distance above when it is a stump —above and below when it is a wound without amputation—with a layer at least five inches thick of cotton batting. Over this he rolls a band very tightly, pressure through the cotton never being sufficient to arrest the circulation, or even to cause pain. In case of an amputation he carefully carries the turns of the band over the end of the stump so as to entirely cover the wadding applied over the wound. When the wound occupies the thigh or arm he carries the dressing as high as the upper end of the limb, or even upon the trunk; and when the injury is of the leg or forearm the cotton is applied at least as high as the middle of the thigh or arm.

By the application of this apparatus M. Alphonse Guérin[1] expects to accomplish two objects—that of preventing air from reaching the wound by means of the occlusion, which seems as if it ought to be complete, and that of exerting compression along the whole length of the limb. At the same time that it may diminish the inflammatory swelling, and perhaps favourably modify the phlegmasia, this compression undoubtedly interferes with the circulation in the lymphatics and superficial veins to such an extent that transport of septic materials is at least diminished, if not entirely prevented. M. Guérin, as I have already told you, leaves this dressing in place for from twenty to twenty-two days. He modifies it sometimes on the second or third day by adding another band if the first seems to be loose, or if it has become soaked with offensive liquids.

Gentlemen, this kind of dressing is still too recent for us to pass final judgment upon it. I do not wish to speak again of its theoretical basis; we could not admit that absorption of atmospherical miasms was the exclusive cause of surgical poisonings. But what of that? We do admit that the presence of air is objectionable, and that it is well to shut it off from the wound. Does M. Guérin's apparatus accomplish this object, and if so, does that suffice to sensibly diminish the chances of septicæmia ?

I believe that it does shut the air out entirely, and I base this belief upon two reasons: it seems to me impossible that the air could penetrate this thick layer of cotton and the band about it, and when it is carefully applied as high up as I said, the cotton is pressed so tightly against the skin that the entrance of air at the upper edge of the dressing seems to me to be equally impossible. Secondly, I was present at the removal of the first dressing from two of M. Guérin's patients, and I have myself removed it on the 21st or 22d day from seven patients whose limbs I had amputated. I was struck in all these cases by the thickness and creamy appearance of the pus, the rosy colour of the wound, and the absence of fetidness. Certainly if the air had penetrated to it the pus would have been altered ; it would have become fetid and ammoniacal, and the wound would have

[1] Alphonse Guérin, Discussion sur l'Infection Purulente. (Bull. de l'Acad. de Méd. 1871, tome xxxvi. p. 328.)

assumed an unhealthy look. I consider the fact, then, as settled beyond question—M. Guérin's dressing prevents the approach of air to the wound.

But is that sufficient to prevent occurrence of traumatic fever or pyæmia? To this I cannot reply so categorically; for while M. Alphonse Guérin, as I myself saw, had a very remarkable series of cures, I have not always been so fortunate.

Of my first series of six amputations on account of wounds received, only one patient survived   That was a young officer whose forearm I amputated near its middle, at the Rothschild Hospital, the twenty-fifth day after gunshot fracture of the carpal and radio-carpal articulations, with burrowing of pus within the sheath of the flexors, and continuous fever which seemed to be leading to pyæmia.   I performed then a consecutive amputation during prolonged traumatic fever, and as I found altered pus and a few eschars in the spongy tissue of the lower ends of the radius and ulna, as, in short, there were signs of putrid osteo-myelitis, I feared that purulent infection might already have begun without having as yet manifested itself by chills.   Happily this fear was not realized.   The fever did not increase after the operation.   It even diminished little by little.   The patient suffered more pain in his stump than the others did ; he was first carried into the garden on the twelfth day.   When we removed the dressing at the end of the twenty-first day we found the wound very rosy, covered with a thick layer of creamy, inodorous pus, which had also soaked into the superficial layers of the cotton ; the bones were covered with granulations, the concomitant erythema was not very marked.   After having cleaned the limb well, I applied another similar dressing, which was equally well borne for twenty days.   At the end of that time the wound, still rosy and covered with laudable pus, had diminished to one quarter its original size.   I applied a simple dressing of cerate, and a fortnight afterwards cicatrization was complete.

The five other patients whose limbs, an arm, forearm, two thighs, and a leg, had been amputated in June, July, and August, 1871, died. But of this I have two explanations to offer.   First, in four of these cases the operation was a consecutive traumatic amputation, and performed a little late, from the twenty-fifth to the thirtieth day after the wound was received.   The fifth patient, whose forearm was amputated, was operated upon rather earlier, but under particularly serious circumstances.   His right hand had been crushed in a printing machine.   The injuries were such that a cure was still possible, and I had, therefore, tried to save the hand.   But on the fourth day there appeared one of those sudden, rapid gangrenes which promptly invade all the tissues and are accompanied by an intense fever, another variety of septicæmia by absorption of the putrid substances which are formed in the neighbourhood of living parts before the vessels have had time to become obliterated.   It is rarely, no matter what you may do, that death fails to follow this gangrenous septicæmia.   Nevertheless, as only twenty-four hours had elapsed since the gangrene began, and in spite of the high fever (pulse 130, temperature 103°), I considered it my duty to propose amputation, and it was accepted. The fever of infection continued, and, as so often happens after intense and prolonged traumatic fever, a violent chill, the sign of pyæmia, occurred on the sixth or seventh day after the amputation; others followed, and the patient died before the cotton dressing had been renewed.

One of the four others had undergone rather late amputation of the thigh for a gunshot wound, involving the synovial membrane of the knee, and followed by suppurative arthritis with rupture of the upper cul-de-sac and effusion of the pus into the deep cellular tissue of the thigh between the femur and the quadriceps. I had proposed amputation on the eighth day, as soon as I had detected the formation and spread of the deep phlegmon in the thigh with very marked febrile movement. The patient had obstinately refused; but about the twentieth day, when the free suppuration of the knee and thigh had exhausted him, when eschars had formed over the sacrum, when the traumatic fever of the beginning had been transformed without interruption into an intense hectic fever, he begged earnestly for the operation, which then offered very slight chances of success. I did it, nevertheless; but the hecticity continued, and the patient succumbed a fortnight afterwards.

Finally, in the other three patients suffering from gunshot wounds, whose limbs I had not amputated at the beginning because I had reason to expect recovery with preservation of them, and because our primitive and consecutive amputations had yielded only failures here at La Charité, an initial chill, apparently indicating pyæmia, had occurred. But this chill had not been seen by the medical attendants, it was rather vaguely described by the nurse and the orderlies, and as there were some doubts of it, and as, furthermore, the local and general symptoms showed that life was in danger, I amputated and applied the cotton dressing. But the chills promptly recurred and purulent infection showed itself distinctly in all three. Death took place a few days after the operation, and at the autopsies we found metastatic abscesses in the liver and lungs.

I am convinced that in these five patients the conditions were unfavourable, and that consequently their death does not justify a judgment unfavourable to the dressing employed. It is evident that no kind of treatment, however well devised it may be, will always preserve from death those who have undergone capital operations; and furthermore that these operations should be performed before the appearance of pyæmia, and even before traumatic fever has lasted long enough and been high enough to preface the way for pyæmia. That will always be one of the great difficulties in practice, for we constantly find ourselves between two dangers: that of performing amputation upon patients in whom traumatic fever has not appeared at all, or only very lightly, and who consequently, if well cared for, are more likely to recover, but of whom a large number might also recover without amputation; and that of waiting long enough to be sure that the limb cannot be saved, and by thus waiting to allow septicæmia to establish a hold which will compromise the success of the operation. As I have told you before, gentlemen, in dealing with this difficult subject we are surrounded by uncertainties; we must allow ourselves to be guided by presumptions drawn from the condition of the injury, the previous health of the patient, and his hygienic surroundings. But these are only presumptions, amid which, while trying to do rightly, we are never certain that we are doing what is best.

To return to the infrequent dressing, I told you that, as regards my five cases of amputation at La Charité, I had another explanation to offer.

In two of them I had the opportunity to renew the dressing once, and I showed you that, as in the cases I saw at St. Louis, and as in the one which I myself amputated at the Rothschild Hospital, the wounds on the twenty-first day looked well, the pus was not fetid, and there were no apparent eschars. At the autopsies I found diffluent pus in the spongy tissue of the bones and in the medullary canal, but it did not smell badly, and was not mixed with either blood or sloughs. There was suppurative osteo-myelitis, but it was not putrid, and I am convinced that the septicæmia of which the patient died occurred before the operation.

Besides, I have a second series of five amputations for pathological reasons: one of the thigh, three of the leg, one through the tibio-tarsal articulation; only one of them, that of the thigh, was carried off by purulent infection, the four others got well.

You saw as well as I that the application and retention of the cotton dressing were not painful, and that the principal objection to it in warm weather was that it had an offensive odour. This we found to be due to the decomposition of organic matter which made its way gradually to the outer layers of the dressing, where it became exposed to the air. But this decomposition did not extend to the deep layers, that is, to the neighbourhood of the wound, where the arrival of the air seemed to me to be impossible. There is one other objection, the moist erythema which is often found extending to a certain distance about the wound, and which is due to the prolonged contact of the pus with the skin. This is a very slight objection, it can be easily overcome by means of starch powder, and has no unpleasant consequences.

In short, gentlemen, notwithstanding the failures of which I have spoken, the results of this infrequent dressing, as I have observed them both upon M. Guérin's patients and my own, justify me in saying to you that it meets more satisfactorily and simply than any other the indication of withdrawing wounds from contact with the air, that it also removes one of the causes of the putrid decomposition which engenders septicæmia, and for these reasons it ought to be employed.

Does this mean that of itself alone it will preserve many patients from grave traumatic fever and purulent infection?

I do not dare to believe so; for, as I have previously told you, the pathogenic problem is so complex that the removal of one of its causes cannot lead to a clinical solution which would amount to absolute preservation. I told you how much influence must be attributed to hygienic and individual conditions; I believe to day that if patients with wounds (surgical or accidental) dressed as I have described, remained in crowded and badly ventilated wards, many of them would still have putrid osteo-myelitis to a degree sufficient to lead to purulent infection. I also believe that this dressing cannot prevent the consequences of previous alcoholism and of unfavourable moral impressions, such as those which follow in most cases of traumatic amputation from the loss of a limb.

To state it briefly, I accept M. Alphonse Guérin's dressing, but in addition I want the patients to be placed in tents, or in isolated and well-ventilated rooms.

Dressings by pneumatic occlusion and by aspiration.—Starting with the idea that decomposition of the pus and other liquids of the wound by the air is the main cause of the toxic complications, M. Jules Guérin likewise thought that the main prophylactic indication was to protect the wounds from contact with the air. With that view he incloses the part in an impermeable sleeve, to which is attached a tube communicating with an aspirating pump which does the work of a pneumatic apparatus. By means of this a vacuum is procured within the sleeve, and the wound is withdrawn from contact with and from the influence of the air. By this method, to which he has given the name of *pneumatic occlusion*, M. Jules Guérin hopes to prevent not only putrefaction but suppuration also, and to obtain what he calls immediate organization, that is, repair without suppuration, similar to that which takes place in solutions of continuity without open wound or with the small ones of the subcutaneous method.

M. Maisonneuve at about the same time made use of a similar apparatus. He did not think of preventing suppuration, and he announced a different intention, that of removing by aspiration all the liquids and even the gases which are found upon the solution of continuity, and thus avoiding the consequences of the absorption which would doubtless take place if these same liquids should remain upon the wound. To obtain this result M. Maisonneuve recommended that the aspiration should be repeated eight or ten times each day, and that from time to time a little water or carbolic solution should be injected, and then removed by the same means.

These two authors have repeatedly published their methods, but not the exact proportion of successes obtained in cases of the kind in which prophylaxis is most necessary, those in which the patients are liable to have acute suppurating osteo-myelitis, and above all they have not told what this proportion was in cases which, while being treated in this way, were obliged to remain in the more or less vitiated air of a hospital ward.

This absence of statistics and the complicated nature of the apparatuses have prevented other surgeons from adopting this method. As for myself, I waited for the publication of favourable results, and this publication not having come I have done nothing about it. Besides, I had other reasons for not using it. It always seemed to me that in order to procure an absolute vacuum about a wound we should have to make very tight constriction over a certain extent of surface, and that this would cause great pain, and perhaps gangrene of the skin. Now, I feared lest these complications, especially the pain, might compensate for the advantages of the vacuum, and add a new cause of poisoning to those which already existed. I said to myself that, if Jules Guérin's and Maisonneuve's patients did not suffer, it was probably because the compression was not very tight, in which case the air would enter between the skin and the apparatus, and thus the intention would not be realized. Let us withhold our final judgment until a sufficient number of successes to compel conviction have been published. While waiting for these let us use M. Alph. Guérin's infrequent dressing if we wish to withdraw our wounds from contact with the air. It seems to me to meet the same indication by much more simple means; and let us not forget that, whatever mode of occlusion is employed, we must still protect the patients from the consequences of vitiated air.

Disinfecting dressings.—If, for one reason or another, the previously mentioned dressings should not be accepted, we could return to an idea which has preoccupied surgeons for a score of years, that of dressing large wounds which expose to traumatic poisoning with substances which have, or are supposed to have, the property of destroying the miasms or toxic principles produced by the decomposition of organic liquids.

I told you in another connection that chlorine water, alcohol, permanganate of potash, and a solution of 1 or 2 per mille of carbolic acid had been employed for this purpose. You have often seen me use a mixture of equal parts of alcohol and a solution of carbolic acid of the strength of one part of the acid to three hundred of water.

I think I may assure you that experience has not shown the efficacy of these different agents, at least from the stand-point which we now occupy. I do not deny that they have a certain value in superficial wounds, or in the superficial part of deep ones, either by retarding the establishment and diminishing the abundance of suppuration, as alcohol certainly does, or by exciting the surface of the wound and provoking the formation of granulations, as Labarraque's chloride of soda does, or by destroying certain of the miasms, although this is not so clearly demonstrated as some seem to believe. But what has never been proved, and what I doubt, is that these agents have the power of preventing eschars and putrefaction in the deep parts of compound fractures, and especially in the cavities and cells of the bones. I admit that they modify the secretion, and, up to a certain point, the alteration of the liquids, but for the present I deny that they prevent the formation of eschars and putrid matter, and the consequences of the contact of air with the mortified parts; and I formulate my opinion clearly as to the use of these different topics in telling you that they have the power of accelerating or retarding cicatrization, but they cannot prevent death by traumatic fever or purulent infection.

You have recently heard recommended a mode of dressing, the value of which is supposed to be due to the disinfecting action of carbolic acid used in a certain way, and in stronger doses than formerly. It is the one called *Lister's dressing*, from the name of the English surgeon who recommended it. It is arranged in the following way: the wound, which has previously been united by sutures (supposing the case to be an amputation), is then covered with lint soaked in strongly carbolized oil (boiled linseed oil 5 parts, solid carbolic acid 1 part). That forms the immediate or permanent dressing, that which is to remain in contact with the wound for two or three weeks. Over this first layer is placed a second, consisting of a paste made of the same carbolized oil and Spanish white (subcarbonate of lime) so mixed as to have the consistency of putty. This paste is put between two cloths, and ought to overlap the permanent dressing a quarter of an inch on all sides. It is to be renewed every two or three days. Lastly comes a piece of oil-silk entirely covering the rest. I should add that energetic compression of the stump is previously made with a band of vulcanized rubber.

I ought to point out to you, gentlemen, that while this dressing may be regarded as a disinfecting one on account of the use of a considerable quantity of carbolic acid, nevertheless it is so arranged as to act in other ways than that of disinfection. Thus, there is a permanent portion which, if I have properly understood it, dries upon the surface of the wound, adheres to it, and preserves it from contact with the air. The paste, although renewed every two or three days, also seems to me to prevent the action of the air. And, finally, there is the compression, which, as in M. Alphonse Guérin's dressing, may easily diminish the chances of absorption. In short, I see mainly in this something which recalls the infrequent dressing; and perhaps Mr. Lister's success, and that of my colleague and friend M. Leon Labbé here in Paris, may have been due as much to occlusion as to disinfection.

The important point, however, is to know if this dressing succeeds. Upon this we should consult foreign sources of information, English chiefly, and French ones. I make a distinction between them because we are especially interested in the cure of the wounded here among us, under the influence of our atmospherical hygiene and the constitution of our patients. Now, I know that M. Lister's statistics show fine results, and that thus far there are no French ones. It is true that the dressing has been but little used in France, but still it has been sometimes, notably by Messrs. Labbé and Cruveilhier. But whether because the trials have not been numerous enough, or because they have not been as satisfactory as Lister's, nothing has been published.

Here, too, another distinction must be drawn. Lister has succeeded chiefly in pathological amputations. In France, for the past year, almost all our amputations have been for traumatic causes. Perhaps that is the reason of our lack of success. We had to deal not only with traumatic lesions, but with men who were fatigued, demoralized, chilled, fated inevitably to suffer the consequences of the overcrowding to which the great number of the wounded exposed them. For these reasons few amputations have succeeded, whatever the dressing employed.

This question of the influence of dressings is then too recent to be definitely answered here in France by the facts. The answer will

18

depend upon future operations performed in pathological cases, and for the traumatisms which surgery allows us to observe in time of peace. Until then I confine myself to the two principal prophylactic measures of which I have spoken: favourable atmospherical conditions, and M. Alphonse Guérin's infrequent and occlusive dressing.

Simple and painless daily dressings, etc.—Remember, gentlemen, that the cotton dressing has not yet been often used for compound fractures, especially for those due to gunshot injuries. 1 should hesitate to recommend it for the latter on account of the need of watching for, and treating the diffuse phlegmons which are always so likely to occur during the first few days. Remember, too, that this kind of treatment, although it has been used, especially after amputations, is not suitable for all of them. If then for any reason you are led to use daily dressings, I advise you to make them so simple that their application and renewal can be made without movement, and especially without pain. In case of a fracture the limb should be placed in a wire splint; after an amputation the stump should be placed upon a slightly raised cushion covered with oil silk. Without seeking immediate union, you should yet place the edges of the wound in the most favourable position possible, and should cover them with two or three compresses wet with a mixture of alcohol and carbolic acid solution, which can be removed and renewed without giving any shock to the limb, and without causing pain and exciting the fear of its daily renewal. I have spoken elsewhere[1] of these simple and painless dressings, and I believe that under favourable atmospherical conditions very good results could be obtained with them.

[1] Mémoire read before the Congrès Médical, 1867.

PART V.

DISEASES OF THE ARTICULATIONS.

LECTURE XXXIII.

DIAGNOSIS OF TRAUMATIC DISLOCATIONS.

I. Generalities upon this diagnosis—Search for deformity and abnormal prominences and depressions. II. Application of these generalities to a dislocation of the shoulder—Search for the subacromial depression and the prominence formed by the head of the humerus. III. Application to a dislocation of the elbow backwards — Depression below the humerus — Search for the olecranon, internal epitrochlear, and radial prominences—Lateral mobility. IV. Application to an iliac dislocation of the hip—Search for the head of the femur and the great trochanter.

GENTLEMEN: I. You see from time to time in the wards patients affected with traumatic dislocations which have remained unrecognized for a longer or shorter time.

In the course of the year two men have been admitted with dislocations of the shoulder; dating in one from twenty-two days, in the other from two months before. I was able to make the reduction in the first, but it was impossible in the other.

Last year I made with the Jarvis apparatus, modified by Robert & Colin, an unsuccessful attempt to reduce a dislocation five weeks old of the right elbow. The patient had been attended by two physicians who had not recognized the lesion, and who contented themselves with putting on leeches and poultices.

I have told you of a consultation to which I was called several years ago in a provincial town, for a supposed non consolidated fracture of the neck of the femur, which was a supra-pubic dislocation unrecognized for more than six months. Errors of this kind are always prejudicial to the patient, for of two things one: either the dislocation is afterwards recognized and reduced—but only after having occasioned useless pain, and, furthermore, associated with the slower and less complete re-establishment of function always found in articulations which have long remained displaced; or else reduction has become impossible; the patient has only the resource of a more or less imperfect pseudarthrosis, and finds himself in a condition of impotence or infirmity which he would have escaped if his surgeon had recognized and treated the dislocation.

The error is sometimes due to insufficient practical instruction,

because the physician during the period of his studies has not sufficiently attended the hospitals, or, if he has attended them, has not
properly noticed what passed, or listened to what was said.

But, it is also due to this, that the subject is more difficult than it
seems to be; and to this, that the precepts of our authors relating to
diagnosis are imperfect, and, as it were, lost amid historical and
anatomo-pathological details.

It is to· protect you in the future from these errors that I wish
to day to speak exclusively of diagnosis; and to give you in a few
short generalities the means, applicable to all regions, of recognizing
articular displacements.

For the diagnosis of dislocations, as for that of many other diseases,
one must look for *rational* and for *absolute* signs. I pass rapidly over
the first, because they do not constitute pathognomonic means. For
pain and difficulty of movement are found as well in contusions,
sprains, and articular fractures as in dislocations.

It is by seeking for *absolute* signs that you must try to make your
diagnosis. Now there are only three for the orbicular articulations:
deformity, abnormal prominences, and abnormal depressions. There
are four for the ginglymoid articulations: the three preceding ones,
and, in addition, abnormal lateral motion. Let us examine a moment
each of these signs and the means of discovering them.

1. *Deformity.*—It is hardly possible for orbicular surfaces to quit
one another without the form of the region and the general attitude
of the limb, which I consider as part of the form, being thereby sensibly modified. It is by the eyes especially that these modifications
are appreciated. But remember this, your eyes may deceive you
when you look only at the injured limb. To appreciate it exactly
you ought to compare it with the other side, if, as is generally the
case, that one is the seat of no lesion.

But a clearly ascertained deformity is only an aid in most cases,
and it must not be depended upon blindly. For in many dislocations it resembles that which may be occasioned by a fracture. And
then, it is sometimes inappreciable; for example, when the patients
are very fat, or when, several hours having passed since the accident,
a swelling, due either to the infiltration of blood or to inflammation,
has appeared. Try, then, to estimate the deformity rightly, but do
not depend upon it alone to make your diagnosis.

2. *Abnormal prominences.*—When you suspect a dislocation, think
at once of the direction in which, according to the facts furnished by
your authors, the displacement may have taken place, and seek the
prominences formed by the articular extremities, especially by that
one which, being the most movable, has abandoned the other. You
may at first use your eyes; but, especially in the enarthroses, you
will rarely be able to clearly see the prominences, the soft parts prevent it. You must then use your fingers, and carry them as deeply
as possible into the regions towards which pathological anatomy
teaches you that the displacement should have occurred. When you
think you have reached an abnormal prominence, do not be satisfied
with the resistance appreciated by the touch; keep your fingers upon

the prominent point and make with your other hand, or by the hands of an assistant, movements of rotation, adduction, and abduction, in order to see if the prominence moves under the hand which examines it. I have often seen this complementary exploration forgotten. It is, however, indisdensable, in order to leave no doubt as to the existence of an abnormal prominence.

3. *Abnormal depressions.*—I do not here mean depressions belonging to that one of the articular surfaces which is more or less hollow, and which, in consequence of the displacement, might be felt through the soft parts. I refer to those which belong to the whole region, and which result from the void left by the abandonment of the articular surfaces. Here, again, you should not depend upon your eyes alone, for if the abnormal depressions are sometimes seen, very often they are not, on account of the volume of the soft parts. It is again to your hands that you must have recourse. Placing them upon the points under which, in the normal condition, you feel more or less deeply a bony resistance, you no longer feel this resistance when the dislocation exists, and you do feel a hollow in its place.

4. *Lateral movements.*—They have no diagnostic signification in enarthroses, since articulations of this kind possess normally all possible movements. But they have a very great one in a ginglymoid articulation, like that of the elbow and those of the fingers ; if, then, by moving the limb outwards and inwards, you find free lateral movements which do not exist at all, or are very limited, normally, there is presumption of a displacement after rupture of the ligaments. It is true that a similar mobility exists in certain sprains, but it is less extensive, and, further, does not coincide with the abnormal prominences and depressions which must always have been found before a diagnosis of dislocation is made.

II. *Application of the general principles to the diagnosis of a dislocation of the shoulder.*—We have just admitted a man, 45 years old, who, having fallen from a ladder yesterday evening, upon his right elbow, felt severe pain in the shoulder, and since then has not been able to use the limb. Let us now consider the explorations which I have made and which are necessary in all cases of this kind.

I removed the patient's shirt in order to compare the two deltoid regions. I satisfied myself that the patient could not move the shoulder, but that he could voluntarily flex and extend the forearm, wrist, and fingers. This last examination is important, for certain dislocations are complicated by paralysis of the forearm and hand, the result of a concomitant lesion of the median, ulnar, and musculo-spiral nerves. It is important to have recognized this paralysis before reducing the dislocation, in order to be very sure that it has not been caused by manœuvres employed during this operation.

Furthermore, I made sure that there was no fracture of the clavicle or of the acromion. I then turned to the deformity and the abnormal prominences and depressions.

1st. *Deformity* —I noticed and pointed out to you the following: Comparing the two upper limbs we saw that the left arm (the uninjured one) descended vertically along the body, touching it at all points. The right arm, on the contrary, was abducted, and the elbow about three inches from the body. I told the patient to bring them together, but he was not able to do it. I then tried to bring them together myself, but felt a great resistance, and made the patient suffer. I could only make the elbow touch the body after an involuntary bending of the latter towards the side corresponding to the injury, and as soon as I let go the limb the position was reproduced. This forced position of the limb in abduction is a variety of deformity which does not exist to so great a degree in all cases of dislocation of the shoulder, but which has a certain value. For if it should be met with in a contusion or a fracture you would be able to correct it, and recognize that, once corrected, it was not reproduced. Here it was only apparently corrected, and reappeared as soon as I abandoned the limb to itself.

You also saw that the shoulder was sensibly lowered, and that the patient supported his forearm with the other hand. This sign has no great diagnostic value, for you find it in all traumatic lesions of this region.

Finally, comparing the two shoulders, you saw that the injured one appeared a little less round than the other.

2d. Carrying then my right hand into the armpit, I felt for the hard *abnormal prominence* which the displaced head of the humerus would form. I at once felt a prominence; the better to appreciate it, I examined the left armpit, and recognized that to feel a bony resistance I had to carry the hand more than an inch higher than on the right side, and further, the resistance which I felt at this depth was that of a much smaller surface. Then again, placing my fingers in the armpit of the affected side, I grasped the right elbow with my other hand, and, rotating the arm, felt distinctly the axillary prominence roll under my fingers; I even discovered that this prominence was regularly rounded. For additional security, and to show you all the useful means of exploration, I asked an assistant to execute these movements of rotation with two hands, and I felt still more distinctly the head of the humerus roll under my fingers. I further looked to see if there was a prominence under the clavicle, behind the pectoralis magnus, as there is sometimes in the so called sub-pectoral dislocations, but I found none.

3d. *Abnormal depressions.*—I had only one to seek, the sub-acromial depression resulting from the removal of the head of the humerus inwards. I have already told you that among the deformities recognized by the eye is a slight flattening of the outer side of the shoulder. I pressed firmly with the fingers of my left hand below the acromion, and recognized, especially by comparing it with the other side, that I had to press very deeply before feeling the bone; the sub-acromial depression, which was scarcely appreciable by the eye, was then very evident to the touch. To be still more certain, I carried the elbow further outwards, so as to relax the deltoid, and then felt the depression still more distinctly. I took care also to make the same manœuvre, comparatively, on both sides.

I admit that in this patient so minute an exploration was not absolutely indispensable for the diagnosis. But in patients who are fatter or more muscular, or in whom the inflammatory swelling is greater, all these explorations, made comparatively on both sides, are necessary, and you should form the habit of not neglecting any of them, so as not to be at fault when you find yourself in the presence of a difficult case.

Enlightened by these symptoms, I did not hesitate; for they are not found all together either in contusion or fracture of the upper extremity of the humerus. I therefore admitted the existence of a subcoracoid dislocation, and reduced it by the method of the heel.

But, as the authors have described quite a large number of varieties of dislocation, you may have been surprised that I did not carry my diagnosis further. On this point, gentlemen, I have a firm conviction: the only important practical distinction among dislocations of the shoulder is that which is founded upon the displacement of the head of the humerus in front of or behind the glenoid cavity. The displacement backward is very rare, it is so exceptional that when dislocation of the shoulder is spoken of, without specifying anything more, it is always understood to mean anterior, or, if you prefer, antero-internal dislocation. As to the distinctions established between the latter, they are perhaps justified by pathological anatomy, but they have no clinical interest, because, on the one hand, they can never be rigorously recognized; and, on the other, the diagnosis would in no way modify the prognosis and treatment.

An antero internal dislocation having been recognized, it should be immediately reduced. Now, with reference to this, there are two categories of dislocations: 1st. Those, and they are the most numerous, which are reduced by simple means, the so-called gentle methods of Malgaigne; for example, the method of the heel; that of Mothe, by elevation; that of Lacour, by outward rotation followed by adduction; 2d. Those which resist the gentle methods, and for which we are obliged to use, after manœuvres of rotation and circumduction, intended either to bring the head of the humerus into a more favourable position or to enlarge the hole in the capsule, forcible methods, such as horizontal traction with ordinary bands and from six to ten assistants, or with India-rubber bands, or with Jarvis's instrument, which, however, is better adapted to old dislocations than to recent ones.

Certainly, if the precise diagnosis of such or such a variety could enable us to foresee a difficulty in reduction, and consequently the urgency of a forcible method, we should have to try to make the diagnosis in spite of the difficulties which it presents. But it is not so. It is not the position of the head a little further outside or a little further inside of the coracoid process, or a little nearer to or a little further from the clavicle, it is not that it is capped in its abnormal position by the subscapularis or by the pectoralis magnus, after a more or less considerable rupture of the latter, which make reduction difficult. This is caused rather by the narrowness and the disposition of the tear in the capsule, or by a peculiar resistance of the muscles, that is to say, by conditions absolutely inappreciable by us which do not belong to a special variety of dislocation, and which are found as well in the sub-coracoid as in the intra-coracoid and sub-clavicular, in the sub-scapular as in the sub-pectoral.

This is why I prefer the diagnosis, axillary or sub-coracoid dislocation. To this diagnosis is attached the indication of a reduction which must not be delayed, because it will be so much the easier as the lesion is more recent. I shall first try one of the gentle methods, and, if it does not succeed, I shall have recourse to one of the forcible ones.

III. *Application of the general principles to a dislocation of the elbow backwards.*—Here, gentlemen, is a woman, 48 years old, quite fat, who fell the day before yesterday, and does not know whether it was the hand or the elbow which received the blow. However that may be, since then she has suffered in the left elbow, and has not been able to move it. She consulted her physician, who could not determine what was the trouble, and sent her immediately to us. I made her undress in order to compare the two arms; and, after having satisfied myself that there is no fracture, either of the humerus or forearm, I shall now make with great care, and applying the general principles which I have formulated, the necessary explorations to discover if there is a dislocation of the elbow backwards. These explorations will take place before you all in the amphitheatre, and I remind you once more how important it is to establish a diagnosis at once, for if there is a recent luxation the reduction will be very easy if made at once; and it will offer greater difficulties the longer we delay.

1st. I first examine the shape of the two elbows; the only difference is that which proceeds from the increased size of the injured one. All the normal prominences and depressions are effaced; this is doubtless due to an infiltration of blood, although thus far there is no ecchymosis. There is nothing characteristic in the attitude. The forearm is in a position midway between flexion and extension, and cannot make any voluntary movement.

From the moment that we find there is no fracture we may presume that the swelling is the result of a dislocation, for it is not so marked in contusions and sprains. But the presumption is not sufficient to justify attempts at reduction. Let us seek then for more certain signs.

2d. I do not see any abnormal prominence, the swelling is too great, but I seek for it with my fingers. Grasping the elbow behind with my right hand, I bring my thumb upon the point where the head of the radius ought to be, and press back forcibly the soft parts in order to feel the bone   I feel something which is more prominent than the radius is when in its proper position. Carrying my finger upwards I think I feel its cup-like depression, but it is not very distinct. Leaving then my thumb upon this prominence, I take the forearm in the other band, and pronate and supinate it; this time there is no doubt, my thumb is upon a prominence which turns, and I also feel the upper depression roll. I make the same manœuvre on the right side, which is uninjured, and do not get the same sensation. I feel the outer part of the radius turn, but I do not feel the whole of its upper extremity, and especially its cup, move as on the other side.

My diagnosis is already advanced. The upper extremity of the radius is dislocated backwards. But is it alone, or is the ulnar also dislocated? The latter is probable, because isolated dislocation of the radius is rare in adults, and is seen ordinarily in children. But this is only probable. Let us look for the prominence of the olecranon. I find it quite easily, and, comparing it with that of the other side, it seems to project backwards, so that the antero-posterior diameter of this elbow seems longer than that of the other. But we must know if this olecranon is higher than it should be, and for that I must discover its position with reference to the internal condyle. I seek the latter by pressing away the soft parts which mask it. Having found it, I leave one of my index-fingers upon it, and, placing the other upon the olecranon, I find that it is a little higher than the condyle. I make the same exploration on the uninjured side, and recognize that there the finger placed upon the olecranon is a quarter of an inch lower than the one upon the internal condyle. There is then no doubt: on the injured side the olecranon is higher and projects a little backwards. Finally, feeling for the inferior extremity of the humerus in front, I find that it is more appreciable by the fingers than the one on the opposite side.

3d. I feel below this inferior extremity of the humerus a depression, that is to say, that in pushing the soft parts backwards I feel a hollow, while on the healthy side the same manœuvre is prevented by a resistance which is nothing else than that of the bones of the forearm.

4th. By the preceding signs my diagnosis is far advanced, but for greater certainty I seek for the lateral mobility which belongs to dislocations of the ginglymoid joints. You see that, fixing the arm with one hand, I can carry the forearm outwards and inwards in a way that is entirely abnormal.

No doubt then is possible: the abnormal prominence of the radius, the olecranon, and the end of the humerus; the depression below the latter; all this, without crepitation, indicates a dislocation backwards of the two bones of the elbow; and you will see that I shall reduce it at once with great facility, by pressing the anterior portion of the humerus against my knee, and making extension and counter-extension with my two hands alone.

The manœuvre has been made. I felt a shock and a cracking which I attributed to the return of the articular surfaces. For greater certainty, and not to allow myself to be deceived by an apparent reduction, I repeat my former explorations, and find neither the abnormal prominences nor the depression. The abnormal lateral movements still exist, but are much less marked. It is then evident that the dislocation is reduced.

I now ask myself if there has not been concomitant fracture of the coronoid process; in which case, if I did not put on a restraining apparatus, the dislocation might be reproduced. To inform myself on this point, I fix firmly the lower end of the humerus with one hand, and, seizing with the other the upper portion of the forearm, I seek to carry it backwards, that is, in the direction in which the dislocation occurred. But I do not produce any displacement, hence I conclude that the coronoid process is not broken, and that a special apparatus is not necessary. Poultices and, in a few days, the compressive cotton dressing will be sufficient to cause the swelling to disappear, and to bring about resolution of the arthritis, rendered inevitable by the ruptures which were caused by the displacement.

IV. *Application of the general principles to an iliac dislocation of the femur.*—The patient who was brought here yesterday evening, and who is lying in bed No. 33 of ward Sainte Vierge, is a labourer, 31 years old. He was caught yesterday afternoon by a slide of earth and rubbish, thrown down violently, and buried under the mass. When taken out he found that he was unable to walk on account of a severe pain in the right hip.

This morning we found the patient unable to move the right limb, and the efforts which he made to do so renewed his pain. Consequently he could not raise his heel from the bed, and, in this respect, resembled patients with fracture of the neck of the femur. As this latter lesion is much more frequent than dislocation, we thought of it at first, but serious doubts were awakened by the fact that the limb, instead of being rotated outwards, was rotated inwards and adducted. Therefore I had to look for a dislocation.

1st. I first called your attention to the shape and attitude of the limb. While at rest in his bed the patient cannot make his two legs perfectly parallel; the leg on the injured side remains slightly flexed upon the thigh, and the thigh upon the pelvis. The foot and the whole limb are turned inwards, and when I tried to turn them outwards with my hands I did not succeed, but only made the patient suffer.

Notice particularly this first symptom. In certain exceptional cases fracture of the neck of the femur is accompanied by rotation inwards; but then you are able easily, with one hand, to turn the limb outwards. Here, on the contrary, that was impossible. I then examined the shape of the hip and of the buttocks, and found them rounder and more prominent than on the other side.

I then measured the length of the two limbs from the anterior superior spine of the ilium to the tuberosity of the inner condyle of the femur, and I found nearly an inch of shortening.

2d. Examining then the great trochanter, I found it more prominent under the skin than it is normally. I then examined its position with reference to the crest of the ilium. I placed one finger upon the most prominent point of the eminence and the other on the crest of the ilium, and I noticed the distance which separated my fingers; I made the same exploration on the unaffected side, and it seemed to me that the distance between my fingers was about half an inch greater on this side than upon the other. I then turned the patient upon the uninjured side, and stretched a string from the right antero-superior spine of the ilium to the most prominent part of the ischion. While an assistant held the string in this position, I placed my fingers upon the highest part of the great trochanter, and found that it was more than half an inch above the string. On the left, the uninjured side, the same investigation showed me that the great trochanter was, as it ought to be in the normal condition, upon the ilio-ischiatic line. This sign, which we owe to M. Nélaton, positively indicates an ascension of the great trochanter, and this ascension corresponded with the shortening which I had previously found.

I had then to seek the abnormal prominence which the head of the femur would form in case of dislocation. I sought this prominence in the groin and near the obturator foramen. I felt sure that I should not find it in these regions; for if there had been a supra-pubic dislocation, the rotation of the limb would have been outwards instead of inwards; and if the dislocation had been into the obturator foramen, there would have been, together with external rotation, considerable abduction of the limb, and not adduction.

I then placed my hand over the external iliac fossa and pressed back as much as possible the mass of the gluteal muscles, and it seemed to me that I felt under them a hard, round prominence. But the sensation was not very distinct on account of the thickness of the soft parts. Therefore, keeping my hand in place, I flexed the thigh upon the pelvis, and then felt the abnormal prominence a little more distinctly. I asked an aid to rotate the thigh a few times, and during these movements I felt very distinctly the round prominence roll under my hand, and could no longer have any doubt of its existence.

3d. It only remained for me to seek an abnormal depression. Theoretically, when the head of the femur is displaced outwards, a hollow ought to be formed in front, over the abandoned cotyloid cavity. I then pushed back with both hands the soft parts of the groin, and it certainly seemed to me that I did not find the same resistance as on the other side. But this sign was not very distinct, and had a certain value only by its coincidence with the abnormal prominence clearly felt in the gluteal region.

To recapitulate, gentlemen: deformity of the hip, adduction and rotation inwards of the limb, shortening, ascension of the great trochanter, abnormal round prominence under the gluteal muscles, abnormal depression in the groin,—all these symptoms, found in a patient who up to that moment had had no disease of the hip, are evident signs of an iliac dislocation, and oblige us to proceed at once to its reduction.

I shall first try, without anaesthesia, the gentle method recommended by Després, flexion of the thigh, and rotation of the limb outwards by the hands of an aid, who will get upon the bed in order that he may, without too much fatigue, combine a certain extension with the movements of flexion and rotation. One or more aids will fix the pelvis, while I myself, standing on the outer side of the limb, will press with the palm of my hand the great trochanter and the whole upper portion of the femur inwards.

If I do not succeed, I shall try, still without anaesthesia, a forcible method, extension and counter-extension by means of straps, and by at least six aids to make extension, and four to make counter-extension. In case a first attempt should not succeed, I would try again after having anaesthetized the patient with chloroform. You know that I have reason to fear the effects of anaesthesia in dislocations.

That is why I do not employ it at first, and why I only use it after one or two unsuccessful attempts at reduction without it. (The reduction was easily obtained by Després's method.)

LECTURE XXXIV.

TRAUMATIC ARTHRITIS OF THE KNEE.

I. Penetrating wound by a piece of glass—Imminent suppuration avoided by the occlusive and compressive cotton dressing—Two varieties of traumatic arthritis: one after wounds, the other without wound. II. Subacute traumatic arthritis after a contusion. III. Subacute traumatic arthritis after a sprain—Reasons for not fearing an articular suppuration—Congestive form—Possible termination by simple chronic arthritis or dry arthritis—Therapeutical indications.

GENTLEMEN : I. *Penetrating wound.*—A young man, nineteen years old, was admitted into the wards two weeks ago, after having been wounded by falling on a piece of glass. He had on the inner side of the right knee a wound about half an inch long, with edges quite smooth and gaping. The accident was quite recent when the patient was brought here during the morning visit. We found upon the skin about the wound a reddish liquid which had the viscid consistency of synovia, and, like it, was sticky. We had to think that this was synovia mixed with a certain quantity of blood. Further, passing a probe very carefully into the wound, I made it enter deeply enough to leave no doubt about its being in the articular cavity. The penetrating wound being recognized, what was there to be done? Exactly the same thing as for fractures complicated with a small wound: close the wound, bringing the edges together as well as possible. You remember that I made this occlusion by means of strips of muslin soaked in collodion and overlapping one another, and I completed the dressing with a thick layer of cotton and a roller bandage drawn tightly over it, extending from the lower third of the leg to the upper third of the thigh. Then the limb was placed in a wire splint.

You have doubtless not forgotten what I then said of the fears which I had for this patient, and of the object proposed in treating him in this way.

I feared articular suppuration, and I sought to avoid it. 1st. Why did I have this fear? Because experience has taught me, as it has taught all other surgeons, that suppuration comes in such a case after a very feverish, acute, or hyper-acute arthritis which greatly affects the health, and when once established it may be complicated by a purulent infection which may carry off the patient, or by a hecticity which may lead to amputation. It has taught me, on the other hand, that, when suppuration does not take place, the consecutive arthritis remains subacute, is accompanied by a moderate fever, or may even remain without fever, does not expose the patient to any fatal accident, and only threatens him with a more or less complete anchylosis.

2d. How did I seek to avoid this acute suppuration which is almost as much to be feared as that of the large, long bones? By the same means and with the same intentions as in compound fractures (see page 105) I wished, by keeping the edges of the wounds together, to favour their immediate reunion or organization, and to protect them from suppurative inflammation which would be very likely to extend to the synovial membrane. I wished also to avoid the entrance of air into the articulation, for this air might have favoured, during the first few days, primitive septicæmia or traumatic fever, by the decomposition of the effused blood and synovia, and a formation by them of septic materials; and it might afterwards have favoured the decomposition of the pus itself, decomposition rendered easy by its retention in a large anfractuous cavity with rigid walls which cannot expel the contents by retraction.

You remember what took place. Our patient suffered very little. His pulse did not rise above 90, nor the temperature above 100½°. The very moderate fever which he had may be considered as a slight traumatic fever by reaction, while, if the arthritis had suppurated, the traumatic fever would have been intense, and probably septicæmic. Twelve days afterwards, I unrolled the band and removed the wadding as well as the strips soaked in collodion. The wound was entirely cicatrized. The articulation was but slightly swollen, and showed neither heat nor fluctuation. Nevertheless, I reapplied a roller bandage.

To-day we have reached the sixteenth day. The general health continues good. The local condition improves. The patient will begin to make voluntary movements while remaining in bed; we shall also communicate some to him every morning and evening. and if he can support this little exercise without a return of acute inflammation, he will get well, and will preserve neither rigidity nor prolonged pains. His age, as I have often told you, singularly aids this favourable termination.

Observe, gentlemen, that if this young man has not had articular suppuration, he has, nevertheless, had an arthritis, and, as this has occurred after a penetrating wound, I am justified in adding that he has had a traumatic arthritis. I shall presently show you other examples of arthritis which deserve this name, but beforehand, I wish to put you on your guard against the signification of this word, which, in the language of some authors, has become the synonym of suppurating arthritis. You have here seen that the arthritis has been neither acute nor suppurating, and yet it is impossible not to recognize that its origin was exclusively traumatic. That simply means that traumatic arthritis may be either suppurating or non-suppurating. Now, as articular inflammations, after the occurrence of external violence, are much oftener suppurating than non-suppurating; this is a reason for not continuing to give the word traumatic arthritis this signification of synovitis about to suppurate. We will distinguish two varieties of traumatic arthritis: one consecutive to penetrating wounds, and for which suppuration is to be feared and to be avoided; the other consecutive to lesions without solution of continuity, and for which suppuration is entirely exceptional.

II. *Contusion and sprain of the knee; Consecutive traumatic arthritis.*— Consider, for example, that which is going on in the two men, Nos. 24 and 46 of Ward Sainte Vierge. The first is a mason, 30 years old, who fell upon his left knee while walking fast. He thinks he did not twist the articulation violently, and we are not justified in believing that there has been the exaggerated tension of the fibrous tissues, which is the initial lesion of a sprain. He has probably had only an exaggerated pressure, that is to say, a contusion which has torn, if not the synovial membrane itself, at least some one of its blood-vessels. The patient has been here for three weeks; you know there have been no general symptoms, and that, as local symptoms, we found at the beginning: All movements impossible, a sharp pain' when the patient tried to make or I sought to communicate any, a little heat felt by the hand on comparing the two knees, and finally a slight swelling and a fluctuation perceived by the manœuvre which I have often had occasion to show you (see page 157). By these symptoms I recognized the existence of a subacute arthritis which I did not hesitate to call traumatic, and for which I told you that I did not fear suppuration, because contusions of the knee are very frequent in the hospital, and because we never see the consecutive arthritis terminate in suppuration.

The second, No. 46, is a teamster, 42 years old, who, jumping down from the back of his horse, fell upon his knee and twisted his leg, as he himself says. He felt quite a loud crack, and was not able to get up. He·was brought to the hospital a fortnight ago. We found in him the same apyrexia as in the preceding case, and the same functional and physical symptoms. Furthermore, making an assistant hold the lower part of the thigh firmly with both ·hands, and taking hold myself with one hand of the lower end of the leg, and moving it alternately to the right and left, I found that lateral movements took place in the articulation. Then, placing one hand above the knee to fix the femur, and the other just below, I pressed with the latter the head of the tibia alternately outwards and inwards, and felt the bone move a little in each direction. No doubt, then, there was abnormal lateral mobility. It was one of those cases of sprain in which the distension of the ligaments, instead of causing an occult or hidden lesion, as so often happens in the foot, had been followed by rupture of the lateral or of the crucial ligaments. In a word, it was a sprain with rupture of the ligaments.

I told you at the beginning that the patient would have a non-suppurating traumatic arthritis, and that in his case we had to occupy ourselves with three principal consequences of the injury: the effusion, the consecutive stiffness, and the lateral mobility. I shall return to these points in a moment, but now I wish to fix your attention upon this, that there was, as in the preceding case, a quite severe arthritis, that this arthritis had no tendency to suppurate, and that, nevertheless, on account of its origin, and to distinguish it from rheumatismal, gouty, and scrofulous arthritis, we are obliged to name it traumatic arthritis. Recall the arthritis of the knee, which you have known to follow fractures of the patella and femur (see pages 142 and 157); they also were traumatic arthritis, sometimes subacute, and sometimes chronic, but having no tendency to suppuration.

I should like to complete this account of the symptoms by that of the lesions which correspond to them; but on this point I am not so well informed as I should like to be, because we do not often have occasion to make an autopsical examination of articulations affected in this way. However, by making use of the notions furnished by experiments upon animals, and those which we have been able to obtain from time to time from our patients, I feel authorized to tell you this.

In arthritis of all kinds there exists a primitive lesion of the syno-vial membrane—injection of the vessels, which we may also call hyperæmia or congestion. This was well seen and described by Prof. Richet,[1] by Bonnet (de Lyon),[2] Panas,[3] and Ollier.[4] Then follows a second lesion, closely associated with the first, thickening of the synovial membrane by the exudation of plastic matter into the con-nective tissue which supports its epithelium, and by the deposit of false membranes on its inner surface. I shall not speak now of the other lesions of arthritis, because they occur rarely in cases of this kind.

In traumatic arthritis especially, I am authorized to believe that the dominant lesion is hyperæmia, that which made Bonnet describe the congestive form of arthritis, and that when plastic and neomembranous thickening occurs it is but slight. This belief is justified by what clinical history teaches us as to the most common mode of termination, and by comparison with what occurs in a certain number of spon-taneous, acute, and subacute arthrites. This termination is complete resolution after a shorter or longer time, especially when the patients are still young. Now, I readily understand this perfect resolution and restoration of movement when there has been only hyperæmia, or when the plastic deposits are not very abundant. Moreover, you will see that this anatomo-pathological problem and the relation of the lesions to the course of the arthrites is the principal difficulty in the clinical study of these diseases.

I wish now to examine before you the question, What will be the duration and the termination of the subacute traumatic arthritis of our three patients? Relying upon what I have just said, and the analogy with the facts of the same kind which I have seen in the

[1] Richet, Mémoire sur les Tumeurs Blanches (Mémoires de l'Académie de Médecine, Paris, 1853, tome xvii. p. 37).

[2] Bonnet, Traité des Maladies des Articulations, Lyon, 1845; Thérapeutique des Maladies Articulaires, Paris, 1853.

[3] Panas, article Articulations du Dictionnaire de Médecine et de Chirurgie Pra-tiques, Paris, 1865, tome iii. p. 268.

[4] Ollier, article Articulations du Dictionnaire Encyclopédique des Sciences Médi-cales, Paris, 1867.

hospitals, I can only say that they will last at least five or six weeks, perhaps much longer, in consequence of the passage of the disease to the condition of chronic arthritis.

As to the mode of termination, it may take place in one of the three following ways :—

1st. In resolution and complete restoration of movements;

2d. By passage to the chronic condition, with possible termination ultimately either in resolution or in anchylosis;

3d. By transformation into that variety of incurable arthritis which we call dry arthritis.

I hope for the first of these terminations, that is to say, cure with restoration of functions, in the first of our patients, in him who had the penetrating wound; for he is young, and from the moment that he escaped suppuration his condition is the most favourable for the complete disappearance of the slight congestion and thickening which undoubtedly have been the principal lesions of his traumatic arthritis.

I may also hope for this termination in our second patient, who has a contusion without sprain. Still, nothing assures me that there will not here be a tendency to pass to that variety of chronic arthritis of which I have often spoken to you in connection with fractures, which leaves for a long time a little swelling, more or less hydrarthrosis, pains while walking, and returns from time to time to the subacute condition, to end finally, after lasting for several months, either in cure, or in a complete or incomplete anchylosis. If he is willing to take care of himself for the necessary length of time, it is probable, since he is not very old and is not rheumatic, that he will escape termination in an infirmity; for I presume that the principal lesion is still congestion, and that the interstitial and neomembranous exudations are not so abundant and have not the same tendency to a definitive organization as in many spontaneous arthrites, and that, therefore, they have a greater tendency to be reabsorbed.

As to the third there is no certainty, for clinical history affords me no means of foretelling the termination of subacute arthrites. But there are more reasons to fear in his case passage to dry arthritis, without anchylosis, which would still be an infirmity. These reasons are, the age of the patient, the rheumatisms which he tells me he has already had several times in the different articulations, the deterioration of his health by the use of alcohol, and the existence of a lesion (rupture of the ligaments) which is sometimes incurable, or which, to be cured, needs prolonged rest, rarely accepted by patients.

You see then, gentlemen, for these patients there is one thing which is certain, that no one of the three will have that which is the most to be dreaded in arthritis, acute or chronic suppuration of the joint; there is another thing which is probable, cure after a longer or shorter time, with restoration of the shape and functions, and behind this probability a little uncertainty as to the possibility of an incomplete anchylosis or a consecutive dry arthritis.

It is now the moment to tell you that suppuration of the large articulations ordinarily takes place under three circumstances: 1st. After a penetrating wound, when suppuration of the external wound has not been prevented, or when there is a concomitant fracture, as in gunshot wounds; 2d. When the patient is scrofulous; 3d. After those dangerous fevers which seem due to an infection, and have more or less analogy with pyæmia, such as puerperal and urinary fevers are sometimes, and such as we see in the course of severe erysipelas and purulent infection, properly so called; and it is because our three patients are in none of these conditions that I am sure they will not have purulent arthritis.

Therapeutical indications.—I have already mentioned these for the first patient, the one with traumatic arthritis due to a penetrating wound. The chief indication was to prevent suppuration. I have told you how it was met.

There remains for him an indication which is the same for the two others—to prevent passage to a chronic state, and termination by an infirmity. For that we recommend, above everything, rest in bed, then compression with the cotton dressing, to be renewed every five or six days. To that we shall add occasional purging. Thus far I see no indication in the sanguinolent or sero sanguinolent effusion. Twice during this year (1872) you have seen me make a puncture and aspiration upon patients, who, after a contusion of the knee, had a considerable effusion of blood. I then gave you my reasons for so doing. I feared that the effusion, on account of its volume, might not be reabsorbed, and that, acting as a foreign body, it might cause permanent irritation and passage to the simple chronic state, or to the form of dry arthritis. I thought that by at once evacuating the liquid, I should remove this cause of prolonged irritation, and put the patients into conditions favouring termination by resolution, rest and compression being also used, as is necessary in all cases of this kind.

In the two patients now before us the effusion is small; it was formed so slowly that I may believe it was composed of as much, and even more, synovia than blood. I count upon the absorption, which is the rule in such cases, and I shall puncture only if, three weeks hence, I find the absorption going on too slowly.

The rupture of the ligaments and the resultant lateral mobility furnish us, in the third patient, the indication to immobilize for a much longer time than in the other two. About two months will be necessary for the consolidation of the ligaments. In order not to condemn the patient to so prolonged a rest in bed, I shall put a dextrine bandage over the cotton dressing at the end of the third week, and leave this immovable apparatus in place for four or five weeks. If, at the end of this time, I still find lateral mobility, I shall renew the apparatus and leave it in place for another month. I do not disguise the fact that this prolonged immobility will favour anchylosis; but that result is far from certain, for anchylosis results from two things: special lesions, which I shall hereafter describe, and immobility. The latter, by itself, would never cause anchylosis. It only favours it by preventing us from employing at a certain moment the movements necessary to prevent its establishment. But, on the one hand, if the lesions which produce the anchylosis are not too marked,

19

we shall still be able, at the end of three months, to use successfully the movements of which I spoke; and, on the other hand, if permanent anchylosis should occur, such a result would be less unfortunate for the patient than persistency of lateral mobility. For the latter exposes the knee, at every moment, to new sprains and, consequently, to renewed arthrites, which are more troublesome than complete anchylosis.

There will probably be, in all three patients, a final indication, that of favouring the restoration of movements and diminishing prolonged rigidity. But as the means appropriate to that are the same as in cases of spontaneous arthritis, I will speak of them when treating of the latter.

LECTURE XXXV.

ACUTE AND SUBACUTE SPONTANEOUS ARTHRITIS OF THE KNEE.

I. First patient affected with acute arthritis of the right knee, gonorrhœal, with contracture of the flexors—Straighteni ng of the limb under ether—Afterwards, discovery of lateral mobility and crepitation—Explanation of these two symptoms. II. Second patient affected with single acute arthritis, probably rheumatic, of the right knee. III. Formation of a complete anchylosis in both cases, notwithstanding the efforts made to prevent it—Study of the lesions—Congestion —Plastic deposits, whence the name plastic or anchylosing arthritis—Explanation of the anchylosis by the establishment of adherences after a struggle between the tendency towards resolution and the adhesive tendency. IV. Therapeutical indications based upon these ideas.

GENTLEMEN: You have seen for more than six months in ward Ste-Catherine two women who have often given me occasion to speak to you of the acute and subacute forms of spontaneous arthritis of the knee. Both are now getting well with anchylosis. As cases of this kind are not rare, and raise thorny questions of science and practice, I propose to-day to recall the principal details of these two observations and the reflections which they have suggested.

I. *Acute arthritis of the right knee, gonorrhœal, with contracture of the flexors.*—One of them, 25 years old, occupying bed No. 24, ward Sainte-Catherine, was admitted the 29th of December, 1871, into the medical service of my colleague M. Pidoux. She had been taken a few days before with sharp pains in the right knee, accompanied by slight fever and loss of appetite. When she was brought to the hospital, the pains were still very severe; not only was she unable to make any movement, but the knee was flexed to a right angle with the thigh, and she was unable to straighten it, the slightest attempt to do so increasing her pain. At the same time the skin was hot, the pulse at 90, and there was sleeplessness, and very little appetite. In a word, the intensity of the local inflammatory symptoms and the persistency of this slight febrile condition indicated that the arthritis belonged to the acute form. Furthermore, M. Pidoux had discovered that this arthritis was single, and that the patient had a purulent urethritis and vaginitis which authorized him to consider the disease as of gonorrhœal origin.[1] The 17th of February, that is, more than six weeks afterwards, the general condition had improved, but the local symptoms remained about the same, and M. Pidoux asked me to take the patient into my service. I then found that the knee was flexed at a right angle, in consequence of which the patient was forced to lie upon the corresponding side, that it was swollen and felt very hot to the hand, and that the least pressure, and of course the slightest attempt to move it, caused very severe pains. When I asked the patient to point out the chief seat of these pains, she always indicated the inner side of the knee, the part which corresponds to the passage of the internal saphenous nerve and to the insertions of the internal lateral ligament. On account of the flexed position of the limb, I was not able at first to determine whether there was any effusion of liquid; however, if there was, it was not very abundant, for I did not find any fluctuation.

I further recognized that for the moment the patient had no other joint affected, and that she was without fever. It was then a single arthritis which had at first been acute, and which, in consideration of the disappearance of the febrile phenomena, might be considered as having passed to the subacute state. Was this arthritis to be called rheumatic? Strictly speaking, yes; for by this rather vague word *rheumatism* we wish to designate a general cause, the essence of which is unknown, which affects the synovial, fibrous, and muscular tissues. Furthermore, gonorrhœa also was present, and whatever may be the way in which the production of gonorrhœal arthritis is explained, it is certain that, in its symptoms and consequences, it resembles certain forms of rheumatic arthritis, especially that in which the disease is single, or very marked and prolonged in one articulation, whilst the others are but slightly affected, and in a very temporary manner. Moreover, if any doubts might have existed as to the rheumatic nature of the affection, they would have been destroyed when, a few months later, in June, we saw this patient affected with pains in several other joints, especially those of the shoulders and left elbow. As to the right elbow, it had long been completely anchylosed by fusion in consequence of a traumatic lesion during childhood.

On making my etiological examination I noticed upon the neck the scars of two ganglionary abscesses, and upon the borders of the eyelids a little alopecia and redness coinciding with slight specks left by keratitis during childhood. The patient, although apparently of a good constitution now, had then the scrofulous temperament. The

[1] I agree with those who think that gonorrhœal arthritis is rheumatic. But clinically it deserves mention and a special description for the following reason, which is absolutely inexplicable: it is localized much more frequently than ordinary acute rheumatism in a single articulation, and there goes beyond the congestive form and takes on the plastic and anchylosing form, of which I shall speak in this lecture.   .

local symptoms do not in any manner authorize me to admit a scrofulous arthritis, but these antecedents might make me fear, in case this acute arthritis should become a chronic one, that it might pass to the fungoid form or white swelling.

However that may be, there was when I first examined this woman one main indication to meet: that of straightening the knee, thus applying the excellent precepts given by Bonnet[1] for the substitution of a good for a bad posture in diseases of the articulations. The patient was then anæsthetized by means of ether, and I straightened the limb very easily by my hands alone, placed it in a wire frame and kept it in place by means of a cushion, an anterior splint, and five straps. Since then the pains have not been so violent. They reappeared however from time to time, especially when the patient moved a little too much, and after we ourselves had made an examination or sought to give motion to the articulation, which we knew to be threatened with anchylosis. At a certain moment during these explorations we discovered lateral mobility, as in the man suffering from a sprain of whom I have previously spoken, and at the same time a loud crepitation which appeared to me to be caused by the friction of the bony surfaces. In a word, after about two months of treatment, the arthritis had passed to the chronic state with the two chief symptoms which I have just mentioned.

To what were these two symptoms due? I again repeat that we do not well understand all the lesions of the beginning of acute and subacute arthritis, because we have not had occasion to study them on the cadaver, and because the only information we possess has been furnished by experiments on animals, and especially by those which Prof. Richet has described in his works on white swelling. Now these experiments probably do not reproduce all the lesions which occur in the living man, and especially those which would explain the symptoms in question. I shall then give you only very probable opinions, warning you that I cannot verify them by direct observation.

As for the abnormal lateral mobility I am disposed to attribute it, like that which I observe after violent sprains, or in patients with white swelling, to a lack of resistance in the lateral ligaments. But I do not disguise from myself that in an articulation where the synovial membrane is thickening and advances, as I shall soon tell you, toward fibrous transformation, it would seem as if the ligaments ought to ollow a similar course, and increase their resistance by a thickening and condensation of their tissue. We should then have to admit that here the ligaments have a tendency, in consequence of the arthritis, to lose in part their fibrous character, while the synovial membrane tends to assume this character. It would be strange; but after all it is not impossible.

And it is because it seems to me strange that I offer you another explanation; perhaps the lateral mobility is caused by the semilunar

---

[1] Bonnet, Traité des Maladies des Articulations ; Lyon, 1845. Thérapeutique des Maladies articulares ; Paris, 1853.

fibro-cartilages being softened, thinned, and about to disappear. For I can understand that if these intermediate bodies were lacking, the two bones would approach one another, the ligaments would slacken and lose the tension which, during extension of the limb, was the principal obstacle to lateral mobility. What authorizes me to offer you this supposition is the fact, that, in all articular diseases which have been a little prolonged, the trouble in nutrition which follows causes, by a mechanism which we do not understand, the destruction of the diarthrodial cartilages. Now as the fibro-cartilages have a similar structure, I presume that, as moreover we see it in white swelling, their cells open, are destroyed, and disappear, and that as the cartilaginous portion is disassociated and absorbed, the fibrous portion either disappears itself by absorption, or is no longer thick and firm enough to fill the space between the two principal bones of the articulation.

I have now to explain the second symptom, the crepitation. I can attribute it to nothing else than to that destruction of the diarthrodial cartilages of which I have just spoken, a partial destruction undoubtedly, but nevertheless occupying the whole thickness in certain points, and thus permitting during lateral motion the rubbing of the bones which we felt. I repeat that this singular destruction of the diarthrodial cartilages, first noticed in white swelling, then in dry, deforming arthritis, seems to occur in almost all arthrites when they have a certain intensity or last for a long time.

I omit, for the moment, the later phenomena which we observed and the present condition of the patient, for, in these respects, she resembles another woman, No. 3, whose antecedents I will now recall, and will then complete the account of the two observations.

II. This second patient, No. 3, is 23 years old, and, like the preceding one, has had no children; she knows no cause to which to attribute the very painful affection of the knee from which she was suffering when admitted to the hospital the 3d of April, 1872. The disease then had lasted a week, and was accompanied by a slight febrile movement. The local symptoms were a notable swelling, a small effusion within the joint, considerable heat felt by the hand, very sharp pain on the slightest movement, and much spontaneous pain during the day and especially during the night. In a word, the general and local symptoms were those of moderate acute arthritis. In her case there was neither the permanent flexion nor the lateral motion which we found in the other. We have treated this woman by immobility in a wire splint, several applications of wet cups, several blisters, purges, opiates, and sometimes, when the pains were very severe, by the subcutaneous injections of the hydrochlorate of morphine. You have noticed frequent renewals of pain and even of fever, which made me fear suppuration; but this has not occurred, and after several weeks all these symptoms were so much better that I have no longer had this fear, and have considered the disease as having passed to the chronic state.

III. Since about the 15th of June the two cases have been so similar that I can complete their history at the same time. Finding myself in presence of a disease which had kept the articulation immovable and threatened to end by anchylosis, I tried to prevent this result and obtain a cure with preservation of the functions. With this object I communicated a few movements to the limb every morning, and ad-vised the patients to do the same. The manœuvre was repeated in the evening by the interne of the service. But see what happened : not-withstanding all their efforts, the patients were not able to bend the knee; their muscles did not contract, and the only movements which took place were in the hip and thigh. As for those which we com-municated during about a minute each time, they were very limited and caused pain which lasted for quite a long time thereafter. At the end of a week these pains increased, so that it became necessary to stop all motion and return to poultices. A few days later we recom-menced, with the same result. I therefore had to give up my attempts and let the articulations rest.

To-day, the end of July, in both patients the patella is united to the femur; the first (No. 24) has lost all movement of the tibia upon the femur; the second (No. 3) has still a few movements, but they are very limited, and I expect to see them disappear entirely. In both of them we shall have subacute arthritis terminating, after passage to the chronic condition, in complete anchylosis. I have shown you, in addition, that since the beginning of the disease the femur has seemed to be tumefied to a great distance above the articulation. To-day, when I compare it with that of the opposite side, I find a swelling similar to that which we have often seen after simple and compound fractures, and after epiphysary osteitis, a swelling which we call hy-perostosis.

Let us now see, gentlemen, 1st, what have been the anatomical lesions in these two women ; 2d, why, in spite of all our efforts, the cure did not take place with preservation of shape and functions.

1st. As for the lesions, it is certain that in the synovial membrane they consisted of a hyperæmia and inflammatory exudations, some of them deposited in the membrane itself and making it rigid, others on its inner surface in the form of fibrinous and neo-membranous flakes, which became vascular and were transformed into a fibro-cellular or fibrous tissue. It is for the sake of better characterizing this capital lesion and to distinguish it from those of fungoid and dry arthrites that you have often heard me employ the expression *plastic arthritis.*

While these lesions are being produced in the synovial membrane, what is taking place in the other constituent parts of the articulation ? That is what autopsies have not yet well cleared up. I presume, as I have already said, that the diarthrodial and inter-articular cartilages are disorganized and thinned, and perhaps have disappeared. It is more than a presumption in the case of the first patient ; for we have not been able to otherwise explain the crepitation which we found in her at a certain time. But is this lesion entirely similar to that which we find in white swelling and dry arthritis, or is it different? Do Brodie's ulcerations and Redfern's velvety change occur here?

Or is it by the histological lesions, the knowledge of which we owe to M. Ranvier, especially by the proliferation of the superficial cells, the segmentation of the fundamental substance, and the opening of the

capsules into the articular cavity, that the supposed destructions commenced? I cannot answer these questions, because the authors I
mention have not made a sufficient number of autopsies to be able
to say whether the lesions which they describe in dry arthritis are also
found in anchylosing plastic arthritis, or at what period of the disease
they appear.

So also for the ligaments; are they softened and destroyed, as we
might have supposed, in the first patient who has had lateral mobility
from the beginning? Are they not, on the contrary, thickened and
rigid, in consequence of their participation in the plastic phlegmasia?
On this point also I am in doubt.

And the bones? I have noticed nothing in the patella or the tibia,
but I told you that the femur seemed notably hyperostosed in both
patients. Is it the periosteum alone which has been invaded by pro-
pinquity, and which has furnished new layers of bone by a periostitis,
likewise plastic? Or has the entire thickness of the bone been affected,
passing to the condition of plastic or condensing osteitis? I do not
know. But on this subject I offer you a final reflection which has
already been mentioned *àpropos* of osteitis. I have often seen hyperostosis follow traumatic and spontaneous arthrites when they had not
taken on the fungoid character and the tendency to chronic suppuration, or, which amounts to the same thing, when the patients were
not scrofulous. I therefore believe that in cases where we have
doubts as to the nature and the tendencies of an arthritis, the certain
appearance of hypertrophying osteitis is an argument in favour of the
opinion that this arthritis is plastic rather than fungoid and suppurating.

2d. How and why was this complete anchylosis established? Two
chief incontestable reasons explain this termination : First, the false
membranes formed adhesions like those we find on serous membranes
after inflammation; these adhesions, becoming more and more firm
and rigid, have diminished little by little the synovial cavity and opposed change in the position of the articular surfaces. Secondly, prolonged immobility has favoured these adhesions. This immobility itself was due both to the pain which permitted neither voluntary nor
communicated movements, and to the muscular insufficiency which
was itself the consequence of these pains. For there are produced
during the course of painful arthrites remarkable physiological and
anatomical modifications of the muscles. They cease to contract voluntarily, and assume a prolonged contracture which completes the immobility in the position either of flexion or of extension. You remember that in one of our patients we had to straighten the knee after having overcome the resistance of the contractured flexors by anæsthesia.
When the first effect, contracture, has lasted a certain length of time
the peri-articular muscles atrophy, then pass to the fibrous and fatty
condition which characterizes retraction. The longer these lesions
of the muscles last, the more do they favour the establishment of the
anchylosis by allowing the formation and organization of the adherences of which I have just spoken.

It is now the moment, gentlemen, to define our opinions upon the influence of immobility in the production of anchylosis. It does not by itself produce it, only when combined with a plastic arthritis. But it may happen that this latter is caused by the immobility itself. Recall in this connection the distinction which I have often made between large and small articulations, at least so far as traumatic articular diseases are concerned. Immobility alone rarely causes plastic arthritis in the large joints, and if the latter occurs it is due to external violence. The contrary is the case in the small articulations. Immobility alone may there cause plastic arthritis and consecutive anchylosis.

These results do not seem to me to agree with M. Charcot's. In his recent works this author has described an arthritis of the large articulations in paralytics ; but the immobility does not seem to me, in such cases, to be the sole cause of the articular phlegmasia. The troubles of the nervous system undoubtedly contribute to a certain extent, and the conditions are not the same as those of immobility after great traumatisms.

But let us return to the mode of production of the anchylosis of the knee in our patients. Is there no reason to lay it to the charge of other causes than those of which I have just spoken? I think there is, but I am not sufficiently acquainted with all the alterations that have occurred, to affirm it. It may be, for example, that the diarthrodial and semilunar cartilages having been completely absorbed, the surfaces of bone thus laid bare and attacked by plastic osteitis have united by a mechanism analogous to that of the formation of a callus. There would then be established an anchylosis by fusion of the bones. It may also be that the cartilages not having been absorbed, fusion has taken place between them, and that thus the anchylosis may be by cartilaginous fusion, a form which is much rarer, but which has been observed, and of which I have seen an example. Or it may be that the cartilages having been preserved, false membranes have formed upon the opposing surfaces, and that solid adhesions have taken place between them. The anchylosis would then be called fibrous.

We are unable to recognize clinically in the living patient with which of these forms indicated by pathological anatomy we have to deal. This would be a source of regret if therapeutics could do anything for complete anchylosis, that in which all movement has disappeared. But I am of those who believe that in such cases nothing should be done. The indication, either to oppose anchylosis itself, or to substitute a good for a bad posture, exists only in those cases in which some movements remain and the anchylosis is incomplete. Now, anchylosis may be incomplete in two ways: first, by the thickening and lack of extensibility of the synovial membrane, consecutive to the cellulo-fibrous, and even fibrous transformation of the plastic materials deposited in it, it is then incomplete anchylosis by rigidity ; second, by the establishment of adhesions which are still extensible and susceptible of resolution between the opposite points of the synovial membrane, in which case the anchylosis is called cellular or adhesive. You understand, finally, that the incomplete anchylosis may be at the same time adhesive and by rigidity.

I now reach the second question, a very interesting one clinically, that of knowing why complete anchyloses are produced. It is first because the arthritis has passed beyond the limits of that which is simply congestive, as happens quite often in the traumatic variety following contusions and sprains, and because by passing these limits it becomes plastic and adhesive. But all plastic arthrites do not end in complete anchylosis: a goodly number end in the rigidity and cellular adhesions of which I have just spoken, and which we finally overcome. What takes place in such cases? The congestion disappears, the inflammatory products infiltrated in the thickness of the synovial membrane, and which have given it its rigidity during a certain time, do not go very far in their fibrous transformation, and may be reabsorbed; the false membranes, if there have been any, are also reabsorbed; the synovial membrane again becomes supple, and the articulation returns to its normal condition.

In our two patients the plastic products, instead of being reabsorbed, have advanced further and further in their organization, have made the synovial membrane fibrous, and have formed adhesions, while at the same time, in all probability, the cartilages and the ligaments have undergone the alterations we have mentioned. The capital difference then is this: the plastic arthritis instead of terminating by resolution, has terminated by adhesion, and consequently, by a profound transformation of the normal anatomical conditions.

But in making this explanation I only move the difficulty back. Why, in fact, this unfavourable termination rather than the first? Here I can no longer answer with pathological anatomy, we must turn to pathogeny, that is, to that which is the most obscure and the most difficult, and yet the most real in our science. These women have got their infirmity because they have had a very intense inflammation of a peculiar kind. The intensity has caused the primitive congestion and the consecutive exudations to be more marked than they are in other cases; the nature or the special mode of inflammation has been such that the tendency has been towards organization rather than absorption of the plastic products. Has there been a special cause? It is probable; but we do not know what it is. We say, since we can do no better, that this cause has been rheumatic; we say, for one of the patients at least, that the rheumatism has been gonorrhœal. But since rheumatism produces also arthrites which are simply congestive, or plastic non-anchylosing arthrites, or still others, it remains to know why it has taken the form which we have observed upon our two patients. Probably we must here accuse, as we are so often forced to do, a peculiar aptitude, an idiosyncrasy behind which lies—we should not hide it—our inability to explain the relation between the etiology, the intensity of the lesions, and the tendency of these lesions to advance in one direction rather than in another.

Let us confine ourselves to the deductions which are applicable to the clinic. These deductions are the following: when you have recognized that an arthritis, whether traumatic or spontaneous, is neither suppurating, nor fungoid, nor dropsical, nor dry, do not forget that it is plastic, and that consequently it has a certain tendency towards anchylosis, a tendency which you must combat by exciting or favouring resolution, and preventing adhesion.

IV. *Therapeutical indications.*—They result from what precedes, and belong to three periods of the disease. In the first, that of the beginning, the intensity of the phlegmasia must be opposed by rest in a good position, antiphlogistics (leeches, cupping) derivatives upon the intestinal canal, narcotics to quiet pain.

In the second, you must try to provoke and aid the absorption of the plastic products. It is still rest and immobility which meet this indication; revulsives upon the skin, blisters, punctate cauterization may also aid it.

In the third, you must try to make the adhesions, which are still thought to be soft, and the rigidity, which is not yet invincible, yield. It is then that it is proper to try massage and communicated movements. But here we find ourselves between two dangers: that of provoking, by these movements, a return of the phlegmasia, and that, by not employing them, of allowing the anchylosis to form. We are obliged to feel our way. If the manœuvres cause only temporary pain it is proper to persevere; if, on the contrary, they provoke continuous pain, with return of the swelling, of the articular effusion, and of heat to the touch, they must be stopped. Perhaps a little later they may be borne; if they are not it is best to abstain entirely and to abandon the arthritis to the chances of anchylosis, as we have had to do for our two patients. At this same period if the articulation has become indolent enough to allow the patient to leave his bed and walk on crutches, baths and douches of sulphurous or thermal waters, such as those of Néris, Bourbonne, and Plombières, would also be very useful.

LECTURE XXXVI.

CHRONIC ARTHRITES OF THE KNEE.—HYDRARTHROSIS.

Dropsical arthritis or hydrarthrosis—Lesions supposed to exist, but inappreciable by physical signs—Probable congestive form—Enlargement of the patella, explained by a hypertrophying osteitis—Prognosis—Long duration, possible relapse—No tendency to suppuration and to anchylosis—Therapeutical indications : 1st curative treatment : compression, blisters, puncture, actual cautery, injection of iodine ; 2d prophylactic treatment.

GENTLEMEN : We have at this moment in the wards several patients suffering from chronic affections of the knee. When passing their beds every morning, I indicate by a word what there is that is characteristic in each one of them, and I recall to you the questions which should always preoccupy us when in presence of affections of this kind : shall we have resolution, anchylosis, suppuration, or the infirmity of dry arthritis? I cannot speak to you of all these patients: I shall take only the three principal types: hydrarthrosis, white swelling, and dry arthritis. I begin with the hydrarthrosis.

Dropsical arthritis or hydrarthrosis.—The patient in No. 20 is a man thirty years old, jeweller, of a medium constitution, but in whose antecedents we find no indications of scrofula. He told us that on several occasions he had pains in the shoulders, arm, and left knee, which however have never been swollen. These pains, although apparently rheumatic, had not been accompanied by fever nor by such an alteration of health that we could explain them by an acute articular rheumatism.

He entered our wards for the first time three years ago for a swelling in the right knee, the cause of which was unknown. He remained six weeks, and left us almost cured, with a rubber knee-cap, which we advised him to wear during the day and to remove at night. He was able to resume work and continue it until a month ago. However, he has always felt at times, especially when a little fatigued and when the weather was damp, pains in this knee. Finally, a month and a half ago, after a long walk, the pain became more intense, more prolonged, a new swelling appeared, and the patient was obliged to return to us.

He has been here four weeks. You noticed at first that the right knee was swollen, that the depressions on each side of the patella were replaced by a tumefaction appreciable by the eye, that the region was not hot to the hand, and that, by pressing with both hands upon the sides, while the index finger of the right hand pressed back the patella, fluctuation was distinctly felt. There was further the sensation that the liquid was not separated from the skin by a thick layer, and on examining the prolongations of the synovial cavity, especially the upper one, we did not feel any thickening.

The diagnosis was not difficult; first, it was certainly an arthritis, since the swelling, the pain, the difficulty in movement, the heat from time to time could be attributed neither to a simple neuralgia,[1] nor to a cancer, nor to any other disease. But we had next to make the anatomical and the etiological diagnosis of this arthritis.

As to the first, the thing was evident; it was certainly a chronic arthritis, but with considerable effusion, so considerable that it was allowable to make use of it to characterize the disease as our authors have done by employing the word *hydrarthrosis.* You have often heard me pronounce this word for the present patient, and for those who have been similarly affected. But I prefer generally the name *dropsical arthritis* or *arthritis with effusion,* because under this name of hydrarthrosis are comprised two things: an essential effusion or one without lesion, like that which is formed during anasarca, and an

---

[1] I have often spoken of patients who, without any anterior disease, or after a traumatic or a rheumatic arthritis, had a very sharp continuous pain in the side of the knee, with exacerbation during walking or without known cause, and without any appreciable swelling. The arthritis had no lesion, or only a congestion inappreciable by our senses; but it was more painful than this simple lesion would have made one suppose. I call it neuralgic arthritis or exaggerated sensibility of the knee.

effusion symptomatic of an inflammatory condition. Now, although we have not often had occasion to make the autopsy of patients dead with hydrarthrosis, yet, in the rare cases where this occasion has been presented, an injection of the synovial membrane has been found, representing Bonnet's congestive form, of which I have already spoken, with a very slight thickening; and as in the other side, the clinic teaches us that most patients affected with effusion in a single knee have at the same time some functional symptoms which can be explained by inflammation, I prefer to make use of the word arthritis, which indicates that in my opinion it is an inflammatory disease.

I sought, in our patient, if there was at the outer and upper part of the articulation one of those indurated nodules which Marjolin and Malgaigne pointed out as sometimes accompanying hydrarthrosis, which may be attributed to a partial thickening of the synovial membrane. But I did not find these nodules, although I have found them upon other subjects.

I have just touched upon another point of the anatomical diagnosis. What are the lessons of this arthritis with effusion? I assure you that the clinic has given no physical sign which could indicate any. If these lesions exist, and I do not doubt it, they ought to be in the synovial membrane, for that is the only way of understanding the effusion. But it does not seem to be thickened, neither as it is in plastic arthritis, nor as it is in fungoid arthritis. I do not deny a slight augmentation of volume like that which sometimes accompanies congestion. I am disposed especially to admit this augmentation in the synovial fringes corresponding to the intercondyloid space; but the lesion is not sufficiently marked to be felt through the skin. I believe much more in the existence of injection or hyperæmia like that which was found in the autopsies of Dupuytren and others, and I believe it, not because it is proved to me by physical signs, but because the effusion and the functional symptoms are those of an arthritis, and because I do not know any other lesion than congestion or hyperæmia which could explain them.

But what must we think of the other constitutent parts of the articulation? I admit that I fear some nutritive trouble in the cartilages; for there is such a solidarity between them and the synovial membrane, that they end habitually by becoming altered when the other has been diseased for some time. Still, there is as yet no physical sign which authorizes me to affirm the existence of a lesion in that quarter. The same is true of the ligaments; if they were softened, and they sometimes are in hydrarthrosis either by excessive distension, or, which seems to me more common, by a concomitant trouble of nutrition, we should have lateral mobility; but I satisfied myself that it did not exist. Moreover, they are not rigid, for all communicated movements are executed almost as they are normally. Voluntary movements also take place, but they are limited by the pain and not by an appreciable material modification of the means of union.

As to the bones, I have noticed nothing in the femur and tibia; the first, in particular, has not shown that hyperostosic swelling with which we were struck in certain plastic arthrites (see p. 295). I point out to you only a very marked transverse enlargement of the patella. We measured it with a compass, and found it nearly half an inch larger than that of the opposite side. This enlargement of the patella in hydrarthrosis was pointed out long ago; but its origin and its signification were not explained. For me, its origin is still in an hypertrophying osteitis, of the kind of which I have so often spoken to you. Instead of affecting the femur and tibia in a manner appreciable during life, this osteitis is confined to the patella, a peculiarity which is utterly inexplicable. Its signification, however, appears to me to be the same as that of femoral hyperostosis in other arthrites, that is to say, since condensing osteitis appears habitually in patients who are not scrofulous and consequently not predisposed to fungoid and suppurating arthritis, the appearance of hyperostosis of the patella would be a reason to dismiss any fear of the occurrence of the latter, even if some physical signs should have given rise to it.

To recapitulate, gentlemen: in making the diagnosis, *dropsical arthritis*, I presume that we have to deal especially with a rebellious hyperæmia or congestion of the synovial membrane, and if I do not use the expression congestive arthritis, it is because this expression does not sufficiently indicate one of the principal things, the abundance of the liquid. And as congestive arthritis may take place without effusion, and as the latter, when it does exist, has a bearing upon the prognosis and treatment, it is better to use an expression which indicates its presence.

As for the etiological diagnosis, I told you a moment ago that it is a rheumatic disease. At least, we can give no other explanation than that. It is an insoluble problem, that of knowing why this same general cause is marked by effects which are so varied, sometimes a plastic arthritis without much effusion, sometimes a simple congestive arthritis, sometimes a congestive arthritis with effusion, and at other times, as you will see, the dry form. But we have nothing better to substitute for this etiology, and we must keep it because it indicates the use of certain curative and prophylactic measures.

Prognosis.—What preoccupies me above all in this patient, is the probability that his affection will last a long time, and the possibility of a relapse after it has been cured. I have but little fear of its terminating by suppuration, because hydrarthrosis, when not symptomatic of a fungoid synovitis, almost never ends this way. Nor do I fear complete anchylosis, because exudations and false membranes do not exist, or exist in too small quantity to bring about this result. Moreover, even if there were false membranes disposed to form adhesions, the interposed liquid would prevent it. If anchylosis should hereafter occur, it would be incomplete and due to rigidity of the synovial membrane following a slight thickening which may now exist, although the physical signs do not clearly show it. But it is probable that such an anchylosis would be temporary, and that resolution would be obtained. It is possible that, if the disease resists our treatment or reappears a certain number of times, dry arthritis may be substituted for the dropsical one. For it is difficult for the phlegmasia to continue without extending from the synovial membrane to the cartilages.

Alteration of the latter leads sooner or later to their destruction, and when they are once destroyed, if the articulation does not become an-chylosed, it is inevitably destined to dry arthritis.

Treatment.—We must distinguish between the curative and the prophylactic treatment.

1st. *Curative treatment.*—Two indications are to be met: to get rid of the synovial congestion, and to get rid of the effusion.

The first needs absolute rest in the horizontal posture; to that we have added since the beginning elastic compression by means of the cotton batting dressing. At the end of a week, not having obtained any diminution, we applied two blisters, and four days later, two others. We interrupted the compression the day the blisters were applied, and renewed it as soon as the epidermis had been opened. Only one purge has been given.

These measures have been sufficient in a certain number of cases, and seemed to act at the same time against the congestion, the start-ing point of the disease, and against the effusion. The patients were able to leave us at the end of five or six weeks, walking quite freely, and having no longer any swelling or fluctuation. In others we needed from six to eight weeks, at the end of which the cure, although temporary, was obtained. In others again, pain on motion no longer existed at the end of this time; the effusion was diminished, but was still quite large. As confinement to the bed fatigued and weakened the patients, I let them get up and walk with crutches, on the condition of always keeping the cotton dressing applied to the foot, leg, and lower half of the thigh. Sometimes I wrapped a band of vulcanized rubber about the outer bandage so as to insure compression.

In this case, after confinement to the bed for four weeks, blisters, and compression, although the sensibility seemed to be diminished, we still found considerable effusion. It is then one of the cases in which we have to turn to the second indication, address ourselves to the effusion itself. I met this indication this morning at the bedside of the patient. I punctured with a very fine trocar and withdrew the liquid by means of an aspirating syringe, making it flow into a vessel in which a vacuum had been made before the faucet communi-cating with the canula of the trocar had been opened. You saw that the liquid escaped very freely, and that I avoided making any pres-sure upon the joint under the pretext of favouring the flow. The evacu-ation ended, I took care to close the small opening with collodion and to replace the cotton bandage. There were about five ounces of liquid. It was sticky, yellowish, and although it did not offer the troubled or gray tint which indicates the admixture of a certain quantity of pus, yet we found a few lecuocytes in it. Still I am not disturbed by this fact, because normal synovia always contains a certain number of these elements, and their augmentation after a slight inflammation by no means indicates a tendency to suppuration, as we understand it in surgery.

But after this puncture, and if we continue the compression, will the patient get well? That depends upon the cause, doubtful for me, of the effusion. There is no doubt but that its starting point was an excess of secretion. It then continued because absorption was insufficient. If now the synovial membrane is so happily modified that equilibrium may be re-established between the secretory and absorbing functions, the puncture will succeed. But if it remains vascularized, its secretory function exaggerated, and its absorbing power diminished, the liquid will be reproduced and not absorbed. It is because no symptom can enlighten me on this point that I cannot determine the consequences of our operation.

If the same quantity of liquid is reproduced, what shall we do? Until recently, we rarely punctured the joints, because we feared consecutive suppuration. But now the facts published by M. Dieulafoy, and those that I have myself observed, authorize us to believe that capillary puncture with aspiration does not expose to this danger. Therefore I should be willing to make a second and even a third puncture if, after two new blisters and the continuation of the compression bandage, the liquid was not reabsorbed.

Perhaps also in this case I shall have recourse to actual cautery. Some surgeons claim to have obtained very good results by this operation, the effect of which is to produce a strong revulsion and cause rigid cicatrices which oppose distension by a new effusion.

If, finally, after five or six months of treatment, I should not have succeeded, which I do not think is very probable, I shall allow the patient to walk while wearing the compressive bandage. Perhaps a little later, and I have seen examples of it, the effusion will end by disappearing and not being reproduced, leaving the articulation its shape and functions.

Perhaps also, the cartilages having disappeared and the synovial membrane having become rigid, the hydrarthrosis may be transformed into an incurable dry arthritis.

If then, after waiting a few months, the effusion persists, or if after having disappeared once or twice it is reproduced; if, above all, I think I see a tendency towards a termination by dry arthritis, I shall propose an injection of iodine, one-third of the tincture of iodine in two-thirds of distilled water. This operation, which was recommended and performed thirty years ago by Velpeau and Bonnet (de Lyon), is now rarely practised. I have employed it only twice. Why this disfavour? Because the injection is followed by a very acute arthritis. In some cases, notably in one of Velpeau's, and in one of Aug: Bérard's of which I was a witness, this arthritis ended in suppuration, purulent infection, and death. In other cases, and this is what happened in my two patients, the arthritis thus provoked remained plastic and ended in complete anchylosis. I believe we cannot count upon a better result, especially upon the substitution for the dropsical arthritis of an arthritis capable of terminating by perfect resolution with preservation of movements, and it is because we cannot count upon this that we should not make haste to advise the injection of iodine. I should however advise it if the relaxation of the ligaments and commencing crepitation made me foresee dry arthritis, for the provocation of an acute arthritis is less to be regretted. I think indeed that with care, and especially by means of immobility and proper compression, suppuration could probably be prevented.

2d. *Prophylactic treatment.*—If we obtain, as I hope, resolution of the effusion and of the congestive arthritis, there will be two indications to meet. The first is that of combating the rheumatic cause, by advising the patient to occupy a dry room which faces the south; to avoid getting chilled, to wear flannel, and to pass, if possible, one or two seasons at one of the thermal springs which I have already mentioned, in short the advice which we usually give rheumatic patients. The second is that of maintaining constantly, while walking or standing, a certain compression upon the knee by means of a laced dog-skin or canvas knee-cap. These appliances are often troublesome bacause they are too tight, or useless because not tight enough. Careful and intelligent patients find it better to wear a flannel band two and a half inches wide and about three yards long, which they apply tightly enough to make the necessary compression without being thereby incommoded.

LECTURE XXXVII.

CHRONIC ARTHRITES OF THE KNEE, Continued.—FUNGOID ARTHRITIS OR WHITE SWELLING.

Non-suppurative white swelling of the left knee in a young man 20 years old—Physical and functional symptoms—Muscular atrophy—Absence of hyperostosis—Increase of local heat—Anatomical diagnosis—Undoubted fungoid transformation of the synovial membrane and the ligaments—Presumed lesions of the diarthrodial cartilages and the ligaments—Rarefying osteitis or simple rarefaction, and fatty condition of the cancellous tissue—Etiological diagnosis—Course, termination, and prognosis; tendency to suppuration; very little tendency to anchylosis—Treatment—Indication to favour anchylosis—Cotton batting apparatus, immovable fenestrated apparatus—General treatment.

GENTLEMEN : The patient who was admitted yesterday, No. 4, ward Sainte Vierge, and who resembles two others who have been here for several months, is a young man 20 years old, a shoemaker, who says his left knee has been affected for about a year. As it caused him no pain, and only a little difficulty in moving, he has thus far done nothing for it. But a week ago, after having walked the day before a little more than usual, he suffered pain, was unable to walk, and was obliged to enter the hospital.

You are at first struck with his puny look. He is small, beardless, pale, and with thin muscles. We find the scars of no abscesses on the neck, but he told us that his childhood had been sickly, and that several times his eyes had been inflamed and there had been a discharge from his ears. Although he has had no hæmoptysis he is subject to colds. His father is still living, but he thinks his mother died of some disease of the chest. He has two sisters who, he says, are pretty well, but he has lost two brothers, one in infancy, the other at the age of 18. In short, his constitution is lymphatic, his antecedents and those of his family show a predisposition to tuberculization.

As for his knee, it presents physical symptoms and functional symptoms.

Physical symptoms.—The knee is completely extended, uniformly swollen, rounded; the lateral depressions on each side of the patella are effaced. Placing the fingers on the outer side, a little above the superior tibio-fibular articulation, I feel a lobe a little distinct from the rest. The swelling is flabby; at certain points it yields a sensation similar to fluctuation. But, if grasping with both hands the lateral portions of the knee, I press the patella backwards with my forefinger, I find that it remains immovable, that it is not pushed towards the condyles of the femur, as it is in hydrarthrosis, and that the fingers placed upon the sides are not raised by the liquid. If we seek fluctuation by placing two fingers on the outer and two on the inner side, we do not find it. There is then no liquid in the synovial cavity; or if there is any it is not abundant enough to give fluctuation. The sensation of this kind which is felt here and there superficially is not furnished by an intra-articular liquid. It is not resistent and not elastic, and is caused rather by very soft tissues than by a collection of liquid. For more certainty I pricked two of these soft points with a pin, and saw no liquid flow except a little blood which evidently came from the prick. When we compare the two thighs we are struck with the difference in their size. The muscles of the left one are evidently atrophied; so too are those of the calf of the leg, but to a little less degree. This atrophy, which is constant after articular diseases of long duration, seems to me to be due, like that which we find after fractures (page 71), to the irregular distribution of the nutritive material between the synovial membrane which uses more and the muscles which receive less. I felt deeply to see if the femur was swollen, it did not seem to be, and, indeed, we have here a chronic disease, in a feeble patient, whose constitution, as I have already told you, does not predispose to general or very extensive hypertrophying osteitis.

As functional symptoms, I showed you an elevation of temperature, easily recognized by placing the palm of the hand alternately upon the two knees. I did not make an examination here with the thermometer, but I have done so upon others who showed the same difference of temperature, and found from two to five and a half degrees (Fahr.) of difference. When at rest, the articulation is not constantly painful; but you heard the patient say that he often felt, especially at night, shooting and throbbing pains, and, like most patients who suffer in the knee, he indicated the inner side as the principal seat of the pains. When asked to flex and extend the articulation, he was unable to do it on account of the pain. I then myself communicated these movements and showed that they were possible; I further found abnormal lateral movements, without crepitation. No general symp-

20

toms, no fever. The chest was carefully examined and showed no physical sign of tuberculization, notwithstanding the fears excited on this point by his antecedents.

Anatomical diagnosis.—We are again authorized here to admit the existence of an arthritis, since it is a disease with swelling, pain, and heat; we may say that this arthritis is chronic, for it began a year ago, and is not accompanied by fever. We may add, on account of the pains which have recently occurred, that it is a chronic arthritis with a subacute inflammatory attack.

We have now to determine by what lesions and by what tendencies this chronic arthritis differs from those of which I have already spoken, and those of which I shall hereafter have to speak.

Among these lesions there is one of which we have no doubt, that of the synovial membrane. It consists in a thick flabby swelling, formed of a grayish tissue, infiltrated with serosity, and moderately vascular, the appearance of which, on section, recalls that of a thin jelly. In its chemical composition there is much fibrine according to Bonnet, mucine according to Paquet; and in its histological composition we find, together with molecular granulations, fusiform and stellate cells and amorphous matter. This singular lesion is that which, since Reimar, has been known as *fungoid substance* or *fungoid synovitis*[1] It may be considered as a profound modification, not of limited portions of, but of the entire, synovial membrane.

When the synovial membrane of an articulation has become fungoid we often find an effusion of liquid into its cavity; in this case I have found none. If there is any, it is not abundant, and is not purulent. For purulency would be accompanied by a notable increase in the quantity, and consequently by a fluctuation which would be easily appreciable.

There is another lesion of which we have scarcely any more doubt. That is the lack of resistance in the ligaments due to their transformation into a similar fungoid substance. Lateral mobility, in our patient, and the frequency of autopsies in which we have found the fungoid condition of the ligaments coinciding with that of the synovial membrane, are the reasons which authorize me to admit the existence of these anatomical disorders.

Other lesions should be suspected, but they are not indicated, like the preceding ones, by physical signs. They effect the diarthrodial cartilages and the bones. They exist, do not doubt it; for auatomopathological studies have abundantly proved that the articular synovial membranes do not become fungoid, without, at the same time, the ligaments, cartilages, and bones being altered, and I have told you that although I have no anatomical documents to prove it, I admitted the same thing in plastic arthritis which had become chronic, aud in dropsical arthritis. There is such a physiological solidarity among all the constituent parts of an articulation that the chief one of them, the synovial membrane, cannot long be troubled in its nutrition, without the nutrition of the others being modified and causing the lesions peculiar to them.

---

[1] Substance fonguense, synovite fonguense.

Here then I do not see, and I appreciate by no special sign the lesions of the diarthrodial cartilages. But it suffices that the articular affection has lasted a year, for me to believe in their existence. What I do not know is the degree which they have reached. Is it only the first degree, that in which the lesion is purely histological and consists, as Drs. Ranvier and Paquet[1] have said, in fatty degeneration of the superficial cells, and then proliferation of the deep cells of the cartilage? Is it a more advanced period, that in which the diarthrodial cartilages present the velvety aspect, that is, an uneven surface formed by a mass of fibrous prolongations instead of the normal smooth and polished surface? Is it not another lesion still more advanced, in consequence of which the cartilages, losing their means of union with the bones, strip off and fall into the articular cavity? Do those solutions of continuity described by Brodie under the name of ulcerations, exist on their free surface with or without decortication? Finally, has that absorption commenced which is so common in these organs and which accompanies or follows the preceding lesions,—is it already quite advanced?

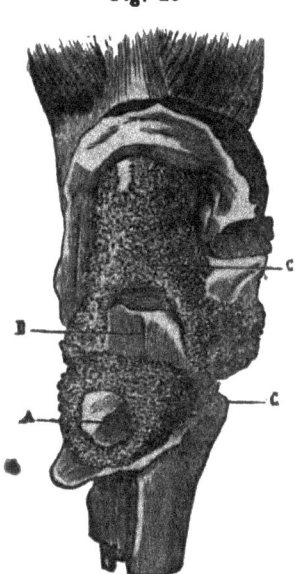

Fig. 20

Fungoid transformation of the synovial membrane of the knee. A. Posterior face of the patella; C. C. Inner surface of the synovial membrane which has become fungoid.

To these questions, and the same ones are to be asked for the fibrocartilages, I do not and cannot reply positively. One single thing is unquestionable: the cartilages are injured and will become more and more so as the affection grows older, until they finally disappear, either by total absorption, or by partial absorption followed by the detachment of some portions, like that of the sequestra of necrosis, into the articular cavity.

Allow me to tell you in passing that lesions of the cartilages are about the same in all diseases of the joints. They are always destructions which are more or less comparable to ulcerations, but which differ from them essentially by the absence of concomitant suppuration; they are velvety change, denudation of the bone, and finally absorption. Modern researches have shown that the histological lesions of the beginning are variable, but the consecutive lesions are not. It seems that when the cells and their capsules are once deprived of their normal conditions and destroyed, the cartilage is always similarly affected and troubled in its nutrition, and that this trouble leads to a total or partial destruction. This lesion is the more important because it is irreparable and has cost the articulation one of the capital conditions of its ability to perform its functions. It is possible that the limited ulcerations heal, like those found in tarsalgia; but exten-

[1] Paquet, Thèse de Paris, 1867.

sive destructions, and still more those which involve the whole cartilage, do not heal.

The same certainties and the same doubts exist for the bones as
for the cartilages. I am sure that the bones are injured, because
autopsies have often shown that they always become injured to a certain degree in fungoid synovitis. I am sure that their cancellous tissue
has not suppurated, for we have neither the external fistulous abscesses
nor the articular suppuration which would be the consequence of this
suppuration. I suppose, for it is very common, that the compact sub-
cartilaginous layer is wholly or in part destroyed and replaced by
vegetations which are continuous with those of the synovial membrane, that the cells of the cancellous tissue have become enlarged,
and their trabeculi fragile, so that a probe or the finger-nail would
penetrate them very easily. Are these spaces filled with a soft, gela-
tiniform, grayish substance similar to the vegetations, and constituting the first period of rarefying osteitis? are they, on the contrary,
filled with that red and very vascular substance which made Bonnet
use the name *splenisation*, or are they filled with fat and not vascular,
which would constitute Cruveilhier's fatty condition, and a variety of
rarefaction, rarefaction without osteitis? Are there not here and
there very vascular points beside others that are hypertrophied and
eburnated, which would belong to the lesion described by Nélaton
under the name of tubercular infiltration, and which for me constitute
a variety of osteitis of the cancellous tissue, an osteitis condensing
and necrotic in some places, rarefying in others? I am not enlightened
upon all these points; and since we have to deal only with presumptions I shall not explain all these lesions, which I shall, moreover,
have occasion to show you whenever we dissect articulations affected
with white swelling, either after amputation or after death.

What I wish to fix to-day in your minds is that we have no doubt
of the fungoid condition of the synovial membrane in our patient, and
that, from the moment when this fungoid condition becomes incontestable, all the other constituent parts, including the bones, are altered
to one of the degrees and in one of the forms indicated by pathological
anatomy, although we are not perfectly informed as to the extent of
these alterations.

There is, however, a point which should detain me a moment.
Our authors have spoken of white swellings, some of which begin in the
soft parts, others in the bones. I presume that in this case the lesions
began in the synovial membrane; for the patient has not had from
the beginning those pains which denote deep osteitis of the cancellous
tissue, and he has not the abscesses by which this osteitis would undoubtedly have ended if the lesion had begun with it. Retain, if you
choose, a few doubts as to the starting point, but have none as to
another which is capital at this moment. If there is osteitis it has not
suppurated, it is not in that condition of rarefaction with suppuration
in the meshes of the cancellous tissue which, for me, constitutes caries;[1]

[1]. We are not all agreed upon the signification of the word *caries;* in my opinion
it ought to be employed to express these two things: rarefying inflammation and
suppuration of the cancellous tissue of the bones. .

nor is it in that state of partial eburnation with peripheral suppuration which constitutes the interstitial necrosis of the cancellous tissue of which I spoke a moment ago, and of which I recently showed you an example.

Etiological diagnosis.—We make that easily by means of the information furnished by observation of a large number of patients. The synovial membrane of the knee becomes fungoid under the influence of that great general cause which we call scrofula, that which gives rise to either ganglionary or pulmonary tuberculosis. The existence of this cause in our patient is indicated by his constitution and his family antecedents. But it seems to have exerted no injurious influence upon the other articulations or upon other organs, especially the lungs. We hope that it will not affect them; but we can have no certainty upon this point.

Course, termination, prognosis.—Do not forget, gentlemen, the serious consequence which results from our diagnosis, fungoid arthritis or white swelling. It is the tendency to articular suppuration after a longer or shorter time. In other words, if the patient is not properly treated, or if the treatment does not succeed, this synovitis will terminate some day by suppuration, with or without suppuration of the accompanying osteitis. The abscesses will open and become fistulous; perhaps, after an intercurrent acute attack, so much pus will suddenly form within the articular cavity that the synovial membrane will rupture in its upper cul-de-sac and let a considerable quantity of this pus pass under the deep muscles of the thigh, an example of which I have lately shown you. In any case the prolonged suppuration, the inaction to which the patient will be condemned, the necessary confinement to the hospital may lead sooner or later to hecticity or to the tuberculosis to which, as you know, his constitution already predisposes him. Again, the difficult passage of the pus from this large anfractuous cavity, and its consequent stagnation and decomposition, might cause a putrid infection and hasten hecticity. A moment, then, will undoubtedly arrive, when, to preserve the patient from one or the other of these terminations, amputation of the thigh or resection will be the only resource.

In case, however, hecticity should not occur, and if the patient should resist articular suppuration, this white swelling might end by anchylosis, the tibia and femur stripped of their diarthrodial cartilages, uniting by a process analogous to that of the callus. It would then be an anchylosis by fusion after suppuration. I admit that I do not count much upon such a result. But I should count more upon it if the patient was younger, if he was a child, if he was in better hygienic conditions.

Nevertheless, if tardy suppuration is the natural termination of the disease, and if it establishes a capital difference between the fungoid arthritis with which we are now occupied, the plastic arthritis of which I have already spoken, and the dry arthritis of which I shall soon speak, yet it is not inevitable, and you should know that all therapeutical efforts should be directed to prevent it.

What will be the course and the termination of the disease if suppuration does not occur? It will not be the return to the not tomical and physiological condition. I do not mean that ▇ is absolutely impossible; it may be that it has taken place i few children, but I do not believe that it has in adolescents ▇ and above all in subjects who belong, as this one does, to class and are unable to obtain all the hygienic resources ▇ bringing about this very rare result—cure of a white swellit knee with preservation of shape and movements.

That is due, gentlemen, to the anatomical and physiologice cations which take place in white swelling. This synovial ▇ transformed into fungoid tissue is too profoundly altered ▇ to recover its normal structure. It no longer has any epith connective tissue; all the abnormal products which infiltrat serosity, the fusiform and other embryonal cells would hai appear and be transformed again into connective tissue cov▇ pavement epithelium, and the necessary condition of such i would be that the state of the organism under the influence the lesion occurred should first disappear. Certainly all th impossible, but you must admit that it is very difficult. formulated it exactly when he said: "The synovial fungoid the product of a bad nutrition, and it has no tendency to be rea▇ I add that it has a very much greater one to suppurate.

What happens sometimes is a very slow transformatio synovial membrane into a more or less fibrous, inextensi rigid tissue. It is a sort of substitution of anchylosing plasti tis for fungoid arthritis threatened with suppuration. The ar also may be incomplete, without bony fusion, and due merel fibrous transformation of the synovial membrane; or it may plete, and by fusion, as I told you that took place sometin preliminary suppuration.

But fusion is too often prevented, either by a displacemer articular surfaces which abandon one another in consequenc softening of the ligaments and form what is called spontane location, or by the nature itself of the osteitis which is not su plastic in these subjects to furnish the materials for a new bon tion.

This difficulty of establishing a complete anchylosis wh has been no suppuration is unfortunate, for this result would desirable after a white swelling of the knee. When this latter to terminate in a fibrous transformation and a lack of extensi the synovial membrane with preservation of motion, there i reason to fear the persistence of some fungoid points and th of the suppurative tendency. When the bones are united sequently a sprain is no longer possible this return is less to b and the synovial, aided by the immobility, completes little its fibrous transformation.

Prognosis.—It is grave and may, in accordance with wha just said, be stated as follows: A disease of long duration ter wards suppuration, and leading almost inevitably to the des of the joint, either because mutilation is rendered necessary ticity and threatened death, or because anchylosis is established; a disease which further threatens to be complicated, one day or another, by pulmonary tuberculosis.

Treatment.—You have already comprehended the indications to be met: to prevent suppuration; to favour the formation of an anchylosis, since we can hope for nothing better; to prevent tuberculization. The means which we have at our disposal to meet these indications have this advantage, that if by chance the patient is in the very exceptional category of those who may get well by the return of the synovial membrane to its normal anatomical character, they favour also this return.

Some of these measures are local, others general.

A. *Local measures.*—I told you that we were in presence of one of those fresh inflammatory attacks to which patients affected with white swelling are exposed. This must first be treated by rest in a wire splint and poultices, sprinkled with laudanum if necessary. If the articulation is bent, as sometimes happens, although it is not the case here, it must be straightened.

As soon as the inflammatory attack is over, rest and compression will be the principal local measures to employ. The patient will remain in bed, and I shall apply the cotton wadding bandage, which I described when speaking of hydrarthrosis, and with which we can make forcible compression without, however, interfering with the circulation. You know that for this purpose we wrap the limb in a very thick layer of wadding, about four inches, and roll a band very tightly about it. It is not necessary at first to envelop the foot. I shall do that a few days later if it becomes œdematous. This bandage will be renewed every six or seven days and we shall see if the swelling and local heat diminish, if an effusion of liquid takes place into the articulation, or if by chance, as sometimes happens, an abscess forms outside the joints, in the external layers of the synovial membrane, an abscess belonging in the category of those which Gerdy "called abscesses by proximity."

After six or seven weeks if no inflammation remains, if no considerable amount of hydrarthrosis has been superadded, if we find no tendency to the formation of abscesses by proximity about the upper cul-de-sac, where they appear most frequently, I shall apply an immovable apparatus, made with dextrine or silicate of potash, after having wrapped the limb in wadding. If there should be any tendency to flexion of the knee I would place inside the apparatus, as you have seen me do several times, a posterior wooden splint of the length which we use for fractures of the leg. This precaution would be useless in this case, for the knee is perfectly extended. My object in substituting the immovable for the movable wadding apparatus would be to allow the patient to walk. For confinement to the bed, which is an excellent means to insure immobility of the knee, has the inconvenience, when prolonged for a long time, and especially when the subject is obliged to live in the midst of other patients, of weakening him and favouring the development, already so imminent, of tuberculosis. With the immovable apparatus the patient will be able,

without any danger of the articulation making any injurious mov
ments, and much more safely in this respect than if the limb was
the cotton bandage, to walk with crutches, go into the garden, breath
a better air, perhaps will even be able to leave us and return to h
family in the country. Another advantage of the immovable appar
tus is that it can remain in place three or four months without tl
intervention of the surgeon unless new pains and inflammation shou
occur.

There are patients in whom the immovable apparatus does not pre
vent pain during walking, whether it be that this pain results fro
some imperceptible movements of the joint, or whether it is due
the pressure of the articular surfaces against one another in the ver
cal posture. Of course in such cases rest in bed must be ordered, ar
continued until new attempts shall have shown that the patient c
walk without pain.

It is not impossible also, as I intimated a moment ago, that aft
walking for a few weeks the patient may be taken with fresh pain
without apparent cause, or after fatigue, or even on account of
change in the weather. For I should tell you, in passing, that lyr
phatic patients affected with white swelling are not exempt fro
rheumatism, and this latter influence, when it exists, may be tl
cause of a return of a pain in the affected joint. In such a case tl
indication is the same, to keep the patient again in bed for a fe
weeks until the sensibility disappears.

The objection has been made against immovable apparatuses th
they hide the affected region and prevent us from observing the ph
sical signs and making use of other local remedies, especially tl
revulsives. You know how I reply to this objection : when the app
ratus has been dry for some time, and I am satisfied that it is st
enough to meet the indication of immobility, I cut out a circular c
about ten inches in diameter over the anterior part of the knee, I the
remove enough cotton to uncover the knee, examine the sides ar
front of the joint, put on fresh cotton, put on the cap, and bind
down tightly by means of an ordinary band, so as to combine the a
vantages of compression with those of immobility.

I have long used this kind of apparatus, to which I gave the nan
immovable fenestrated ; we often have in our wards patients who we
it, and from time to time you see others who having returned to the
families come back to see us, either to tell us how they are, or to as
if their bandage needs to be changed, for they have to be renewe
every three or four months to prevent their deterioration.

Whatever may be the usefulness of this dressing, it does not pr
vent the long duration of the disease, nor does it inevitably preve
suppuration. Among the old patients who came back to see us th
year (1872) I showed you a stout, young man 26 years old, whom
began to treat at the Hôpital de la Pitié in 1866, upon whom I hav
placed the immovable fenestrated apparatus twelve times for a whi
swelling of the left knee, who has sometimes been able to walk f
several months with a cane, and sometimes has been laid up f
several weeks with sharp pains, the seat of which seemed to me to l

in the tibia rather than in the synovial membrane, who, however, has had neither articular nor ossifluent abscesses, and who, in short, has reached the complete anchylosis which we sought and hoped for. I showed you also a young girl 23 years old, in whom I placed ten times, in the space of five years, the immovable fenestrated apparatus, made sometimes with plaster, sometimes with dextrine, sometimes with silicate of potash, and who, notwithstanding an incomplete spontaneous dislocation and slight flexion of the knee, has also reached anchylosis.

On the other hand you doubtless remember two of our patients in whom, notwithstanding the use of the apparatus for two and three years, suppuration and hecticity occurred and necessitated in one re-section of the knee, in the other amputation of the thigh, both of which were successful.

I shall then place upon our present patient the immovable fenestrated apparatus. I shall open the fenestra every other day to apply tincture of iodine, and I shall take care each time to renew the appa ratus and the compression in the way I indicated. If I always find the knee hot, if I hear of pains which oblige the patient again to keep his bed, I shall make through the fenestra, as you saw me do two weeks ago to the patient in No. 6, a punctate cauterization. If an abundant effusion forms I shall apply blisters, still without removing the bandage. Finally, the apparatus will be removed every three or four months, and each time I shall see if the anchylosis which I desire is forming. We shall continue thus for as many years as may be necessary. Of course if suppuration should set in and should open directly outwards or through the deep muscular interstices, and hecticity should occur, I should consider, after a fresh examination of the chest and determination of its proper condition, the question of amputation or resection, a question which I cannot now discuss.

B. *General treatment.*—It ought to consist in the use of all the tonics which we have at our disposal in the hospital: cod-liver oil, antiscorbutic syrup, quinine, wine, iron, strengthening nourishment, and moderate exercise according to the conditions which I indicated.

If he was a private patient and in a social position which permitted it, we should add the much more powerful resources of a visit to the country, to the seaside, to the bromine and iodine thermal springs, especially those of Salins.[1] Perhaps then we should be more likely to prevent suppuration and obtain anchylosis. I also repeat that perhaps, if it was a child, we might exceptionally, by the combined use of these local and general measures, obtain a cure with preservation of the movements.

[1] See Duraud Fardel's Dict. des Eaux minerales, Lebret and Lefort, Paris, 1860.

LECTURE XXXVIII.

DRY ARTHRITIS OF THE KNEE.

I. Case of a patient affected with dry arthritis of both knees. II. On the left the arthritis is at the same time dropsical and deforming, knock-kneed—Anatomical explanation of the symptoms by synovial congestion, probable wearing away of the cartilages, absorption, after rarefaction, of the cancellous tissue of the outer condyle of the femur—Ultimate course of the disease; its incurability— The name dry arthritis is the only one we have to express this group of symptoms. III. In the right knee, considerable increase in size of the end of the femur, very marked lateral mobility, loud crackling—Subluxation of the tibia —Explanation of these symptoms by the formation of osteophytes, destruction of the ligaments, eburnation of the articular surfaces. IV. Cases of other patients affected with dry arthritis of the knee—Principal varieties of this disease.

GENTLEMEN: I. We have at No. 25, ward Ste. Vierge, a man 58 years old, whom we shall not keep very long, although both his knees are diseased, for we cannot cure him. He has been suffering for seven years, without apparent cause, or at least without his being able to attribute it to any traumatic lesion. He only knows that his left knee has often been swollen, and that he has been treated for dropsy of it. The right one does not appear to have been the seat of a similar effusion, but the patient has also suffered in it almost constantly, sometimes a little more, sometimes a little less, without the pains having ever been excessive and accompanied by fever; but the patient has often been obliged to enter the hospitals, leaving them, after a month or two, ameliorated but not cured. He has walked with more and more difficulty, and finally was no longer able to do it without the aid of crutches, and even then with much difficulty and fatigue. We find the following condition of affairs.

II. In the left knee, a very evident effusion, without enlargement of the patella, without hyperostosis of the femur, without appreciable thickening of the synovial membrane, without movable or immovable foreign body; no lateral mobility; voluntary movements but slightly limited, notwithstanding the pains; communicated movements of flexion and extension almost as free as in the normal condition; perception by the hand and ear of very marked cracklings during both voluntary and communicated movements; finally we find that deformity which is known by the name knock-knee, and which consists in the deviation of the leg outwards, and in the very marked prominence of the inner condyle of the femur.

What is the anatomical explanation of these symptoms, what will be the ultimate course of the disease, and what name should we give it?

I explain the effusion, as I did in simple hydrarthrosis, by a congestion of the synovial membrane with exaggeration of its secretory function, and diminution of its power of absorption. But I suppose, for autopsies have shown it in several cases of this kind, that the congestion
is not general, and that it occupies more particularly the folds known
as the synovial fringes.

I attribute the sensation and sound of crackling to a lesion which
has often been found in the autopsies, that is, the loss of polish and
the partial destruction of the diarthrodial cartilages. I do not know
exactly to what degree this destruction has advanced, but recalling
the lesions described by Redfern and M. Broca, lesions which I have
already had occasion to mention when speaking of the other varieties
of arthritis, I believe that the arrangement in parallel fibres which
constitutes the velvety condition, and its coincidence with a partial
disappearance of the cartilage, cause the crepitation which now occupies us. I know that pathological anatomy leaves a gap here, for I
have never had, and no one, so far as I know, has ever had the
opportunity to dissect subjects in whom this symptom had predominated, and to see exactly what lesion had produced it. Moreover you
might raise the objection that I have already spoken of—possible
velvety change in patients who had offered no crepitation. That undoubtedly was due to this, that the movements, limited by the pain,
by the rigidity of the synovial membrane, by commencing adhesions,
and above all by muscular contracture, were not sufficiently extended
to cause this loud friction; for I now call your attention to the fact,
as I shall undoubtedly do again, that one of the characters by which
this patient's arthritis differs from those of which I have heretofore
spoken, is that the muscles are not contractured and immovable, or
are so to a much less degree.

As to the deformity, we must not consider it congenital, as the
knock-knee often is. For the patient tells us that his knee was
always well shaped, and that the deformity appeared only five or six
years ago and has increased little by little. It is then accidental, and
I cannot explain it otherwise than by a rather vaguely described
lesion of which I, for my part, have not thus far been able to give an
anatomical demonstration. I refer to the sinking of the outer condyle caused by absorption of its substance, absorption undoubtedly
prepared by rarefaction. I have already often spoken to you of rarefaction of the cancellous tissue; I told you that it sometimes accompanied one of the varieties of osteitis, but that it might also occur without osteitis, that then it coincided with an infiltration of fat, and that
it was a result of age. I spoke to you of fractures made possible by
this rarefaction, but I have not yet had occasion to show you the
concomitant disappearance of a large part of the rarefied cancellous
tissue. It is precisely that which seems to me to have taken place
in this patient. The same thing probably occurs in other patients
affected with this or some other accidental deformity, hence the name
deforming arthritis used by some authors.

What will be the ultimate course and termination of this disease?
Observe well two principal things: 1st. The arthritis, although it has

lasted a long time, has not suppurated; 2d. It has not caus
chylosis, even incomplete. Now by the phenomena which we
found, by what has taken place in the right knee, of which
presently speak, by the age of the patient, by what the clin
pathological anatomy have taught us about this subject, I ar
vinced that the disease will go on in the same way. The a
will persist, without terminating either by suppuration or by
losis. Why so? Because there is, in the phlegmasia of this ar
tion, a nature, a mode, as they still say, a tendency, as I hav
said, which does not lead to these results. The articulation w
suppurate, because it is not fungoid, and because the patient's co
tion is not scrofulous; it will not anchylose, because there is
the rigidity by thickening, nor the false membranes which cha
ize plastic arthritis, and perhaps also because, as the muscles co
to act a little, the movements, slight as they may be, will p
the rigidity and adhesions from establishing themselves to the
necessary to produce anchylosis. I can carry the explanati
further. It is evident that here we touch upon the question
intimate nature of the disease, and, as in all questions of this ki
are stopped by the unknown.[1]

    And now what name shall we give this affection? After
have just said, it will be neither that of congestive arthriti
that of plastic arthritis, nor that of fungoid arthritis. It might,
ly speaking, be that of dropsical arthritis, for there is liquid
articulation. But no, I shall not employ this expression eith
it would give you false ideas upon the prognosis and treatmen
fact, to these words, dropsical arthritis and hydrarthrosis, is att
the idea of curable anatomical lesions, of temporary physiol
troubles, of probable cure, in a word, and of efforts to be me
the surgeon to obtain this cure. But here you have a cong
which has become permanent, and perhaps subsequent inappre
transformations into cartilaginous tissue about the synovial fr
you have irremediable lesions of the diarthrodial cartilages a
epiphysis. None of that will disappear. The tendency is not
well, but rather to get worse by the development of other dis
of which the present lesions are only the prelude, and of whi
right knee will show us examples.

    There is only one word, in the present state of surgery, to e
both the lesions and the very curious nature of this disease—it
of dry or deforming arthritis. Undoubtedly it will seem stra
you that I call dry arthritis a disease which has an effusion f
of its manifestations. But I have to use a word which will mak
feel that it is not an ordinary hydrarthrosis, and I have no

¹ An apparent contradiction may be found between the characters whicl
to dry arthritis of the knee, and those which' I gave, page 54, to the arthriti
tarsalgia of adolescents. But there I made only a comparison; I did not
establish a complete identity. If the tarsal arthritis of adolescents resemb
arthritis by the lesion of the cartilages, it differs from it by its accompanying
upon the muscles, by possibility of anchylosis, and by its curability after p
repair of the ulcerated cartilages.

than those I have just used. But I shall say more upon this point after having spoken of the right knee.

III. The physical symptom of the right knee which first strikes us, is a considerable increase in size, affecting especially the lower extremity of the femur which at the same time is rounded. Placing your hand upon this swelling you find it very hard, and, as it were, lobulated, all the hard points have the consistency of bone and are evidently united with the femur. There are similar, but much fewer, roughnesses upon the tibia. The patient can make a few movements of flexion; but it is not a muscular resistance which limits them, for, taking the limb in both hands, you can give it these movements very easily; at the same time you feel and hear a loud crackling; very extended abnormal lateral movements can also be made; and, finally, by analyzing carefully the situation of the tibial epiphysis, we see that it is placed too far behind, that it cannot be brought forward, in a word, that it is in that state of displacement which is often called subluxation.

I ask for this knee the same three questions as for the other. And first, what is the anatomical explanation of the different symptoms? Of course the idea may at first occur that the swelling of the femur is due to an osteo-sarcoma. But if it had been that disease, during the time it has lasted it would have extended to the shaft of the femur and would have softened. Is not then this hardness that of a hyperostosis? I have avoided using this word; for hyperostosis, as we understand it, occupies the shaft and the whole thickness of the compact portion of the long bones, while here the bony swelling corresponds to the cancellous extremity, and seems to occupy the external layers rather than the parenchyma of the epiphysis. Now, we have here, gentlemen, a special lesion with which the labors of modern pathological anatomy have made us acquainted, that is, ossifications of the edge of the cartilage and the neighbouring periosteum, perhaps even of that portion of the synovial membrane which covers the latter. These ossifications are analogous to those which, in the same variety of arthritis, we sometimes find upon the inner face of the synovial membrane in the place of the fringes, and to those which sometimes become loose in the articulation and form a variety of movable foreign bodies. In a word, these are rounded concretions or stalactites, osteophytes, as they are still called, of complex origin, due to an abnormal ossifying power of the articular cartilages and of the synovial membrane. What makes them very remarkable and uncommon in this patient is that they are much more abundant and agglomerated than they generally are in cases of this kind.

Figure 21, for example, which I borrow from M. Duplay, represents osteophytes much less agglomerated than those of our patient.

As for the crackling, I explain that also by a lesion of the cartilages; I think even that it is no longer a question here either of the velvety condition, or of the wearing away indicated by Prof. Cruveilhier in 1824.[1] I think there is a more advanced lesion, an extensive destruction of these same cartilages, and friction of the bony articular

---

[1] Cruveilhier, Archives de Médecine, 1824, 1re serie, tome ii.

surfaces which have become hard and eburnated. This eburnation is perhaps explained, as M. Ranvier admits, by calcification of some of the cartilaginous cells, and more probably by a hypertrophy limited to the compact sub-cartilaginous layer, which, instead of disappearing, as in fungoid arthritis, has undergone a process of condensation, in which, however, neither the parenchyma of the cancellous nor that of the compact tissue has participated; this would be the continuation of the process of ossification which takes place at the periphery, without, although for absolutely unknown reasons, the participation of the interstitial portions of the bone. In any case, you recognize here a peculiar lesion which has been described by Cruveilhier[1] under the name of eburnation or eburexostosis of the articular surfaces.

Fig. 21.

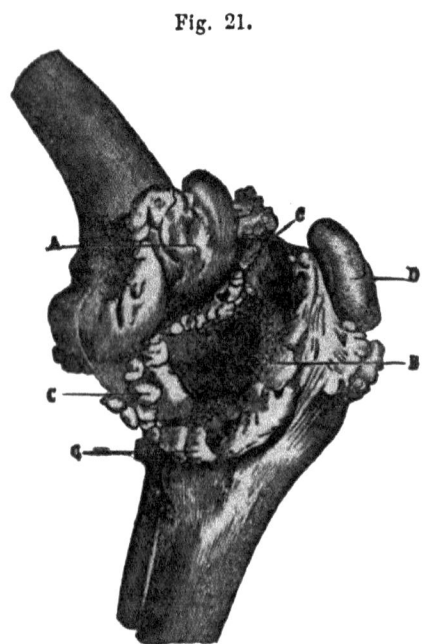

Osteophytes. A. Condyles of the femur. B. Articular surface of tibia. C. C. C. Osteophytes. D. Patella.

But should we not also attribute the crackling to lesions of the synovial membrane? I told you that there was no effusion. Might there not then be a condition of dryness which, during movement, would give crepitation? I admit that, studying the origin of this word dry arthritis, I have examined specimens which have been shown me, to see how far the synovial membrane participated in the dryness indicated; but I have never found it dry enough to account for the crackling. Indeed there was always enough humidity on its inner surface to make the expression seem to me unjustified.

Are there no other lesions of the synovial membrane in such cases? I do not speak of the congestion which probably occurred at the beginning, and which undoubtedly has now disappeared. I allude only to the fibro-cartilaginous and even bony transformations which have been pointed out as possible in the synovial fringes. If such transformations have taken place we can understand that they might contribute to the production of crackling. But there is no sign which authorizes me to affirm the existence of this lesion.

Lateral mobility is too marked in this patient for me to think of seeking its explanation, or at least its sole explanation, in the destruction of the semilunar fibro-cartilages. I do not doubt the softening and perhaps destruction of the lateral and even of the crucial ligaments. But has it been a simple absorption, or a fatty degeneration?

[1] Cruveilhier, Bulletins de la Société anatomique, 1826, tome i. p. 195.

This point has not been thoroughly studied. I only know that M. Duplay[1] makes fatty transformation of the ligaments an almost constant lesion in diseases of this kind.

As for the subluxation, it is also explained by the weakening of the means of union, and especially of the posterior ligament which would have been affected by lesions the same as those of the lateral and crucial ligaments.

In short, gentlemen, we have the explanation of the symptoms in a series of lesions affecting all parts of the joint, and consisting in: congestion of the synovial membrane, destruction of the ligaments, new ossification by means of certain points of the synovial membrane, of the articular surfaces, and of the periosteum, without false membranes leading to anchylosis, without any tendency to suppuration, without condensing osteitis of the adjoining diaphyses.

What name then shall we give the disease? As before, I am not authorized to use any of the denominations which I employed in the precedent lectures. I need one which indicates these three principal characteristics: no anchylosis, no suppuration, long duration and incurability (for there is still less reason to hope for a cure in this latter knee than in the other, because there is a too profound modification of the normal anatomical condition). I still have only the name dry arthritis to express all this. This name has the advantage of indicating a real characteristic, the persistence of an inflammatory condition which from time to time becomes subacute. It has certainly the disadvantage of exaggerating a symptom, the dryness of the synovial membrane, and of not sufficiently indicating the three characteristic tendencies I mentioned. I use it, however, because I have no other, and because I should not easily find one which would better express all the negative and positive characteristics of this variety of arthritis.

IV. Observation of the two knees of this patient has already shown us that dry arthritis presents different degrees or characters. Recall the patients I have shown you at different times in the lectures of this and the preceding years, and you will see that there are still other varieties.

We often see at our consultation, and sometimes in our wards, patients verging on old age, whose only symptoms are articular pain and cracklings. I have often pointed out arthrites of this kind after fractures of the thigh, contusions and sprains of the knee, after subacute rheumatisms, and almost always in patients who are more than fifty years old.

I showed, in 1868 and 1869, ward Ste. Catherine, No. 19, a woman 46 years old, whose left knee, following an attack of rheumatism with hydrarthrosis, had been painful for several years and the seat of an infirmity, the principal cause of which was an excessive mobility which seemed to indicate a destruction of all the means of union. You remember that the lateral mobility was very great, and that I was even able with my hands to move the tibia outwards, inwards, forwards and backwards, so as to produce a subluxation in these

[1] Folliu et Duplay, Traité de Pathologie, tome ii.

different directions. You remember that all these movements caused
a dry sound which was heard by those standing about the bed, and
which must have been caused by the contact of very hard surfaces,
probably the eburnated articular ones. At that time the hydrarthrosis
was slight. It should be noted also that I had made, a few months
before, an injection of the tincture of iodine, which, strange to say,
had not caused acute arthritis, or, consequently, the anchylosis I
sought, as if the articulation had lost, at the same time with its principal anatomical dispositions, its aptitude to inflame under the influence
of a severe irritation. The name dry or deforming arthritis was then
the only one that I could give to this disease.

Hence I concluded that, clinically, we have to distinguish at least
four varieties of dry arthritis: a first and very common one, in which
the crepitation and the moderate but habitual pains are the dominant
phenomena, and in which, doubtless, the lesions affect only the synovial membrane, which is congested, and the diarthrodial cartilages,
which are eroded and scratched; a second, in which a temporary or
permanent synovial effusion is added to the preceding lesions and
symptoms; a third, in which there is lateral mobility and more or less
subluxation indicating the destruction of the lateral ligaments; and
a fourth, in which, with or without destruction of the lateral ligaments, we find osteophytes, either in the synovial membrane, or about
the diarthrodial cartilages; furthermore, different degrees of deformity
by partial osteo-malacia of the articular extremities may be found in
all these cases.

Etiology.—I have carefully questioned the old man, the present
patient, and have found no cause to which I could refer the affection
of his knees. But as both articulations were attacked at the same
time, and as we are always disposed to explain multiple arthritis by
a rheumatic diathesis, I am willing to admit, although the patient has
had no other rheumatic manifestation, that the disease is due to this
general cause. I should, however, tell you that you must expect to
see dry arthritis appear in subjects who are not rheumatic. In those
cases where it is absolutely single a certain complaisance is needed to
admit the rheumatic diathesis. Also when it follows a traumatic
lesion, a wound, a contusion, a sprain, a fracture, this same cause
cannot be invoked. That is why I am still obliged to appeal to an
unknown cause in those cases in which rheumatism cannot be legi-
timately admitted. Is it not also necessary, even in those cases where
the latter is admissible, to suppose a particular form of the diathesis
which gives rise to these manifestations so special and so different
from those by which rheumatism generally betrays itself?

On account of what precedes, I regret that our learned colleague,
M. Charcot, has given the anatomical description of dry arthritis under
the title of chronic rheumatism.[1] On the one hand, the arthritis in
question is not always rheumatic; and, on the other hand, rheumatism,
as I have told you, gives rise to other forms of curable chronic arthritis (plastic and dropsical). There is then a disadvantage in giving

[1] Charcot, Leçons sur les Maladies des Vieillards et les Maladies chroniques.
Paris, 1868.

a description of chronic rheumatism, which leaves the impression that this disease leads inevitably to the incurability of dry arthritis.

If you wish to confine yourselves to the information furnished by the clinic, do not forget, gentlemen, that dry arthritis of the knee, of which thus far the anatomical characteristics have been studied far more than the symptomatology and the etiology, presents, with reference to its origin, two forms: it is primitive or consecutive. When it is primitive, it may be rheumatic, as I told you, or of another nature which remains unknown to us. But most frequently it is consecutive to one of the forms, with which you are acquainted, of acute, subacute, or chronic arthritis. You see it, I repeat, after neighbouring contusions, sprains, fractures, which have given rise to one of the arthrites which I have just mentioned. You see it also after pure rheumatic arthritis, which at first takes on the characters of plastic arthritis, and then terminates by the lesions of dry arthritis instead of by resolution or anchylosis. Finally, you see it after arthritis, which has been at first purely dropsical. You may also see it, as M. Charcot's work testifies, after gouty arthritis, that in which the initial lesion is the invasion of the cartilaginous cells, and the other constituent parts of the articulation, by an excess of uric acid and urate of soda contained in the blood.[1]

You will more rarely see fungoid arthritis followed by dry arthritis, because, as you know, it tends rather to terminate by suppuration and sometimes by anchylosis, and also because it belongs to the youthful period of life, and because there is one almost necessary condition for the development of dry arthritis, that is, senility.

Indeed, gentlemen, and it is with this final consideration that I shall terminate the etiology, the tendency of arthritis to end neither by resolution, nor by anchylosis, nor by suppuration, and to be accompanied in certain cases by ligamentous destructions and osteophytes, is rarely seen before the age of fifty years, and developed especially in old age. But it happens in this, as in the rarefaction of the cancellous tissue, that certain subjects have this pathological aptitude a little earlier, say from forty to fifty years of age, and in consequence of a premature local senility.

Treatment.—I have nothing useful to say about the treatment. We have only to treat the new inflammatory attack by rest and poultices. As soon as it ends we shall advise compression of the dropsical knee with a flannel band, and a roller bandage, including a posterior splint for the right knee, which is so movable, and we shall let the patient resume the use of his crutches, without which he cannot now get along. If he asks, on account of his infirmity, which is only too real, admission to Bicêtre,[2] I shall obtain it for him.

---

[1] While normally only traces of uric acid exist in the blood, from 5 to 17 centigrammes are found in 1000 grammes of blood during an attack of the gout.
[2] Hospital for indigent, infirm, and incurable old men, situated just outside Paris.

LECTURE XXXIX.

GENERAL CONSIDERATIONS UPON ARTHRITIS IN THE OTHER ARTICULATIONS.

Arthritis is traumatic or spontaneous. I. Traumatic arthritis is with or without a wound—Arthritis without wound is congestive or plastic, and ordinarily gets well by resolution—The elbow an exception in children—It goes on to chronic arthritis and to dry arthritis in old people—Examination of the question with reference to the upper limb and to the lower limb. II. Spontaneous arthritis is multiple, or mono-articular—Examination of the varieties : 1st for the large articulations of the lower and of the upper limbs ; 2d for the small articulations —Assimilation of nodosity of the joints to dry arthritis—Difference of origin between gouty arthritis and rheumatic arthritis ; analogy of the ulterior lesions.

GENTLEMEN : It would be interesting and useful to do for each one of the other articulations what I have done for the knee, that is to say, to point out to you the different clinical forms under which arthritis may appear in them ; but I should not have a sufficient number of examples to show you, because these arthrites are not so frequent as those of the knee, and because certain varieties are treated rather in the medical than in the surgical service; and further-more it would involve much repetition.

It will suffice to offer you a few generalities upon the subject; and these generalities will be simple and short, for we shall have to deal with the same questions of etiology, pathological anatomy, and prog-nosis, as in the knee.

In all the articulations the arthritis is either traumatic or spon-taneous.

I. *Traumatic arthritis.*—In all of them traumatic arthritis is threatened with suppuration when its origin is a penetrating wound; but the smaller the articulation, the less intense and the less danger-ous are the general effects of this suppuration when it takes place. As for traumatic arthritis without wound (that is to say, after fracture, dislocation, contusion, sprain), the form which you see it take most often is, at the beginning, the subacute form, congestive and plastic, with or without effusion of blood or of synovia, and afterwards the chronic form tending to terminate by resolution and return of the normal functions, sometimes by complete or incomplete anchylosis, sometimes by dry arthritis. The differences depend upon the articu-lation or upon the age of the subject. One word upon these differ-ences.

A. *Articulations of the upper limb.*—Traumatic arthritis (without wound) ordinarily gets well by resolution in children, adolescents, and adults; termination by complete anchylosis is the exception. But after the age of fifty years, and consequently in old people, termination by rigid incomplete anchylosis and by dry arthritis is quite frequent.   I have often shown you that, after dislocations of the shoulder, movements are re-established very well in young patients, but that they long remain slow, difficult, and painful in subjects who are advanced in age.

As for the elbow, there is this that is peculiar to it and very strange: children, up to the age of adolescence, are much exposed to anchylosis after traumatic arthritis, even after causes that are apparently slight.   You should know this in order not to condemn children to a too prolonged rest.   By exercising the joint early you can prevent the establishment of adhesions, or break up those which have already begun.

In the wrist traumatic arthritis has less tendency to anchylosis, and much to end by complete resolution; but after the age of fifty years anchylosis by rigidity alone or by adhesions, prolonged arthritis, and incurable dry arthritis are quite frequently seen.   I have often explained this subject when speaking of fractures of the lower extremity of the radius.

In the digital articulations we must distinguish between direct traumatic arthritis, that is to say, that which is consecutive to lesions of the articulation itself which becomes affected, and indirect traumatic arthritis, or that which invades the digital articulations in consequence of the treatment by immobility of a traumatic lesion situated above, in the forearm, elbow, arm, or shoulder.   I have told you that in such cases I admitted arthritis by immobility.   Although I have had no occasion to make an autopsy, I presume, from facts observed upon the living patient, that these digital arthrites are congestive and slightly plastic.   In general they get well by resolution after some weeks or months of care; but we should have to fear, especially in old people, incomplete anchylosis by rigidity, and even complete anchylosis, if we did not have the affected joints moved frequently.

B. *Articulations of the lower limb.*—There is traumatic arthritis, without wound, of the hip as of the shoulder.   It is congestive and slightly plastic, and tends always to terminate by complete resolution in young subjects, by prolonged chronic arthritis and incurable dry arthritis in old people.

The same is true of the tibio-tarsal articulation and those of the foot.   It is by the age alone that we can foresee whether the arthritis will get entirely well, or whether it will pass to the incurable condition of dry arthritis.

In short, in subjects who are still young, traumatic arthritis, although it be congestive and plastic, is rarely sufficiently so to cause anchylosis, and the treatment by movements communicated every day has the advantage of opposing this tendency successfully, and almost always without bringing back the inflammatory conditions which I mentioned when speaking of spontaneous arthritis of the knee, and which trouble us so often in spontaneous arthritis of the other articulations.

II. *Spontaneous arthritis.*—There is a very common variety, the acute or subacute polyarticular arthritis, which you know under the name of articular rheumatism, and which you see more often in the medical wards than in ours. It offers these remarkable peculiarities, that it is ordinarily limited to a little effusion in every articulation affected by the congestive form, and complete resolution is the rule. I shall then have to make special reference to the acute and subacute mono-articular arthritis and to some forms of multiple chronic arthritis. Here I need no longer take the articulations one by one; it will be sufficient to describe the large and the small ones of the upper and the lower limbs.

1st. In the upper limb the large articulations rarely become the seat of single acute arthritis, either gonorrhœal, or simply rheumatic. We have, however, met them in those of the shoulder and of the wrist. As for the shoulder, I have been struck with the facility with which, in spite of all our care, this arthritis ends in complete anchylosis. The indication is to oppose this tendency by means similar to those I mentioned for the knee. But it will often happen, as I reminded you a moment ago, that you will not be able to continue the use of communicated movements, on account of the return of acute inflammation.

Among the chronic arthrites there is one variety which you will rarely find in the large articulations of the upper limb, it is hydrarthrosis. You see, on the other hand, fungoid arthritis quite often at the elbow and at the wrist. At the elbow, termination by suppuration is frequent and comes quite rapidly. This fungoid arthritis terminates more often by anchylosis, without preliminary suppuration, in the wrist than in the elbow, and for both these articulations, as for the knee, the indication is always to strive, by all the local and general means at our disposal, to substitute anchylosing, plastic arthritis for fungoid arthritis, which tends to suppuration. It is always the best termination that we can hope for; the means which enable us to obtain it would moreover give a cure by resolution, if the patient was in the very exceptional category of those in whom, after a commencement of fungoid transformation, the synovial membrane can resume its normal, anatomical, and physiological condition.

Primitive and consecutive dry arthritis is sometimes seen in the large articulations of the upper limb, but it is less common there than in those of the lower limb; it prevents the same anatomical varieties.

2d. Among the large articulations of the lower limb the coxo-femoral is rarely affected with acute and subacute plastic arthritis, or if it is affected, the symptoms, on account of the depth of the joint, are so difficult to distinguish from those of the fungoid synovitis called coxalgia that they are easily confounded. For me, when I see after several months anchylosis succeed a disease which has been considered coxalgia, I am disposed to believe that it has been, not a fungoid synovitis tending to suppuration, but a plastic synovitis.

The tibio-tarsal articulation is, after the knee, that which is the most often affected with solitary acute arthritis, and especially with that which has a gonorrhœal origin. The termination there by anchylosis is quite common, and takes place by the mechanism which I described for the knee.

If the articulation of the hip is not frequently affected with acute arthritis, it is in return much exposed to chronic arthritis, especially to the fungoid form in young subjects, and to the dry form in old people. You know that the first description of the arthritis which we call dry, was given for the hip, at the beginning of this century, under the name of *morbus coxæ senilis*.

The tibio-tarsal articulation is less often affected with white swelling and dry arthritis than the knee and the hip, still we see them there quite frequently.

To recapitulate, gentlemen: among the large articulations that of the knee, first because it is the largest and then because it belongs to the lower limb, is the most exposed to all the varieties of single acute, subacute, and chronic arthritis. It is for this reason that I took my principal types from it. But the etiological, anatomo-pathological, and clinical details into which I entered apply to all the large articulations. By placing in relief these four principal forms—plastic, dropsical, fungoid, and dry—the natural tendencies of each one, and the consequent therapeutical indications, I wished to give you the means of directing your conduct at the bedside of the patient whenever you should be called upon to treat an arthritis. But I want to tell you, in closing, that in the large articulations these forms are sometimes mingled and cause difficulties in diagnosis and prognosis rather than in treatment. It will happen to you especially to hesitate long before deciding if a chronic arthritis is simple and still curable, or if it has passed to the condition of incurable dry arthritis, and especially to the variety in which there are as yet no appreciable osteophytes and eburnation. Remember that it is the age above all which ought to enlighten you, and that in any case there is no disadvantage in admitting at first that which is most favourable to the patient, that is to say, curable arthritis, and to make your prescriptions correspond.

3d. As for the small articulations, you will rarely see single acute and subacute spontaneous arthritis in the upper limb, that is to say, in those of the hand and fingers. You will more often see multiple chronic arthritis, that is to say, the simultaneous invasion of several phalangeal articulations, and sometimes of all, by an essentially chronic disease, of probably rheumatic nature, which you hear called *rheumatic arthritis*,[1] and, for the articulations of the last two phalanges, *Heberden's nodosities*. I do not know why they have given these special names to these digital arthrites. Perhaps it was because their ideas were not sufficiently well established as to the varieties of arthritis in the rest of the economy to establish a relationship between those of the fingers and those of the other regions. This relationship seems to me to-day very possible. The clinic has taught us that rheumatic arthritis does not suppurate, and that sometimes it anchyloses by fusion, sometimes it persists indefinitely without anchylosing.

---

[1] Rheumatism noueux.   Rheumatic arthritis, nodosity of the joints.

In the first case, it is a plastic rheumatic arthritis, in the second a dry arthritis. I admit that a rigorous diagnosis, so long as the anchylosis is not established, is a little difficult, as is also the case in the large articulations, but I repeat that that has not a great importance practically. Always try to cure your patient. If after a year or two of treatment you have not succeeded and anchylosis has formed, your diagnosis is made. If anchylosis has not formed, and your patient is old (it is almost always old persons who have rheumatic arthritis), be sure that you have to deal with incurable dry arthritis, with more or less deformity, produced either by bony deposits or by muscular retractions, deformity of which M. Charcot's book offers you very fine plates.

As to Heberden's nodosities, I think they have honoured this physician too much in giving his name to a disease which he has the merit of having distinguished from gout, but which he described without sufficiently knowing the French works of Cruveilhier, Deville, and Broca on dry arthritis. For the little lumps which he found in the dorsal face of the second phalanx, near its articulation with the third, are nothing else than the osteophytes of dry arthritis; they coincide, as M. Charcot has well seen, with some of the other lesions of this disease, especially with eburnation and other osteophytes. It is then simply a dry arthritis in a small articulation

The small articulations of the lower limbs are also affected with the chronic forms of this rheumatic arthritis of old people. You will also sometimes find there acute gouty arthritis, especially at the metatarso-phalangeal articulation of the great toe, and gouty chronic arthritis. I share fully the opinion of Garrod, and that which Charcot has so well formulated, upon the essential difference which exists between gouty arthritis and rheumatic arthritis. I admit very willingly with them that the initial lesion of gouty arthritis is the invasion of the diarthrodial cartilages and the other constituent parts of the articulation by uric acid and the urate of soda. But this initial lesion once established, the anatomical characters of ordinary arthritis are added, simple synovial congestion, with or without effusion, in the acute and subacute varieties; thickening and false membranes in the slower varieties, tendency to complete anchylosis when the patient is old, prolongation under the form of congestive and still curable chronic plastic arthritis, and finally the dry form, with coincidence of the tophic deposits peculiar to gout and the special lesions of dry arthritis. In a word, notwithstanding their special etiology and their peculiar anatomical beginning, gouty articular affections are arthrites, the lesions and ultimate course of which are analogous to those of other articular inflammations, and especially to those caused by rheumatism. That is the reason why they were authorized to consider gout and rheumatism as the same disease, at the time when they did not know the real cause and mode of formation of the gouty arthritis.

PART VI.

PHLEGMONS, ABSCESS, FISTULA.

LECTURE XL.

ABSCESSES OF THE HAND CONSECUTIVE TO SYNOVITIS OF THE FLEXOR TENDONS.

I. Autopsy of a subject whose death was caused by a contused wound of the little finger followed by inflammation of the synovial bursa of the flexors—Putrid infection—Presence of pus in the synovial sheath of the flexor tendons of the little finger—Spread of the inflammation behind the bundle of tendons in the palm of the hand—Its extension to the synovial sheath of the thumb—Integrity of the synovial sheaths of the other fingers. II. Tendinous synovitis of the flexors, partly suppurative—Inflammation starting from the little finger—Abscesses of the thenar and hypothenar eminences, without concomitant palmar abscess—Explanation by a combination of plastic synovitis with suppurative synovitis—Deep diffuse phlegmon of the forearm; its termination by resolution.

GENTLEMEN: I. I place before you an anatomical specimen coming from a man 55 years old who occupied bed No. 38, ward Sainte-Vierge, for about twelve days (from the 23d of December, 1868, to the 5th of January, 1869).

You remember that this man had had the end of the little finger of his left hand crushed by a stone, which had caused a contused wound, occupying the palmar face of this finger between the middle of the ungual and the middle of the second phalanges, and accompanied by fracture of the first of these bones and denudation of the extremity of the flexor tendons.

A suppurative inflammation had been developed and had gained the deep parts of the hand and forearm. Three weeks had already passed since the accident when the man was brought to the hospital. The most prominent symptom then was a most serious general malaise, characterized by frequency of the pulse, prostration, dryness of the tongue, yellowish subicteric tint of the skin, profound alteration of the countenance, and finally a tranquil and almost continual delirium. According to the information which we have obtained, the patient was not given to drink.

As local symptoms we found a very marked swelling and redness of the forearm and hand. The thumb and the little finger were much more swollen than the other fingers. All these parts presented

PHLEGMONS, ABSCESS, FISTULA.

doughiness and deep œdema. We did not find superficial fluctuation, but by pressing steadily with one hand upon the palmar surface of the wrist, and slowly pushing back the soft parts of the forearm an inch or two above with the other, I felt that the fingers of the first were pressed up. You noticed the position which I gave the limb in order to avoid all chances of error when I made this examination; I raised the hand and rested its dorsal face together with the whole length of the forearm upon a pillow. I thus gave the limb a support which prevented it from being pushed back by my exploratory manœu-vres, and after having demonstrated several times the existence of deep fluctuation by sending this wave alternately up and down the arm, I was sure that we had to deal with one of those deep and diffuse ab-scesses of the forearm which are due to the propagation towards this region of inflammation starting from one of the fingers, and much more frequently from the thumb and little finger than the others.

Notwithstanding the intensity of the general symptoms and the gravity of the prognosis, I at once made a deep incision in the fore-arm. I divided layer by layer along its centre, for a distance of about three inches, the skin, the subcutaneous cellular tissue, and the deep fascia. I then tore with my finger, so as to avoid hemorrhage, the cellular tissue of the first inter-muscular space which I found, and thus reached a deep collection of pus limited behind by the pronator quadratus and the interosseous space. A considerable quantity of good phlegmonous pus escaped. A few days later a second abscess was opened on the inner side of the little finger.

The escape of pus from the forearm remained difficult, notwithstand-ing the bunches of lint and the drainage tubes which I employed successively. The febrile condition continued, and the 29th of December the first chill took place; others followed, the patient grew weaker and weaker, and died.

I expected to find metastatic abscesses, as they sometimes form after these deep abscesses, the pus of which escapes with difficulty on account of the obstacle offered by the muscles which overlie them. But there were none, and I had to suppose that the patient had suc-cumbed to one of those putrid infections, bastard septicæmia, which are due at the same time to severe traumatic fever and pyæmia.

But it is not upon this point that I wish to speak to-day. What I want you to notice particularly is the seat and the extent of the suppuration.

Look first at the little finger, the starting point of the affection. We have opened the sheath of its palmar tendons; you find pus in it covering on the one side the parietal layer of the synovial mem-brane, and on the other the tendons which are also softened and dis-associated. Follow the collection towards the hand, and you see that it passes behind the bundle of the flexor tendons, and continues with-out interruption or line of demarcation as far as the middle of the forearm. Let us now look for the lower limits of the collection in the palm of the hand. It stops above the metacarpo-phalangeal ar-ticulations, and does not extend into the tendinous sheaths of the index, middle, and ring fingers, but on the outer side the pus continues in the sheath of the thumb, even to its very end. This anatomical disposition of the purulent collection recalls to those of you who have sufficiently studied anatomy that of the synovial bursa of the flexors in the palm of the hand. You know that in some subjects this bursa is double: there is an inner one which corresponds to the palm of the hand and the little finger, and an outer one which is destined solely for the long flexor of the thumb. But in most people the cavity is single and is composed: 1st, of a central portion which stops at the lower part of the palm of the hand, and consequently does not extend to the extremity of the three middle fingers, in which the flexor tendons have separate sheaths; 2d, of two lateral prolongations which accom-pany the flexor tendons of the little finger and thumb to their ex-tremities.

You see, then, that here the suppurative inflammation starting from the little finger must have been propagated along the inner surface of its sheath to the common portion of the great synovial bursa, and thence to the prolongation of the thumb. At its upper extremity the great synovial bursa is largely open and communicates with the deep cellular tissue of the forearm, to which the inflammation has been transmitted either by a propagation of the phlegmasia itself or by an effusion of pus coming from the synovial bursa after ulceration or rupture in consequence of distension.

Consequently there existed at the same time in this patient sup-purative synovitis and deep abscess of the forearm. The latter was consecutive to the former, and it is probable, although it has never been possible to demonstrate it either by the symptoms or by the autopsy, that the deep layers of the forearm have suppurated after opening of the synovial membrane, which had itself already suppu-rated, just as in suppurative synovitis of the knee we often see deep abscesses of the thigh begin by the effusion of synovial pus into the deep cellular tissue of the limbs.

I do not mean to say that things always occur exactly in this way, and that all suppurations, starting from any point of the synovial membrane of the flexors, will end in deep suppurating phlegmon of the forearm. First, contused wounds of the thumb are not followed by this propagation as frequently as are those of the little finger. That is probably due to this, that, in the subjects affected, the outer portion of the bursa is independent and closed, as I told you was sometimes the case. Secondly, it is not impossible that the propagated inflammation may remain plastic and adhesive, although it was sup-purative at the starting-point.

II. *Synovitis of the flexors, partly suppurative; Recovery with defor-mity of the fingers.*—In No. 20 is a woman 28 years old, whose occu-pation as burnisher obliges her to work a great deal with her hands, who shows on the palmar face of her fingers a great number of calluses and cracks. A fortnight ago there appeared at the end of the little finger of her right hand an inflammation, which soon spread to the hypothenar eminence and thence to the palm of the hand, the thenar eminence, and the thumb. This inflammation terminated rapidly in partial suppuration; the first collection opened spontaneously at the upper portion of the thenar region: yesterday there was another in the hypothenar eminence, which was opened with the bistoury. A probe introduced into either of these two openings passes far up in a cavity, which is doubtless nothing else than the great synovial bursa of the flexors. From the course followed by this inflammation this must be a phlegmasia which occupies the common synovial membrane of this region.

I think, however, I can show you a notable difference between this synovitis and the preceding one. In the other the whole synovial bursa had suppurated; in this one I showed you that although the palm of the hand was swollen, pressure exerted upon it did not cause pus to flow from the orifice of the thenar nor from that of the hypothenar eminence. Moreover the quantity which escapes spontaneously is much less than it would be if the collection occupied the whole bursa. Of two things one: either the abscesses have formed by proximity outside of the great synovial membrane, the cavity of which has been the seat of an adhesive inflammation; or else the abscesses have formed within circumscribed portions of the bursa, the rest of which is filled with false-membranous products, the synovitis having remained plastic in the centre while it has become suppurative in the lateral portions.

I cannot determine by clinical signs with which of these two varieties we have to deal. The important point for me is, that there is at this moment a mixture of non-suppurative with a partially suppurative synovitis or abscesses by proximity.

If things remain in this condition life will not be compromised. But you know that this inflammation is easily propagated to the deep cellular tissue of the palmar side of the forearm: if it suppurates it causes at this point a deep abscess which is very serious, because it may be complicated by erysipelas, purulent infection, or putrid infection. Our patient's forearm is much swollen and doughy, but it is not red, and is not the seat of that pain and tension which indicate a deep diffuse phlegmon; moreover, the general phenomena which characterize the latter are entirely lacking. There is then here a synovitis, but one which has not suppurated, in and beyond the palmar portion of the synovial membrane. What still remains serious in the case is this, that this disease will probably end by adhesions which will interfere with the motions of the fingers: that is, the small accessory sheaths of each of the tendons are probably the seat of a plastic inflammation, which will result in the formation of adhesions and the abolition or diminution of the movements, the fingers remaining more or less flexed, and flexion itself being very limited by this sort of anchylosis of the tendons.

I had occasion to show you recently, at the consultation, a patient who had been treated by a seton for one of those affections of the great synovial bursa of the flexor, to which the name of crepitant dropsy has been given. Suppurating synovitis had been the consequence of this treatment. The patient had recovered with the adhesions of which I have just spoken, and came to us with all his fingers half flexed and incapable of being extended, in short, in the condition described as the claw hand.

Now, if suppurating synovitis of the flexors habitually produces this result, do not forget that a simply adhesive or plastic synovitis may also do it. You have had quite recently an example of this in a man in whom the synovitis starting from a contused wound of the thumb, had suppurated in it and in the thenar eminence, but not in the palm of the hand and the little finger. Nevertheless, the movements of flexion and extension were very limited, and, as the affection had commenced two months before, I expressed the fear that the adhesions were too solid to yield to the frictions and sulphur baths which I prescribed.

To return to our patient, I describe her situation in reminding you that she has to-day a tendinous synovitis in the thenar and hypothenar eminences which has suppurated, and the beginning of a diffuse phlegmon propagated to the deep layers of the forearm.

Therapeutical indications.—They result quite naturally from the possible consequences of the synovitis which I have described.

We should first try to keep the phlegmasia within its present limits, that is, prevent it from invading in a suppurative form the whole of the synovial bursa, if, as I have reason to think, the suppuration still occupies only a part of it, and if the inflammation, originally plastic, has produced adhesions in the centre of the cavity which have prevented the pus from filling it. We must then make every effort to get resolution of the phlegmon which is beginning in the forearm, and, finally, if we obtain these first results we shall have to combat the deformity and the functional lesions caused by the adhesions.

This then is what we shall do. The openings will be dressed with cerate; then we shall envelop the hand and forearm in cotton·and apply a moderately tight band. In a word, we shall treat the diffuse phlegmon by compression. The patient will keep the bed, the limb will be kept immovable upon a chaff bag, the hand a little higher than the elbow.

The compressive bandage will be renewed every day on account of the suppuration, and to see if deep fluctuation appears in the forearm.

Afterwards, if things go on happily, we shall prescribe sulphur baths, and have prolonged frictions made with lard or beef marrow, morning and evening, together with movements carefully communicated to all the fingers, so as to favour resolution of the plastic materials which form the adhesions. We shall employ, in short, treatment analogous to that of incomplete articular anchylosis.

(The suppuration remained limited to the points which it occupied at the beginning. Resolution took place in the forearm; but flexion and extension of the fingers were still very incomplete when the patient left the hospital after two months' sojourn in it.)

LECTURE XLI.

SUPERFICIAL AND DEEP DIFFUSE PHLEGMON OF THE FOREARM.

I. Two cases of subcutaneous diffuse phlegmon of the forearm, one with erysipelas, the other without erysipelas—Termination with rigidity, probably temporary, of the fingers and the hand. II. Deep or sub-aponeurotic phlegmon of the forearm, consecutive to a suppurative synovitis of the flexor tendons—Two theories to explain the propagation of the phlegmasia : that of synovitis, and that of deep lymphangitis—Termination by recovery with the deformity known as the claw hand.

GENTLEMEN : I. I spoke to you a few weeks ago of two patients affected with subcutaneous diffuse phlegmon of the back of the hand and dorsal face of the right forearm. One of them, 32 years old, occupying No. 38, ward Sainte-Vierge, had seen his affection develop in consequence of an insignificant scratch upon the back of his hand. He came to us, ten days after it had begun, with swelling, redness, and heat extending from the extremities of the fingers to the shoulder. Upon the back of the hand and forearm was the doughiness which characterizes the first period of diffuse phlegmon. The doughiness of the arm, where the redness occupied the entire circumference, was much less, and the appearance was rather that of a slightly œdematous erysipelas than that of a diffuse phlegmon. As moreover the intense febrile movement which characterizes erysipelas existed, I presented the patient to you as offering an example of phlegmonous erysipelas, or, if you prefer, of diffuse phlegmon with erysipelas, pointing out at the same time that the diffuse phlegmon occupied the hand and forearm, and the erysipelas chiefly the arm. The ultimate course of the affection confirmed my first opinion. Suppuration set in upon the dorsal face of the hand and forearm ; I made several long incisions there, from which you saw an abundant quantity of pus flow, followed a few days afterwards by gray and whitish membranous strips composed of mortified cellular tissue. I showed you, however, that the suppuration was under the skin, and that it had not passed through the deep fascia; that no abscess had formed upon the palmar face of the limb, but that the inflammation had terminated there by resolution, at the same time that the erysipelatous redness had disappeared from the arm.

To-day, five weeks after the beginning of the disease, the general condition is excellent, and the wounds left by my incisions will soon be cicatrized. I have advised the patient to begin now to move his fingers, either with the corresponding muscles or with his other hand, for the articulations of these fingers have become rigid through their prolonged immobility, and their participation to a certain extent in the morbid process which was developed in their neighbourhood. If we should do nothing for it, this rigidity would last for a long time, perhaps indefinitely, and we should thus have an infirmity succeeding to the affection. I hope that by the aid of spontaneous and communicated movements, to which we shall soon add a little massage, this rigidity will not last more than two or three months, and I have the more reason to hope so because the patient is still young, and, as I have often told you, articular rigidities, especially those of the small articulations, are less rebellious as the patients are younger.

Not far from this patient is another one, in No. 41, sixty years old, who presents an example of a similar affection, that is to say, of a subcutaneous diffuse phlegmon of the dorsal aspect of the left hand and forearm. But in him we find this difference, that the phlegmon has been neither preceded nor accompanied by erysipelas propagated to the arm and body, that the febrile symptoms have not been intense, and that as the suppuration was limited to the lower third of the forearm and the back of the hand, we have had to make fewer incisions, and the suppuration has been less prolonged. This patient also is recovering; but the articulation of the fingers are stiff, and I fear, on account of the age of the patient, that this rigidity will last longer than in the preceding case.

II. The patient in No. 29, a baker's boy, 24 years old, hurt the palmar face of the little finger of his right hand near the articulation of the first and second phalanges with a saw a week ago. To what depth did the tooth of the saw penetrate; was the articulation opened? We do not know. Is the synovial membrane of the flexor tendon interested? It is probable, but we have no proof of it. The patient continued to work for three days; on the fourth a swelling appeared in the little finger, the palm of the hand, the thumb, and the forearm; at the same time general symptoms set in: insomnia, due to the pain, and fever. The patient, however, had no chills. To-day we see a suppurating contused wound occupying the middle of the little finger, a swelling of the thenar and hypothenar eminences, of the palm of the hand, and of the palmar face of the forearm extending nearly to the elbow; still the swelling of the hand is small. The forearm is the seat of a redness which is intense but which cannot be called erysipelatous, because at the beginning there were none of the general symptoms which precede this affection: violent chill, intense fever, vomiting. The redness appeared only after the swelling; and then it does not extend very far, and is limited to the phlegmon. If it had been a real erysipelas it would undoubtedly have extended beyond the tumefied and phlegmonous parts. The dorsal face of the hand and forearm does not present, so to speak, any swelling, differing in this respect from the other two patients.

Can we detect fluctuation? In the hypothenar eminence there is a soft swelling, but it is without elasticity. The thenar eminence presents a considerable swelling; if we compress it with one finger we feel a mingled sensation of elasticity and softness; if we place the two fingers at a certain distance from one another and make pressure with one while the other remains immovable, we feel a sensation which resembles that of fluctuation. But it must be remembered that this region gives, in the normal condition, false fluctuation, and we might almost say that, in phlegmasia, the presence of pus here is only certain when fluctuation is no longer as marked as it is normally.

This is the eighth day of the accident, but the fourth of the inflammation: it is not probable that there is yet any pus; still, in order to be certain, I made three punctures with a pin, and without any result; no pus came.

Is there any fluctuation in the forearm? I have not found the slightest sign of it.

This then is a phlegmonous inflammation which has not yet suppurated, and, as it is extensive, we may call it a diffuse phlegmon. In the preceding patients also the affection was a diffuse phlegmon, but it was subcutaneous, while here it is deep, sub-aponeurotic.

My reasons for this opinion are the following: There is a considerable swelling, without the superficial doughiness which is seen at the beginning when the phlegmon is subcutaneous. We see at the wrist the raised lines formed by the tendons, and in the middle of the forearm we have that peculiar sensation of softness given by the muscles through the skin; but these muscles are slightly tense, and as if raised by something behind them. All these signs indicate a deep inflammation; and another argument in favour of this opinion is the propagation to the forearm of the phlegmasia starting from the hand. It is evident that in the latter the inflammation is not superficial; for by pressing upon the wrist we can feel the annular ligament and the tendons, notwithstanding the enormous swelling; now, if the swelling was subcutaneous these parts could not be felt, and we should find a superficial tumefaction which would mask the rest. For a moment I asked myself if it was not the muscular hypertrophy' which is often found in bakers, but the other arm shows nothing similar. It is certain then that it is an inflammation: now, so soon as we decide that the inflammation is not superficial, we have to admit that it is sub-aponeurotic and submuscular, and that it is situated between the pronator quadratus and the deep layer of muscles.

Is this development of an inflammation in a finger, and its propagation to the deep parts of the hand and forearm, an unusual occurrence? Not at all. I have had occasion to show you several similar cases, and a year never passes without our having two or three examples of it here. You have not forgotten the explanation which I gave of these facts: the suppurative inflammation starts from a finger (the thumb or little finger) to the extremity of which the main synovial bursa of the palm of the hand extends. It is propagated to the latter, and thence to the deep cellular tissue of the forearm, by virtue of a peculiar aptitude possessed by the subcutaneous and tendinous synovial bursa to transmit to the surrounding connective tissue the phlegmasiæ, and especially the suppurating ones, of which they become the seat. I remind you also that I showed in this amphitheatre a specimen in which the course of the suppurative inflammation within and beyond this tendinous synovial bursa was very evident (page 327). It is true that since I showed you that specimen another

explanation has been offered. Prof. Dolbeau[1] thinks that the starting
point of these deep phlegmons of the forearm is a lymphangitis of
the deep lymphatic vessels which accompany the arteries. He bases
his opinion upon this incontestable fact, that the suppuration sometimes appears in the forearm without at the same time occupying the
hand and the whole length of the finger in which the affection began.
I have sought, on other occasions, to explain this peculiarity by telling you that the inflammation propagated from a finger to the synovial bursa and to the deep cellular tissue might remain plastic or
adhesive at some points and might suppurate at others.

Furthermore, I offer four objections to Professor Dolbeau's theory:
1st. It cannot be proved anatomically. 2d. It supposes that the sub-
aponeurotic abscesses must be along the course of the radial and
ulnar arteries, that is, not very deep, for it is there that we find
the principal sub-aponeurotic lymphatic vessels. The abscesses which
we see in these cases are very much deeper; they are found in front of
the pronator quadratus, of the inter-osseous ligament and of the bones,
which are sometimes denuded in consequence of the participation of
the periosteum in the disease; now, at this depth there are very few
lymphatic vessels, only those which accompany the interosseous
artery, and they are very small and too few to cause such large
phlegmons and abscesses. Notice what occurs after superficial
lymphangites. The affected lymphatic vessels are very large, and
yet only circumscribed abscesses form about them. 3d. M. Dolbeau's
theory does not explain why deep abscesses of the forearm occur so
habitually after deep wounds of the thumb and especially of the little
finger, and only very exceptionally after wounds of the other fingers
whose synovial sheaths are independent of the main synovial bursa of
the wrist and palm of the hand. 4th. Finally it does not enlighten us
upon the causes of the gravity of the prognosis in these cases, of the
adhesions of the tendons, the insufficiency of the movements of the
fingers, the claw hand; all those phenomena which can hardly be
explained except as phenomena consecutive to a tendinous synovitis.

I willingly believe, for it agrees very well with what we see in the
superficial layers of the limbs, that a deep lymphangitis intervenes in
cases of this kind, that it is one of the means of extension of the
phlegmasia, that perhaps even it is that which propagates it sometimes to the main synovial bursa. But I want you to admit at the
same time the existence of a synovitis, either plastic or suppurative;
I consider it important, because with this notion, proved to be true
by autopsies, is associated that part of the therapeutics the object of
which is to combat the tendinous rigidities as soon as possible, and
to diminish, if it can be done, the deformity and the functional trouble
which their persistence occasions.

At the present moment, then, two things preoccupy us in this case:
1st. The imminence of a deep or *intermuscular* suppuration in the
hand and forearm, and the possibility of a septicæmia; 2d. The con-

[1] Dolbeau, Mémoire sur les Abcès profonds de l'Avant-bras, conséoutifs aux bles-
sures des doigts (Bulletin de Thérapeutique, 20 Février, 1872).

secutive deformity, a deformity all the more serious since it will occupy the right hand.

As for the treatment, I can hardly have recourse to anything except rest, poultices, and narcotics. I thought of making compression, but the swelling and redness are so great that I fear it might cause strangulation and gangrene. Moreover I must examine this swelling every day and open it soon as I find fluctuation.

The young man in No. 29, who had had the little finger of the right hand wounded by a saw, presented, 48 hours after I had spoken about him, distinct fluctuation in the anterior part of the hypothenar eminence. The next morning I felt a deep fluctuation in the forearm, a fluctuation the limits of which were the radio-carpal line below, the junction of the lower and middle thirds of the palmar aspect above. I sought carefully to see if the wave could be sent from the forearm to the palm of the hand, as should have been the case if the purulent collection occupied both the tendinous bursa of the wrist and the deep cellular tissue of the forearm. I did not find it to be so. Furthermore, pressure upon the forearm did not cause pus to flow from the opening made in the hypothenar eminence, nor from that made by the injury in the little finger which still suppurated. It seemed then that we had three separate suppurations. This circumstance was favourable to M. Dolbeau's explanation by deep lymphangitis, along the course of which the abscesses might form here and there without communicating with one another. Admitting propagation by synovitis, I presume that, in this case also, the synovial membrane has not suppurated on its inner face, and has been the seat only of a congestive and plastic inflammation, but that the cellular tissue of the hypothenar eminence and of the palm of the hand, to which it has transmitted the inflammation, has taken part in the suppuration.

However that may be, experience having shown us that these deep abscesses, when once formed, have more tendency to burrow and spread along the deep layers than to approach the skin, from which they are separated by very thick muscular and aponeurotic layers, I told you that we must not temporize, and that as soon as fluctuation could be felt, an incision must be made.

Still, as it was necessary, in order to reach the collection, to traverse the superficial and deep layers, I completed my diagnosis by means of puncture and aspiration with the Dieulafoy syringe. After I saw the pus flow into the aspirator I anæsthetized the patient with ether and made, layer by layer, an incision two and a half inches long along the middle of the forearm. M. Dolbeau, in the article of which I have spoken, advises two incisions to be made, one along the course of the radial artery, the other along that of the ulnar, that is, in the points where the lymphatic vessels are to be found which are the starting-point of the abscess. But as this collection was much deeper than the arteries, as it corresponded much more to the centre than to the sides of the forearm, as, on the other hand, I wished to be sure of avoiding hemorrhage, I made my operation as upon other patients, and notably as upon the one of whom I spoke last year (page 328), that is, I used a bistoury to get through the fascia, and then my fingers to tear through the muscular interstices. The following days I had some difficulty to get a free escape for the pus, notwithstanding the use of bundles of lint and drainage tubes. Every morning and evening I had to separate the muscular interstices and make injections of carbolized water, as much to prevent the stagnation of the pus as to disinfect the deep pouch.

We had no dangerous general symptoms. After the fourth day the flow was freer, but I continued the injections morning and night. The patient was sustained by nourishment and tonics. During the treatment I often tried if pressure upon the palm of the hand would make the pus flow from the openings, but it never did so, and I continued to think that the synovitis had not suppurated in the palm of the hand, as is quite often the case in cases of this kind.

In this connection, I remember an old woman whom I treated at the Hôpital Cochin, and who also had a deep phlegmon of the hand and forearm originating in a wound of the little finger. She succumbed to a putrid infection, and I found suppuration, not only of the great tendinous synovial membrane of the wrist and forearm, but also of all the carpal articulations, to which the suppurated phlegmasia starting from the tendinous bursa had been propagated.

To-day all is cicatrized, and our patient is cured of his suppuration, but he has not recovered the use of the limb; the tendons of the fingers, bound down by adhesions, no longer permit either flexion or extension except within very narrow limits. You saw that the fingers were half flexed and that the patient could not extend them: he cannot complete this imperfect flexion and cannot close the thumb entirely against the other fingers. In short, he presents the claw shape of which I have spoken several times.

Will this condition of things disappear? I hope that it will diminish, because it seems to me that the adhesions ought to be less numerous and less rebellious when the inflammation has remained plastic, at least over a great extent of the synovial membrane, than when it has become suppurative and the membrane has granulated. I hope so, especially if the patient will follow our prescriptions, that is, will take sulphur baths, make prolonged frictions, massage, and communicated movements. I make all these recommendations, but am not able to oversee them myself, for he is tired of the hospital and intends to leave us in a few days.

22

LECTURE XLII.

DENTAL ABSCESSES AND FISTULÆ.

I. Suppurated submaxillary adeno-phlegmon—Mode of formation—Commencement by an adenitis consecutive to a lymphangitis either of the pulp of the tooth or of the alveolo-dental periosteum—Obscurity upon this point because anatomists have not sufficiently studied the dental lymphatic vessels. II. Phlegmon and dental abscess under the gum of the upper jaw—Probability of consecutive alveolar necrosis—Utility of the removal of the decayed tooth. III. Cutaneous dental fistula kept up by caries of the second upper molar of the right side with an indurated course extending from the fistula to the tooth. IV. Submasseteric abscess of dental origin—Quite extensive consecutive alveolar necrosis—Peculiar gravity of these abscesses—Their possible prolongation to the temporal region—Consecutive purulent infection—Necessity for large openings and washing out.

GENTLEMEN: We have recently had four patients affected either with abscess or fistula consecutive to caries of a tooth, and it will be sufficient to mention them to fix in your minds the principal varieties of suppuration of dental origin.

I. *Suppurated submaxillary adeno-phlegmon.*—The patient who is now in No. 20 shows you a quite common type. She is twenty-four years old, blonde, slightly lymphatic, generally enjoys good health, and has never had any scrofulous manifestation. She is not pregnant, and has never had any children. She knows that she has caries of the second molar of the left side of the lower jaw, and she has sometimes suffered from it, but never enough to decide her to have the tooth drawn, or, what would be better, to have it filled. More recently she has again suffered some pain in it which has prevented her from chewing her food upon that side; then, five days ago, she felt a rounded and painful tumefaction at the upper part of the neck under the edge of the lower jaw, and a little in front of its angle. This swelling increased and was accompanied by a febrile movement which compelled her to enter the hospital.

You found at first a uniformly rounded swelling of the superhyoid region, rosy in colour over a great extent, and of a deeper red at one point where the consistency was less than at others. There was heat appreciable by the hand, spontaneous shooting pain, and pain on pressure. The jaws were kept closed by a contraction of the muscles which prevented examination of the teeth.

After a few days fluctuation could be felt; I made as small an incision as possible, about half an inch long, not wishing to cause a large cicatrix. A small quantity of good phlegmonous pus escaped, but there still remained a pasty tumefaction formed by a considerable part of the inflammatory swelling which had not yet advanced to suppuration.

The following days, while the pus flowed from the wound, the lips of which were kept apart by a strip of frayed linen, this swelling diminished and terminated by resolution. To-day, the seventeenth day since the operation, the cicatrice is formed, there is no fistula, the patient can separate her jaws and eat. By placing her before a well-lighted window, I could easily see a carious loss of substance in the second lower molar. As it would be difficult to fill the tooth, I advised the patient to have it drawn, and warned her that if she did not consent she would be exposed to a renewal of the suppuration. But, as she does not suffer, she refused for the present to follow my advice, and I did not urge it.

Permit me now to explain the mode of formation and the course of this abscess, in what points it resembles the others of which I shall presently speak, and in what it differs from them.

It resembles them, first, in its starting-point, which was evidently the affected tooth. I do not mean by that to say that all inflammatory submaxillary abscesses are caused by carious teeth. There are some, and I have shown you examples of them during the year, which are consecutive to an affection of the mouth, others which start from a sore throat, that is to say, they may be caused by inflammation of any of the parts which, like the teeth and gums, send their lymphatic vessels to the submaxillary ganglions. In this case I believe in the dental origin, because it is the most common, and because I found no inflammation in the throat.

It differs in its mode of formation: for, among the phlegmons of dental origin, there are some which, having begun in the periosteum, confine themselves to the neighbouring cellular tissue, and sometimes to that which is more or less distant, and the lymphatic vessels have no part in the development. There are others, on the contrary, in which the inflammation first affects one or several lymphatic ganglions and then is propagated to the cellular atmosphere surrounding them, as takes place in other regions, and especially in that of the groin, during the formation of most of the acute bubos consecutive to non-infectious chancres.

It is with this latter form, which you have often heard me designate by the name of adeno-phlegmon, that we have to do here. For the affection did not commence on account of the proximity itself of the tooth, as is the case in phlegmons of periosteal origin; it commenced at a distance in the suprahyoid region, which I also call the sub-maxillary, there where, you know, lymphatic ganglions are found in considerable numbers, most of which are inclosed within the sheath of the submaxillary gland, and receive lymphatic vessels from the cavity of the mouth, and especially those of the teeth and gums of the lower jaw.[1] Further, the trouble began by a rounded, rolling, painful lump, like those formed by acute adenitis; then, in a second period, this rolling tumour was found enveloped in a uniform mass, which was the surrounding phlegmon.

[1] The lymphatics of the gums and teeth of the upper jaw communicate with the deep parotid ganglions.

This abscess differed, also, from others by its mode of term
It has left neither fistula nor necrosis. You remember that
after the incision I introduced a probe into the wound, and
felt no denudation of the jaw at any point. I should undo
have felt it if the starting point had been an osteo-periostitis;
such a case, the periosteum is almost always destroyed or ε
off, and the naked bone can be felt. The ultimate course corres
to this examination, for there remained no fistula, such ε
persists after denudation, fistula due to the non-reproduction
periosteum and consequent necrosis of the maxilla.

Events proceeded as follows in this patient. The dentε
became inflamed about the caries. If I were sure that this p
lymphatic vessels, I should say that they had transmitted the
mation to one of the submaxillary ganglions, and that this
mation had been propagated to the surrounding cellular tiss
become phlegmonous, and taken on the suppurative form.

But there is here a *nescio quid* which often intervenes in patl
Many subjects have carious teeth without having adenitis;
have simple adenites which do not become phlegmonous,
suppurate, and terminate by resolution. Some indeed, and w
lately had an example of it, have the adeno-phlegmon, but it
nates by resolution instead of suppurating. Now, we are nev
to find the particular cause, under the influence of which the
mation, starting from the pulp of the tooth, transmits to the gai
an inflammation of one form rather than of another. It is alwι
question of individual aptitudes, varying with the subject, aι
the moment in the same subject; a question which is surrι
with obscurities which render it everywhere insoluble.

Next, to admit a starting-point in a lymphangitis of the ι
the tooth, we must be certain that lymphatics exist in this pulι
for myself, I have never seen them, and I do not know if other
seen them. M. Sappey, the most competent of our anatomist
this point, does not describe lymphatic vessels of the teeth; b
tions only those of the gums, and, according to him, those
lower jaw empty into the submaxillary ganglions, those of the
jaw into the deep parotid ganglions. I admit that I am never
disposed to believe in the existence of lymphatics of the pulp, ι
ing to the facts furnished by the clinic. The submaxillary gaι
become painful so easily and so promptly after caries of the
teeth that it seems to me difficult to explain without a lymph
originating in the pulp. If it is not the latter which is at ι
must then be the lymphatic network of the alveolo-dental perio
which is better demonstrated, I believe, than that of the pul
perhaps it is that of the gum to which the affected tooth maι
transmitted its inflammation; but I should then be surprised
so often submaxillary adeno phlegmon without appreciable gin,

And, since the occasion has presented itself, I point out ι
another peculiarity. We very rarely see adeno-phlegmon cau
affections of the upper teeth. Is it because the lymphatic ne

either of the pulp or of the alveolo-dental periosteum, is too small?
or is it for some other reason? I do not know.

But let us return to the practical standpoint. My principal object
in insisting upon this subject has been to make you understand,
gentlemen, that, among the abscesses of dental origin, there are some
which are not followed by denudation, necrosis, or fistula, and which
may get well without removal of the tooth which caused the affection.
For, if I advised this woman to have her tooth drawn, it was not to
cure the abscess or its consequences; it was only to protect her from
a return of the same trouble, or from another of the same kind.

II. *Subgingival dental phlegmon and abscess of the upper jaw.*—
You saw yesterday at the consultation a man who had had pain for
several days, about one of those fragments of a carious molar which
we call stumps, and in whom a painful swelling of the gum over
this stump had appeared. As the swelling of the gum was tense and
distinctly fluctuating, I at once cut it, taking the necessary precautions
not to wound the lips with the blade of the bistoury while doing so.
I opened it freely, because wounds of the mouth have a great tendency
to close too soon, and there was reason to fear, in case cicatrization
took place before the occlusion of the pouch, that the latter would
again fill up.

The pus which escaped was mixed with blood and had a fetid odour,
which is quite common in abscess of the cavity of the mouth.

This abscess resembles, by its origin, the one previously described.
It was certainly an inflammatory process, starting from a carious
tooth, that caused it. But with respect to its position, it differs in
two ways: first, it was not developed so far from its starting-point;
and, secondly, it did not begin by the lymphatic element. In this
connection I wish to remind you of one remark: dental adeno-phlegmon arising in the lower teeth is not rare in the lower jaw; we see
it arise much less frequently from the upper teeth. When caries of
the latter gives rise to it, the inflammatory swelling ought to appear
in the parotid region. But the clinic has not enlightened me very
much upon this subject, because, in the rare parotid adeno-phlegmons
with which I have met, with the exception of one case in which it
was certainly due to caries of an upper wisdom-tooth, I was never
able to determine positively if the starting-point of the initial lymphangitis had been in the teeth or in the mouth.

In this case it is probable that the inflammation starting from the
affected tooth first gained the alveolo-dental periosteum, then the external periosteum, and the cellular tissue between it and the mucous
membrane of the gum. It is then a subgingival and periosteal phlegmonous abscess. It is, however, possible that the pus may have
formed under the periosteum, and that consequently the abscess has
been subperiosteal. This is all the more probable because, after having made the incision, I passed in a probe and found part of the
upper maxillary bone denuded. Still, I do not know, and fortunately it is without much importance, whether the periosteum has
been destroyed because the abscess formed below it, or consecutively
to the suppuration of its outer surface. It is the same here as in

acute subperiosteal abscesses of the large long bones; we know
periosteum disappears or is stripped off in consequence of these phl
masiae, but we do not know exactly which of these lesions has be
produced, nor, above all, what has been the course and the success
of the phenomena.

The denudation warned us of one thing, that necrosis was possible
I say possible, and not certain, for in such cases we sometimes
the bone cover itself again and continue to live. But if the decay
tooth remains in its place, it causes another abscess after a cert
length of time, a new denudation, and, if the necrosis does not th
take place, it does on the third or fourth attack. It is to be remark
moreover, that in these cases of gingival abscess the necrosis is gen
ally limited to a circumscribed point of the alveolus, and is nev
very extensive; and that at the same time the concomitant ostei
does not become hypertrophic in the neighbourhood, as you know tl
it does in the long bones.

What will.this abscess become? If the osteitis is not yet necro
it will close, and everything will resume the condition in which
was previously, that is, the patient will keep his stump and w
almost inevitably have the relapse of which I have spoken. If, ho
ever, necrosis has already occurred, and elimination must take pla
in the form of dust or of a splinter, suppuration will be kept up a
the fistula will last until this result is obtained; now this does r
take place, or at least it is not definitive, until the affected tooth l
been removed from its cavity, a process which is always slow wh
it goes on spontaneously. We have recently seen at the consultati
a woman who has had for nearly a year a fistula of this kind (gingi
dental fistula) kept up by a very limited spot of necrosis on t
lower jaw corresponding to a carious and loose canine tooth.

These fistulae, which are very common, are not serious; but th
keep up an unclean and inconvenient suppuration in the mouth.

To relieve the patients of these inconveniences: return of the a
scess, slowness of elimination, and persistence of the fistula, there
only one useful advice to give them, and that is to remove the too
or the stump which is the cause of the trouble. Whether it be tl
the operation itself removes the necrosed alveolar portion, or that t
opening of the alveolus prepares an easier way of elimination, it
none the less true that after the removal of the tooth the suppurati
and the fistula, if there is one, disappear promptly. I have giv
this advice to our patient, and he has followed it. The root of t
carious tooth has been removed, and I consider the recovery assure

III. *Cutaneous dental fistula kept up by the second upper molar on*
right side, with a callous band between the fistula and the tooth.—In c
nection with the preceding case I spoke of gingival, and consequent
intra-buccal, fistulae consecutive to abscesses starting from decay
teeth and the alveolo-dental periosteum, with imminence of necros
But it happens sometimes that abscesses of this kind, instead of pr
jecting simply under the mucous membrane, open through the sk
and cause cutaneous fistulae which are much more disagreeable to t
patients, since they occasion an ugly deformity. You will meet wi

these osteo-periosteal abscesses followed by cutaneous dental fistulæ upon the upper jaw as well as upon the lower. In the first case they open upon the cheek, in the second upon the outer face of the lower jaw. Generally the concomitant necrosis·is still very limited and will promptly disappear after removal of the tooth, removal which will always be the principal means of treatment. But in some exceptional cases, the necrotic osteitis having spread very far, you will have a more extended and slower necrosis, the elimination of which will only take place long after the removal of the carious tooth.

In the case which we have just seen at No. 6, ward Sainte Vierge, the cutaneous dental fistula is made remarkable by the existence of a very hard callous band which cleared up the diagnosis, and by the opposition which the prolonged contracture of the muscles which close the jaw offered to the examination of the teeth and the necessary removal of one of them.

It is a man 33 years old, very subject to toothache, who seems to have had gingival abscesses on several occasions. Seven weeks ago a new abscess opened spontaneously on his left cheek in front of the masseter and at the outer portion of the canine fossa, and remained fistulous.

You saw that the orifice, depressed in its centre, was surrounded by vegetations, and that it yielded a small amount of serous pus. This liquid was not as limpid and did not flow in as large quantities when he was eating, as it would if it had been a salivary fistula. A probe introduced into the fistula passed towards the upper jaw, and although I strongly suspected necrosis I did not find the characteristic hard and sonorous point.

The fistulous canal was about an inch long. By placing a finger in the mouth upon its course, I felt an elongated induration, which certainly corresponded to it. Seizing the cheek between the thumb and forefinger, one of them·being placed within the mouth, the other upon the skin, I still better appreciated the elongated, hard, evidently callous cord, extending from the cheek towards the hindermost part of the upper alveolar arch. I called your attention especially to this callous cord; I told you that it was found almost always in cases of cutaneous dental fistula, that it was not very appreciable when the course was short, but that it was much more so when it had a certain length. I added that it was a great help to the diagnosis, because it indicated the certain existence of a carious tooth and necrosis, and the point where these lesions were to be found.

This double indication was all the more precious in our patient, because the probe did not reach the necrosed bone, and the exploration of the mouth was rendered impossible by the constriction of the jaws. This constriction, which is seen rather during the acute period of dental phlegmons than during the chronic and fistulous period with which we have to deal here, is more often met with when the last two teeth are involved than when the others are. In the absence of certain signs, all the others—the existence of a callous tract, its direction towards the posterior portion of the upper alveolo-dental arch, contraction of the muscles—united to make me believe in the existence of an alveolo-dental lesion corresponding either to the wisdom-tooth or the second upper molar.

The indication was precise; to open the month, examine, and remove the tooth that was found to be affected. I should have temporized if the inflammation had still been in the acute state, for, at such a time, the attempts to separate the jaws by force sometimes cause an exacerbation of the phlegmasia, and, moreover, it is difficult to succeed, because the muscles are too firmly contracted. But in this case there was no acute inflammation, it was probable that the resistance was not great, and it was necessary to prevent the contraction, which was still curable, from giving place to an incurable retraction.

That is why I first took a spoon and passed its handle, on the flat, between the two rows of teeth, and then tried to turn it on its edge, so as to separate them. I did not entirely succeed, but I obtained a separation of a few lines. I told the patient, who for some time had been able to eat nothing but soups, and was anxious to have the functions of his jaws restored as quickly as possible, to use the spoon in the same way, five or six times during the day.

The next day I found the separation a few lines larger, and then substituted for the spoon the conical screw of boxwood, which I first introduced myself, so as to show the patient how to use it. At the end of three days enough separation had been obtained to allow me to discover, with the aid of a dental mirror, a deep caries behind the second upper molar, which was a little loose, and whose alveolus suppurated. I did not see the point which was necrosed, but the intra alveolar suppuration left me no doubt of its existence.

The tooth was then drawn. Four days afterwards the cutaneous fistula closed. To-day, the callous tract commences to grow smaller, and I count upon a definitive recovery.

IV. *Submasseteric phlegmonous abscess of dental origin. Necrosis of the lower jaw.*—Gentlemen, a young man, 23 years old, who was for a long time in No. 43, ward Sainte Vierge, and who returns to consult us from time to time, came to see us again this morning. On examining the interior of his mouth, I found, in the place of the second molar of the right side of the lower jaw, which I had removed two months ago, an alveolar cavity full of pus, with a denudation and sonority of the whole cavity and of the internal and external faces of the maxillary bone, over a surface of about one-third of an inch. There is then necrosis, but it has been preceded by a peculiar variety of abscess, of which I will now recall the principal details.

When he entered the hospital, about two months ago, this young man had had for seven days a painful and quite hard swelling of the right cheek, without redness and with a little fever.

He was unable to open his mouth, on account of a prolonged contraction similar to that of the preceding patient. At first I was not able to determine the condition of his teeth. But I felt with the finger a few asperities and inequalities upon the crown of the first and second molars of the lower jaw; I had, moreover, recognized that the wisdom-tooth was well out, and that consequently this was not of those affections which are sometimes caused by the difficult and laborious evolution of that tooth. Examining as well as possible the posterior portion of the entrance to the mouth, I saw pus flow from the neighbourhood of one of the last molars, and I thought that it was a deep gingival abscess, the opening of which announced the approaching termination in a definitive cure or in necrosis. Still there remained a considerable swelling of the region of the masseter, and pressure exerted upon this region caused a good deal of pus to flow from the opening in the gum. We had then a deeper and more extensive abscess than those which we ordinarily see open in the neighbourhood of the gum, and I had to suppose that the spontaneous opening was not sufficient. Not only was it not sufficient, but it even closed in a few days, and then the swelling became greater in the region of the masseter and advanced evidently towards the temple. Then deep fluctuation became apparent in the first of these regions; I then made a transverse incision an inch long, parallel to and below Steno's duct, and, also parallel to the principal branches of the facial nerve, some of which I should certainly have cut if I had carried the bistoury vertically. I divided, layer by layer, the skin and the whole thickness of the masseter, and it was only when the deep face of the latter had been divided that we saw a large amount of fetid pus escape; pressure exerted upon the temporal region, which was tumefied even then, did not cause pus to flow from the opening, thus proving that the phlegmon, although propagated to that region, had not yet suppurated there. The probe introduced through the wound reached the outer face of the branch of the inferior maxillary bone, but did not allow me to detect any denudation. After this operation, the pouch, which was kept open by means of strips of frayed linen, emptied itself little by little, the temporal swelling disappeared, and the jaws could be opened, thanks to the aid of the conical screw. Meanwhile, the opening in the gum was re-established, and suppuration persisted on that side, while it ceased and cicatrization took place in the cheek.

What was there peculiar in this patient, and in what did his dental abscess differ from those of which I have already spoken? It differed in this, that, starting from an affected tooth and its alveolus, the inflammation was propagated along the periosteum, as in gingival phlegmons; but instead of stopping in the gum, or burrowing in the submucous and subcutaneous cellular tissue, it made its way along the outer part of the jaw as far as the deep face of the masseter, and further to the sheath of the temporal muscle, moving along the coronoid process to the outer and perhaps the inner face of this muscle. The phlegmon thus propagated became submasseteric and temporal, although I cannot say whether, at this latter point, it was subtemporal or was limited to the connective tissue placed between the muscle and the aponeuroses. Then the submasseteric abscess formed, and, at the same time, the temporal portion of the phlegmon terminated by resolution. Finally, the submasseteric abscess terminated without fistula, and without necrosis of the branch of the maxilla. Only the portion of bone adjoining the carious tooth necrosed. We recognized, afterwards, that this affected tooth was the second lower molar, and we removed it.

This was not the first time I had seen deep temporo-submasseteric phlegmon follow dental caries. In two of my private patients the suppuration invaded not only the submasseteric p   , but also the subtemporal portion of the phlegmon. I considered it necessary to make two incisions, one through the temporal, the other through the masseter muscle, and to pass a drainage tube from one to the other, in order to assure the evacuation of the collection. In one of the patients, the incision of the temporal muscle occasioned a flow of arterial blood, which rendered a rather laborious ligature necessary. Both patients recovered without necrosis of the branch of the maxilla, and did not even have the alveolar necrosis which we observed in our last patient.

Things did not pass so happily in a man whom I treated at La Pitié in 1867. After the submasseteric collection had been opened, purulent infection occurred and caused death. I did not find the maxilla denuded to a very great extent, nor its parenchyma in suppuration; the purulent infection seemed to me to have been caused by septicæmia consecutive to the decomposition of blood and of pus in the deep pouch.

The possibility of this complication authorizes me to tell you that the indication in abscesses of this kind is to open early and freely, and in both regions (of the masseter and temporal), when fluctuation can be sent from one to the other; in one alone, the first, when the collection remains exclusively submasseteric. Stagnation, and consequent decomposition, of the pus in the bottom of the foyer must be afterwards avoided by means of repeated washings.

As for the patient, we have only to wait for the elimination of the necrosis of the lower jaw, which is more extensive than usual, but still quite limited, and to advise frequent washings of the mouth, so as not to allow the pus to be swallowed.

INDEX.

348   INDEX.

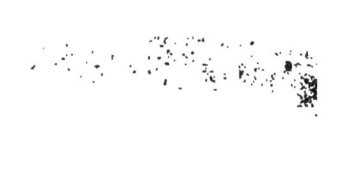